The
RESPONSIVE
PSYCHOTHERAPIST

The
RESPONSIVE
PSYCHOTHERAPIST

Attuning to Clients in the Moment

Edited by
Jeanne C. Watson and Hadas Wiseman

 AMERICAN PSYCHOLOGICAL ASSOCIATION

Published by
American Psychological Association
750 First Street, NE
Washington, DC 20002
https://www.apa.org

Order Department
https://www.apa.org/pubs/books
order@apa.org

In the U.K., Europe, Africa, and the Middle East, copies may be ordered from Eurospan
https://www.eurospanbookstore.com/apa
info@eurospangroup.com

Typeset in Charter and Interstate by Circle Graphics, Inc., Reisterstown, MD

Printer: Gasch Printing, Odenton, MD
Cover Designer: Gwen J. Grafft, Minneapolis, MN

Library of Congress Cataloging-in-Publication Data

Names: Watson, Jeanne C., editor. | Wiseman, Hadas, 1956- editor.
Title: The responsive psychotherapist : attuning to clients in the moment /
  edited by Jeanne C. Watson, Hadas Wiseman.
Description: Washington, DC : American Psychological Association, [2021] |
  Includes bibliographical references and index.
Identifiers: LCCN 2020052795 (print) | LCCN 2020052796 (ebook) |
  ISBN 9781433834011 (paperback) | ISBN 9781433834028 (ebook)
Subjects: LCSH: Psychotherapy. | Psychotherapist and patient.
Classification: LCC RC475 .R47 2021 (print) | LCC RC475 (ebook) |
  DDC 616.89/14—dc23
LC record available at https://lccn.loc.gov/2020052795
LC ebook record available at https://lccn.loc.gov/2020052796

https://doi.org/10.1037/0000240-000

Printed in the United States of America

10 9 8 7 6 5 4 3 2 1

To our mentors,
Laura Rice and Irene Elkin,
innovators, sources of inspiration and
leaders in psychotherapy research

Contents

Contributors   *ix*

Acknowledgments   *xi*

**Introduction: Exploring Responsiveness and Attunement in
Psychotherapy**   3
Jeanne C. Watson and Hadas Wiseman

I. THE CASE FOR RESPONSIVENESS   13

1. **Responsiveness in Psychotherapy Research: Problems and
   Ways Forward**   15
   William B. Stiles

2. **Responsiveness, the Relationship, and the Working Alliance
   in Psychotherapy**   37
   Robert L. Hatcher

3. **Attachment Theory as a Framework for Responsiveness in
   Psychotherapy**   59
   Hadas Wiseman and Sharon Egozi

4. **Responsiveness to Ruptures and Repairs in Psychotherapy**   83
   Catherine F. Eubanks, Joey Sergi, and J. Christopher Muran

II. RESPONSIVENESS IN DIFFERENT THERAPEUTIC APPROACHES   105

5. **Responsiveness in Psychodynamic Relational Psychotherapy**   107
   Orya Tishby

6. **Responsiveness in Control-Mastery Theory**   133
   George Silberschatz

7. Context-Responsive Psychotherapy Integration Applied
   to Cognitive Behavioral Therapy   151
   Michael J. Constantino, Brien J. Goodwin, Heather J. Muir,
   Alice E. Coyne, and James F. Boswell

8. Responsiveness in Emotion-Focused Therapy   171
   Jeanne C. Watson

9. Responsiveness and Therapeutic Collaboration in Narrative
   Therapy   195
   Eugénia Ribeiro, Miguel M. Gonçalves, and Dulce Pinto

10. Therapist Responsiveness in Attachment-Based Family
    Therapy for Sexual and Gender Minority Adults and Their
    Nonaccepting Parents   219
    Gary M. Diamond, Rotem Boruchovitz-Zamir, and Ofir Nir-Gottlieb

11. Therapist Responsiveness in Treatments for Personality
    Disorders   237
    Ueli Kramer

12. Enhancing Therapist Responsiveness in Dialectical Behavior
    Therapy   257
    Jamie D. Bedics and Holly J. McKinley

13. Responsiveness in Integrative Therapies   277
    James F. Boswell, Brittany R. King, Carly M. Schwartzman,
    Rachel H. Wasserman, and Michael J. Constantino

III. INTEGRATION AND CONCLUSIONS   297

14. Meeting the Challenge of Responsiveness: Synthesizing
    Perspectives   299
    Jeanne C. Watson and Hadas Wiseman

Index   323
About the Editors   345

Contributors

Jamie D. Bedics, PhD, ABPP, Graduate School of Psychology, California Lutheran University, Thousand Oaks, CA, United States

Rotem Boruchovitz-Zamir, MA, Department of Psychology, Ben-Gurion University of the Negev, Beer Sheva, Israel

James F. Boswell, PhD, Department of Psychology, University at Albany, State University of New York, Albany, NY, United States

Michael J. Constantino, PhD, University of Massachusetts Amherst, Amherst, MA, United States

Alice E. Coyne, MS, University of Massachusetts Amherst, Amherst, MA, United States

Gary M. Diamond, PhD, Department of Psychology, Ben-Gurion University of the Negev, Beer Sheva, Israel

Sharon Egozi, PhD, Department of Social Work, Tel-Hai College, Upper Galilee, Israel

Catherine F. Eubanks, PhD, Ferkauf Graduate School of Psychology, Yeshiva University, Bronx, NY, United States

Miguel M. Gonçalves, PhD, School of Psychology, University of Minho, Braga, Portugal

Brien J. Goodwin, MS, University of Massachusetts Amherst, Amherst, MA, United States

Robert L. Hatcher, PhD, Graduate Center – City University of New York, New York, NY, United States

Brittany R. King, MA, Department of Psychology, University at Albany, State University of New York, Albany, NY, United States

Ueli Kramer, PhD, Department of Psychiatry, University of Lausanne, Lausanne, Switzerland

Holly J. McKinley, PsyD, Minneapolis VA Health Care System, Minneapolis, MN, United States

Heather J. Muir, MS, University of Massachusetts Amherst, Amherst, MA, United States

J. Christopher Muran, PhD, Gordon F. Derner School of Psychology, Adelphi University, Garden City, NY, United States

Ofir Nir-Gottlieb, MA, Department of Psychology, Ben-Gurion University of the Negev, Beer Sheva, Israel

Dulce Pinto, PhD, School of Psychology, University of Minho, Braga, Portugal

Eugénia Ribeiro, PhD, School of Psychology, University of Minho, Braga, Portugal

Carly M. Schwartzman, MA, Department of Psychology, University at Albany, State University of New York, Albany, NY, United States

Joey Sergi, PsyD, Therapists of New York, New York, NY, United States

George Silberschatz, PhD, Department of Psychiatry and Behavioral Sciences, University of California San Francisco, San Francisco, CA, United States

William B. Stiles, PhD, Miami University (Emeritus), Oxford, OH, Appalachian State University, Boone, NC, United States, and Metanoia Institute, London, United Kingdom

Orya Tishby, PsyD, Department of Psychology and the School of Social Work; Director of the Freud Center for Research in Psychoanalysis, Hebrew University, Jerusalem, Israel

Rachel H. Wasserman, PhD, Private Practice, Albany, NY, United States

Jeanne C. Watson, PhD, Department of Applied Psychology and Human Development, OISE/University of Toronto, Toronto, ON, Canada

Hadas Wiseman, PhD, Department of Counseling and Human Development, Faculty of Education, University of Haifa, Mount Carmel, Haifa, Israel

Acknowledgments

This book originated from a shared interest in psychotherapy that led us to York University to work with our mentor, Laura Rice, almost 40 years ago. At that time, she and Les Greenberg were advancing the patterns of change paradigm in psychotherapy research. Since then, our friendship has been sustained from graduate school onward through our involvement with the Society for Psychotherapy Research (SPR), where, with Laura's encouragement, we presented our work as graduate students and subsequently as full members culminating in us serving in succession as presidents of SPR in 2014 and 2015. This project was an opportunity to revisit our roots as process researchers, listening for markers and describing productive episodes of therapy to facilitate understanding of the change process in psychotherapy. We acknowledge the inspiration of luminaries in psychotherapy research and are grateful especially to David Orlinsky, the cofounder of SPR, and our colleagues and friends for their inspiration, support, and spirit of collaboration.

Projects like these do not materialize without the support and assistance of many collaborators. We would like to express our thanks to all the people at the American Psychological Association (APA) who provide the support and infrastructure to nurture ideas and realize them in print. Special thanks to Susan Reynolds of APA Books, whose support, encouragement, and faith in us when we proposed the idea at the SPR meeting in Toronto, Canada, in 2017, helped bring it to fruition. Thanks, too, to David Becker, who provided guidance and support toward the end of the project, as well as to the many others who work behind the scenes and screens to support our efforts. We are grateful to our collaborators for their willingness to share their ideas and provide opportunities for new learning as well as for their responsiveness throughout the project.

Our gratitude, too, to our clients and students throughout the years who have challenged and taught us the lessons on attunement and responsiveness, that we have shared with you. Finally, we cherish our respective families' ongoing love and support.

The
RESPONSIVE
PSYCHOTHERAPIST

INTRODUCTION

Exploring Responsiveness and Attunement in Psychotherapy

JEANNE C. WATSON AND HADAS WISEMAN

Responsiveness in psychotherapy is recognized as a ubiquitous characteristic of therapist–client interaction and dialogue (Kramer & Stiles, 2015). Synonyms for responsiveness include *openness, alertness, sensitivity, approachability,* and having positive reactions toward another, whereas being nonresponsive is described by words such as *sluggish, slow, sleepy, unaware,* or giving no response. The synonyms for responsiveness convey the quality of being fully present and available in the moment, whereas the antonyms convey an absence or lack of attention and disregard for the other. Responsive therapists are attuned, fully alive, and present with their clients, letting go of their own concerns and conflicts to mobilize all their resources to focus on what the client is bringing to the session and how to respond most appropriately in the moment. Like Rogers's (1980) therapeutic conditions—empathy, acceptance, warmth, and genuineness—responsiveness is an attitude, a way of being with another characterized as a willingness or capacity to be flexible and fluid to align with and be attentive to their goals and needs. Indeed, responsiveness is key to all interpersonal interactions, the aim of which is to foster connection and build relationships to promote positive outcomes, the primary goals of most psychotherapy approaches.

https://doi.org/10.1037/0000240-001
The Responsive Psychotherapist: Attuning to Clients in the Moment, J. C. Watson and H. Wiseman (Editors)

RESPONSIVENESS AS KEY TO RESEARCH AND PRACTICE

Responsiveness in psychotherapy has come into focus as research accumulates with respect to the complex relationships among emotional development, right brain functioning, psychopathology, and treatment options. Schore's (1994, 2003, 2019) work on the neurobiology of emotion highlighted the role that negative life experiences, including neglect and emotional and physical abuse, play in the emotional development of individuals. According to Schore, negative life experiences have a significant impact on the right brain—the seat of emotional learning—and its connections with the body, the autonomic nervous system, and the hypothalamic–pituitary axis. Research has highlighted that emotional learning is implicit and procedural rather than declarative and language based and thus less amenable to change with insight, rational knowledge, and thought processes alone. Facilitating change in emotional learning requires therapists to be highly attuned and responsive to clients' cognitive, emotional, and behavioral processes in the session to promote and encourage the acquisition of new emotional learning, interpersonal experiences, and memory reconsolidation in clients.

The landmark book *Psychotherapy Relationships That Work* (Norcross, 2002) broke new ground by focusing renewed and much-needed attention on the substantial research behind the crucial, but often-overlooked, client–therapist relationship. Subsequent editions have elaborated this focus to include a review of research on the effective elements of the therapy relationship and the particular aspects of treatment that support therapists to maximize their responsiveness and tailor their treatments for each patient (Norcross & Lambert, 2019; Norcross & Wampold, 2019). The evidence from the meta-analyses indicated that the client characteristics that are important to consider to fit treatments to particular individuals include attachment, coping styles, cultural adaptations, gender identity, preferences, reactance level, religion, spirituality, and sexual orientation, as well as clients' readiness to change. The identification of these variables as salient represents the state of the art in terms of those variables that are important to consider when tailoring treatments and being responsive to clients' intersecting identities and issues. However, these are higher order variables to guide practice and do not provide a fine-grained description or understanding of what therapists do in the session as they make moment-by-moment decisions and alterations to treatment manuals and principles to be maximally responsive to their clients.

Research shows that therapists' capacities to be responsive and tailor interventions and specific techniques to their clients' cognitive and affective states as they encounter them at different points in the session and across the course of treatment can make important contributions to treatment outcomes (Baldwin et al., 2007; Zuroff et al., 2010). Therapists' capacity to attune in the moment is key to enhancing optimal responsiveness and is essential to balancing the needs of clients with treatment procedures and techniques, as well as other process variables that compete for attention at any one moment in the therapy hour and across the treatment trajectory. Being responsive entails a complex type of responding that attends to and tracks shifts in clients' moment-to-moment process. It is much more than adherence to treatment protocols or the correct and adequate implementation of specific techniques. Rather, it requires sensitive, perceptive attention and a quality of listening that is alert to micro-shifts in clients' moment-to-moment behavior in the session, including their emotions, nonverbal behavior, and the content of their narratives, to facilitate access to their unconscious, implicit, and procedural knowledge. Access to implicit and procedural knowledge provides clients with opportunities for new learning in therapy.

With the increased recognition of the importance of responsiveness to treatment outcomes across different therapeutic approaches, along with ways of optimizing it to enable therapists to work more effectively with diverse clients by responding appropriately to the unique needs of each, we invited expert research clinicians from different approaches to share their expertise about what they attend to in the moment to steer the therapeutic process and be optimally responsive to their clients. We hoped that they would share their implicit procedural knowledge and make it more explicit to guide practice and research. Our aim was to highlight specific client and therapist processes along with specific signals or markers that alert clinicians to shifts in client process to be maximally attuned in the session and optimally responsive moment to moment in psychotherapy. Contributors were asked to discuss responsiveness within their approach and provide clear illustrations of what they attend to in the moment and to elaborate on the implications of responsiveness in terms of issues related to diversity and training to advance the understanding of the concept in practice and research.

Thus, the primary focus of this book is on therapist and client processes and the identification of specific signals that alert clinicians to shifts in clients' process and behavior in the therapy hour and over the course of therapy to be maximally responsive to their clients. It is recognized that therapists' responsiveness is important to facilitate new emotional learning and reconsolidate emotional memories to promote change in psychotherapy. In addition, to improve treatment effectiveness and work with diverse groups of clients with multiple intersecting identities, it is important for therapists to be able to monitor their interventions and ways of working to effectively tailor their interventions to clients' needs and objectives. We hoped to identify ways to enhance therapists' capacities to use the tools of psychotherapy more effectively. The book is written for both new and experienced therapists, with applications across a broad range of therapeutic approaches and issues pertinent to psychotherapy. We believe that meeting the challenge of responsiveness is crucial both for those involved in practice, training, and supervision, as well as for psychotherapy researchers in order to explore and design new research methods that will advance our understanding of responsiveness in relation to process and treatment outcomes.

OVERVIEW OF THE CHAPTERS

The book is composed of three parts. Part I provides an overview of the concept of responsiveness, including issues related to its definition and its differentiation from the working alliance, client engagement, and other constructs related to the therapeutic relationship. Part II focuses on the role of responsiveness in different therapeutic approaches, including psychodynamic therapies (psychodynamic relational psychotherapy and control-mastery theory), cognitive behavior therapy (CBT), emotion-focused therapy, narrative therapy, systemic-experiential psychotherapy, dialectical behavior therapy, and integrative therapy, as well as two approaches that focus on responsiveness in treatments for specific populations, including personality disorders and sexual and gender minority adults. To provide a common framework, contributors were asked to discuss the definition and conceptualization of responsiveness within their approach and identify signals or markers that therapists attend to in the moment to guide them in the session, along with clinical examples.[1] They were also asked to address the implications of responsiveness in their approach to issues of diversity and training. Finally, Part III integrates and synthesizes the different approaches to provide a rubric of the different signals and procedures that these research clinicians have identified as they try to meet the challenge of responsiveness. By pulling together the expertise of these research clinicians and developing a common lens through which to approach the concept, we hoped to elaborate our understanding of responsiveness, expand our clinical lexicons, offer support for training, and provide inspiration for further research.

---

[1]The identities of the clients in the case examples throughout this book have been disguised either by changing identifying information or using composites.

Part I. The Case for Responsiveness

The first two chapters of the book present the formulation of responsiveness and its implications for research and practice. In Chapter 1, Stiles, who first defined and posed the responsiveness problem for psychotherapy research (Stiles et al., 1998), provides an updated overview of the theoretical and methodological underpinnings of the issue of responsiveness (Stiles et al., 1998). Stiles defines responsiveness as behavior influenced by emerging events, such as therapists being influenced by and responding to what clients do, and as something that occurs on all time scales (from months to milliseconds) in the human context. In this chapter, he discusses how responsiveness undermines psychotherapy research and proposes and elaborates on the suitability of existing evaluative measures to reflect appropriate responsiveness. He discusses the work on responsiveness in terms of the six ways that psychotherapy researchers have engaged conceptually and empirically with the problem (Kramer & Stiles, 2015) and concludes with three suggestions for future research: "unpack evaluative measures, focus on immediate effects, and build an explanatory theory."

In Chapter 2, Hatcher provides a wide lens to explore and critique the concept of responsiveness and deciphers its place in relation to the working alliance and related therapeutic relationship concepts, collaboration, and engagement. He offers an astute and expanded view on responsiveness as studied within the science of relationships (Reis, 2014) and in Bacal's (1998) writing on optimal responsiveness in psychoanalytic psychotherapy. He reviews relevant types of research (e.g., feedback on routine monitoring of treatment process and outcome, personalized approaches to treatment) that have implications for developing professional training that seeks to enhance therapists' responsiveness and suggests new directions for training and research.

The next two chapters in Part I present two pantheoretical frameworks that have been developed to inform and enhance responsiveness in the client–therapist relationship. In Chapter 3, Wiseman and Egozi present Bowlby's (1962/1982) attachment theory as a pantheoretical framework for conceptualizing responsiveness in clinical research and practice. They reference research on infant–parent interactions that has demonstrated the centrality of responsiveness in infant–parent bonds and discuss its implications for therapists, especially the importance of providing a secure base for clients to facilitate engagement and productive outcomes. These authors suggest that to enhance attunement and responsiveness, therapists need to regulate an appropriate distance in the therapeutic relationship tailored to clients' attachment styles and needs. The challenges faced by therapists in their efforts to regulate optimal distance tailored to their client's needs are illustrated through relational narratives that represent markers of lack of responsiveness and misattunement, as well as appropriate responsiveness and attunement.

In Chapter 4, Eubanks, Sergi, and Muran examine responsiveness in rupture–repair cycles in the therapeutic alliance as a pantheoretical construct, viewed through a two-person perspective. These authors view therapist responsiveness as essential to the development and maintenance of a positive working alliance in therapy and as beneficial to treatments at any stage. In their chapter, they highlight the role of therapist attunement and responsiveness in successfully repairing alliance ruptures and demonstrate how the latter can occur as a result of failures in therapist responsiveness. State-of-the-art research on alliance rupture and repair cycles is presented along with context-dependent rupture resolution strategies for how clinicians can be more optimally responsive to achieve and maintain productive working alliances.

Part II. Responsiveness in Different Therapeutic Approaches

The second part of the book examines responsiveness within different therapeutic approaches. In the first two chapters in this part, therapist responsiveness is considered within two contemporary psychodynamic approaches. In Chapter 5, Tishby defines and explores responsiveness in psychodynamic relational psychotherapy, highlighting key concepts in relational thinking such as two-person psychology, which sees the individual in the context of dyadic interactions with other subjects, mutual recognition, and implicit relational knowing. She provides illuminating clinical vignettes illustrating how relational therapists are attuned and responsive to the state of the alliance, ruptures and repair, the transference–countertransference matrix, enactments and patient's dissociated self-states, and subtle shifts in patient and therapist affect, as well as clients' nonverbal communications.

In Chapter 6, Silberschatz uses principles from control-mastery theory, an integrated cognitive–psychodynamic–relational theory, to elucidate the concept of therapeutic responsiveness. According to the plan formulation method, an approach to case formulation, therapist interventions that are compatible with the patient's plan are considered optimally responsive because they help to disconfirm the patient's pathogenic beliefs, thereby increasing feelings of safety, relaxation, and useful therapeutic work. The author discusses the implications of this approach for training and presents preliminary data showing that training in the plan formulation method enhances therapist responsiveness and plays an important role in the process and outcome of psychotherapy.

In Chapter 7, Constantino, Goodwin, Muir, Coyne, and Boswell discuss context-responsive psychotherapy as applied to CBT. The authors make a strong case for paying attention to the therapists' responsivity across the course of treatment, referred to as the treatment "lifespan." The first step in being responsive focuses on getting off on the right foot, which is followed by during-session responsiveness, defined as doing more of the same or engaging in marker-driven departures. The authors provide research findings that support contextual responsivity, propose directions for future research, and offer strategies for training to maximize clinicians' responsiveness in a manner that applies not only to CBT but that can also be applied more pantheoretically within other approaches.

The next three chapters share an experiential–process view of responsiveness within a specific approach. Watson, in Chapter 8, examines responsiveness in emotion-focused therapy (EFT). In this approach, the therapeutic relationship, characterized by therapists' responsively attuning to clients' moment-by-moment process and moving between leading and following, is seen as an active ingredient of change. The author proposes a developmental model of the self, consisting of certain client capacities reflective of specific therapeutic zones of proximal development (TZPD), to guide therapists' responsiveness. Markers, located within therapists, clients, and the interpersonal process, are identified to guide therapists' attention and optimize their responsiveness in the session and across treatment. Suggestions for being responsive with clients from diverse backgrounds and multiple intersecting identities are presented, and the implications of responsiveness for EFT research and training are discussed.

In Chapter 9, Ribeiro, Gonçalves, and Pinto describe responsiveness and the therapeutic collaboration model in narrative therapy (TCM). Using the TCM, they offer a micro level perspective on responsiveness, focusing on the interactions in the therapeutic dyad moment to moment in the session. Appropriate responsiveness is viewed as an inherent property of therapeutic collaboration, which in turn is bounded by clients' TZPD, which is influenced by clients' characteristics, beyond diagnosis or the specific problems that clients bring to therapy. These concepts are illustrated in a session from narrative therapy at a moment-to-moment level. The authors review a number of studies that support their conceptualization of therapeutic responsiveness based on being sensitive and alert to clients' TZPD.

In Chapter 10, Diamond, Boruchovitz-Zamir, and Nir-Gottlieb focus on therapist responsiveness in attachment-based family therapy (ABFT), a manualized, experiential, emotion- and relationship-focused treatment designed for families in which parents have difficulty accepting their adult child's sexual orientation or gender identity. These authors delineate appropriate responsiveness as therapists using sensitive and effective interventions in the context of specific treatment tasks, including building a working alliance with the young adult, corrective attachment and identity episodes, and collaborative problem-solving, the client's characteristics, and the client's immediate, emerging behavior. Therapist responsive task interventions for this targeted population are illustrated and training issues are discussed with respect to applying ABFT in a responsive manner.

The next two chapters focus on responsiveness in treatments of personality disorders and, more specifically, borderline personality disorder. Kramer argues in Chapter 11 that treatment for clients with personality disorders represents a particularly fruitful context to demonstrate responsiveness effects, to find a context-appropriate definition of therapist responsiveness, and to show which interventions work with which client behavior to help therapists make productive use of opportunities that arise in the therapy process. He identifies three operationalizations of therapist responsiveness—generic, disorder specific, and individualized—and reviews studies using these operationalizations to examine the progression of the therapeutic alliance and outcome in borderline personality disorder.

In Chapter 12, Bedics and McKinley focus on enhancing therapist responsiveness in dialectical behavior therapy (DBT; Linehan, 1993), a cognitive behavior therapy initially developed for the treatment of suicidal behavior and later expanded for the treatment of borderline personality disorder with co-occurring Axis I disorders. These authors describe responsivity in the overall framework of delivering DBT (i.e., defining treatment goals and modules of interventions) and outline relevant principles guiding effective responsivity within DBT in outpatient individual psychotherapy.

In Chapter 13, the final chapter in Part II, Boswell, King, Schwartzman, Wasserman, and Constantino describe responsiveness as the raison d'être of integrative psychotherapies as therapists and clients use emerging information and contexts to modify their behavior in the service of optimizing therapy outcomes. They focus on two complementary meta-frameworks that can inform responsive integrative practice: the common principles of change framework that builds on common clinical strategies and putative mechanisms of action to guide clinician behavior and context responsive psychotherapy integration, an if–then framework supporting evidence-based clinical responsiveness in the form of matching therapist decision making and strategy to therapy contexts and clients' needs. Clinical examples of responsiveness are provided, and the intersection of the two meta-frameworks in responsive integrative psychotherapy is discussed.

Part III. Integration and Conclusions

In the quest to meet the challenge of responsiveness in theory, practice, and research, in the final chapter of the book (Chapter 14), we offer readers an integrative, pan-theoretical rubric of the different signals and markers used to guide therapists moment to moment in the session and provide possible directions for further research and training. First, an overview of the conceptualization of responsiveness across different approaches is provided, followed by a compilation of signals. The signals, garnered from the different therapeutic approaches, are classified in terms of whether they originate in the therapist, the client, or the interpersonal process. Finally, responsiveness in relation to working therapeutically with diverse populations, implications for training, and directions for research are considered, amalgamating the wisdom and suggestions of each of the contributors. It is our hope that this text will prove useful to clinicians and researchers as they continue to explore this new frontier in psychotherapy.

It is only fitting that we mention the unusual context of the COVID-19 worldwide pandemic, during which the final stage of the book was completed. Being a responsive therapist became even more challenging given this unfamiliar terrain and the chaos surrounding the pandemic, as well as other issues that claimed our attention on the world stage. We hope that readers will find the ideas presented in this book valuable as a guide to *doing the right thing at the right time.*

REFERENCES

Bacal, H. A. (Ed.). (1998). *Optimal responsiveness: How therapists heal their patients.* Jason Aronson.

Baldwin, S. A., Wampold, B. E., & Imel, Z. E. (2007). Untangling the alliance-outcome correlation: Exploring the relative importance of therapist and patient variability in the alliance. *Journal of Consulting and Clinical Psychology, 75*(6), 842–852. https://doi.org/10.1037/0022-006X.75.6.842

Bowlby, J. (1982). *Attachment and loss: Vol. 1. Attachment* (2nd ed.). Basic Books. (Original work published 1962)

Kramer, U., & Stiles, W. B. (2015). The responsiveness problem in psychotherapy: A review of proposed solutions. *Clinical Psychology: Science and Practice, 22*(3), 277–295. https://doi.org/10.1111/cpsp.12107

Linehan, M. (1993). *Cognitive behavioral treatment of borderline personality disorder.* Guilford Press.

Norcross, J. C. (2002). *Psychotherapy relationships that work.* Oxford University Press.

Norcross, J. C., & Lambert, M. J. (Eds.). (2019). *Psychotherapy relationships that work: Vol. 1. Evidence-based therapist contributions* (3rd ed.). Oxford University Press.

Norcross, J. C., & Wampold, B. E. (Eds.). (2019). *Psychotherapy relationships that work: Vol. 2. Evidence-based therapist responsiveness* (3rd ed.). Oxford University Press.

Reis, H. T. (2014). Responsiveness: Affective interdependence in close relationships. In M. Mikulincer & P. R. Shaver (Eds.), *Mechanisms of social connection: From brain to group* (pp. 255–271). American Psychological Association. https://doi.org/10.1037/14250-015

Rogers, C. R. (1980). *A way of being*. Houghton Mifflin.

Schore, A. N. (1994). *Affect regulation and the origin of the self: The neurobiology of emotional development*. Erlbaum.

Schore, A. N. (2003). *Affect regulation and the repair of the self* (Vol. 2). Norton.

Schore, A. N. (2019). *The development of the unconscious mind*. Norton.

Stiles, W. B., Honos-Webb, L., & Surko, M. (1998). Responsiveness in psychotherapy. *Clinical Psychology: Science and Practice, 5*(4), 439–458. https://doi.org/10.1111/j.1468-2850.1998.tb00166.x

Zuroff, D. C., Kelly, A. C., Leybman, M. J., Blatt, S. J., & Wampold, B. E. (2010). Between-therapist and within-therapist differences in the quality of the therapeutic relationship: Effects on maladjustment and self-critical perfectionism. *Journal of Clinical Psychology, 66*(7), 681–697. https://doi.org/10.1002/jclp.20683

PART **I** THE CASE FOR
RESPONSIVENESS

1

RESPONSIVENESS IN PSYCHOTHERAPY RESEARCH

Problems and Ways Forward

WILLIAM B. STILES

Things weren't working for researchers. Psychotherapy outcome research seemed unable to identify the most effective treatment approach. Since 1936, the Dodo's verdict had been that "everybody has won, and all must have prizes" (Carroll, 1865, p. 34); that is, each of the many alternative psychotherapies appeared about as effective as any of the others (Luborsky, Singer, & Luborsky, 1975; Rosenzweig, 1936; Stiles et al., 1986; Wampold & Imel, 2015). This seemed not just disappointing but also unbelievable to advocates of particular approaches, and they continued to conduct comparative trials, with different controls and improved methods, but with similar results. Could all psychotherapies really be equivalent?

Things were also problematic in process research. Investigators developed elaborate systems for coding therapeutic techniques and other processes (Elliott et al., 1987; Greenberg & Pinsof, 1986; Kiesler, 1973; Russell & Stiles, 1979). But, except for broad evaluative variables like the alliance (more about that later), comparisons with treatment outcomes failed to confirm the value of psychotherapy's key technical ingredients (Stiles & Shapiro, 1994; see also Orlinsky & Howard, 1978, 1986; Orlinsky et al., 1994, 2003). Are the main tools that psychotherapists are trained to use inert or worthless?

https://doi.org/10.1037/0000240-002
The Responsive Psychotherapist: Attuning to Clients in the Moment, J. C. Watson and H. Wiseman (Editors)

An explanatory concept that made sense of these puzzling and frustrating results for me is responsiveness. I have been writing about responsiveness for quite a while (e.g., Kramer & Stiles, 2015; Stiles, 1987, 1988, 2009, 2013, 2020; Stiles et al., 1998; Stiles & Horvath, 2017). This chapter highlights and elaborates points I have argued previously in explaining this concept as it applies to psychotherapy and psychotherapy research.

The first two major sections of this chapter describe how responsiveness has been a problem for psychotherapy research. This may seem negative, but I think understanding the problem is a prerequisite for solving it. The final section briefly reviews how researchers have investigated responsiveness and argues that its resistance to conventional research designs opens opportunities for thoughtful creativity.

RESPONSIVENESS IS PROBLEMATIC FOR PSYCHOTHERAPY RESEARCH

Responsiveness refers to behavior being influenced by emerging context (Stiles et al., 1998). It means people behave differently depending on what happens around them, such as what other people do. Paying attention and being polite are responsive. If I open the door for you or answer your questions or repeat something when you look puzzled, I'm being responsive. If mothers repeat the sounds or expressions their babies make, they are being responsive.

People are responsive on time scales from months to milliseconds. They save for retirement in response to their current income and what they expect the future to hold. They choose what clothes to wear in response to the weather and the occasion. They adjust the car's steering wheel and the pressure on the accelerator depending on the road and the traffic and where they want to go. Since different things happen around people all the time, people respond differently all the time.

Responsiveness isn't necessarily benign; it just means that people's actions depend on the circumstances. People can be responsive with malicious intent, for personal gain, or for any reason. But psychotherapists generally have good intentions. They generally aim to help their clients, and they respond to do that in ways consistent with their approach's principles. We can call this *appropriate responsiveness*. To be appropriately responsive means: *Do the right thing*. In general, therapists try to do the right thing—that is, they try to be appropriately responsive.

Therapists' main skills and activities involve appropriate responsiveness. That is, they try to do the right thing in treatment assignment, treatment planning, active listening, timing, staying on topic, turn-taking, attunement, and adjusting interventions already in progress. They customize treatment to fit clients' requirements. Arguably, therapists are effective because they are appropriately responsive, that is, because they consistently do the right thing, providing each client with a different, individually tailored treatment (Stiles & Horvath, 2017).

Treatment theories, descriptions, and even treatment manuals emphasize appropriate responsiveness. They instruct therapists to establish rapport, to frame and time interventions to fit the client's progress, to push where it moves (pursue a line of intervention that seems to be having the intended effect), and to adapt interventions to client resources. Supervisors and supervisees review session recordings and verbal accounts of what happened, seeking the optimal response for each situation. What they seek is not mastery of a standard (if complex) task but rather sensitivity to what the client brings and flexibility and resourcefulness to adapt a repertoire of skills to emerging requirements.

Formulating the Responsiveness Problem

Perhaps researchers should have seen earlier that the Dodo verdict and the process–outcome disappointments were aspects of the same problem. After all, in practice, treatment approaches are packages of process components. The concept of responsiveness offers an explanation, but formulating the problem has taken a long time.

For me, the issue began to take shape around a paradox regarding client self-disclosure. Passages representing good psychotherapeutic process tended to include substantially higher proportions of client disclosure than passages representing poor process (Stiles et al., 1979). However, clients whose sessions had higher proportions of self-disclosure did not tend to have better outcomes (McDaniel et al., 1981). A clue to the explanation of this seeming paradox was that the clients who were distressed tended to use high levels of disclosure (McDaniel et al., 1981). Perhaps the relation of disclosure to psychological distress is analogous to the relation of a fever to infection (Stiles, 1987): Just as fever is an adaptive response to physical infection but not a good predictor of physical recovery, client self-disclosure is an adaptive response to psychological stress or distress, and hence an important component of good process, but it is not a good predictor of psychological recovery. That is, the people with the most serious infections or the greatest distress are not the ones most likely to recover. In retrospect, we could say that a client's amount of disclosure is responsive to the client's need to disclose, a need that psychotherapy is designed to meet.

A parallel argument can explain why therapist verbal techniques that are frequently used and that are important theoretically and clinically (e.g., interpretations, questions, exploratory reflections, treatment directives) nevertheless show negligible correlations with improvement (Stiles & Shapiro, 1994). If clients' requirements for, say, interpretations or Socratic questions vary, and therapists adjust their use of the technique to match clients' requirements, then all patients get what they need. An appropriately responsive therapist approximates an optimum level of such techniques, which is different for different clients and occasions. There is no reason to expect use of the technique to correlate with outcome even though the technique is appropriate and helpful. That is, if every client receives just the right level of the technique, then its expected correlation with outcome is zero (unless clients' optimum levels predict outcome for some other reason). It wouldn't help to do more or less than optimum. As a result, process–outcome correlations are misleading (Stiles, 1988, 2013).

Therapists may even compensate for experimental manipulations of specific process components by responsive adjustments in other components. For example, Cox, Holbrook, and Rutter (1981; Cox, Rutter, & Holbrook, 1981) manipulated interviewer style in diagnostic interviews with mothers of referred children. Interviewers using four contrasting styles (directive vs. nondirective crossed with active vs. passive) elicited similar levels of information and feeling, but they did so by different paths as they responsively adjusted to the experimental manipulations. A therapist instructed to ask fewer questions might elicit information by using more reflections or remaining silent, allowing clients more space to talk.

How Responsiveness Undermines Psychotherapy Research

Thus, appropriate responsiveness actively defeats the process–outcome model because therapists respond appropriately to clients' differing requirements. The null hypothesis in statistical tests of process–outcome relations requires the assumption that the process components (e.g., verbal techniques) are delivered randomly—that what therapists say and do is independent of what their clients say or do or need. No human conversation is like that.

To dramatize the point, assume that interpretations are an important active ingredient in psychodynamic psychotherapy. Different clients require different numbers of interpretations. Perhaps some see the point quickly and apply what they learn, whereas others require rephrasing or more extensive exploration. Therapists respond to these differing requirements, offering fewer when clients require fewer, more when clients require more. Yet despite the therapists' best efforts, the quicker clients may have better outcomes than the slower clients. In process–outcome research this yields a negative correlation between interpretations and outcome (as observed in a classic study by Sloane et al., 1975). Reviewers could conclude that interpretations are useless or even harmful, even if (as assumed) interpretations are an important active ingredient in the therapy.

Responsiveness also distorts dose-effect relations, which in psychotherapy usually means the relation of the number of sessions to the amount of improvement (Howard et al., 1986). In naturalistic settings, rather than improving with the number of sessions, outcomes tend to be similar no matter how many sessions a client receives (Barkham et al., 1996, 2006; Robinson et al., 2020; Stiles, Barkham, & Wheeler, 2015). This may seem surprising if the treatment is considered as an experimental manipulation. But it is clinically sensible if clients and therapists are considered as responsively ending treatment when their requirements have been met. Clients change at different rates and achieve a good-enough level of gains at different treatment durations. When they've had enough, they stop.

Positive dose-effect relations may appear in randomized trials of different treatment durations, where experimental specifications override the normal responsiveness. For example, in the second Sheffield psychotherapy project, depressed clients were randomly assigned to receive either eight or 16 sessions. Those who received 16 showed a bit more improvement (Shapiro et al., 1994), perhaps because some in the eight-session group ended too early, while some in the 16-session group improved beyond their good-enough level. But even in this experimental study, clients and therapists appeared to adapt by accelerating key processes responsively (Reynolds et al., 1996), muting the effect of the manipulation.

As noted, responsiveness undermines tests of differential treatment outcomes (Stiles, 2009, 2013). In trying to be appropriately responsive, therapists are working to eliminate precisely the differences between techniques and treatments that researchers are trying to discover. Therapists do their best to adapt treatment to their clients' needs and resources, so each client receives a different treatment, responsively crafted to work as well as participants know how. Within the limits of resources and therapists' abilities, then, clients tend to have optimal outcomes in all bona fide treatments, as the Dodo has been reminding us for 8 decades (Rosenzweig, 1936; Wampold & Imel, 2015).

As a further consequence, the independent variables are not independent of the dependent variables. Outcome affects process; that is, therapeutic improvement affects techniques as therapists responsively adapt their treatment approach to emerging client requirements. Therapists monitor progress and shape the treatment depending on how well things are going. Thus, the delivered treatment (the independent variable) is dependent on improvement or lack of it (the dependent variable). This lack of independence violates a central assumption of the statistical techniques used to analyze results.

Responsiveness even undermines the terminology. Because therapists and clients respond to ever-changing circumstances, no two minutes of therapy are the same, much less any two courses of treatment. Thus, the levels of the independent variable (i.e., the treatment conditions) in outcome research are never the same twice. Treatments with the same name (e.g., cognitive, psychodynamic, person-centered) are not stable, so the names themselves lose meaning. Saying, for example, that all clients in the cognitive therapy group received cognitive therapy is misleading because none of those treatments was the same and none could be reproduced except in an abstract sense. It is not clear what a conclusion that, for example, "cognitive therapy was more effective than treatment as usual" might mean scientifically.

Appropriate responsiveness is an integral part of all treatments; it is not a confounding or extraneous variable, not a source of noise or bias or intrusion that obscures or distorts the effects. Training and supervision are designed to teach therapists how to establish rapport, frame and time interventions to fit the client and the occasion, listen actively, and so forth. Even treatment manuals call for such appropriate responsiveness. Because responsiveness is part of the therapy, it cannot be eliminated by more careful specification, and it cannot be overcome by randomization.

EVALUATIVE MEASURES ASSESS APPROPRIATE RESPONSIVENESS

If appropriate responsiveness is so central in psychotherapy and in training and supervision, you might expect psychotherapy researchers would have found ways to measure it. I think they have done so, albeit not explicitly, in the form of evaluative process measures.

Evaluative Process Measures Reflect Appropriate Responsiveness

Evaluative variables concern whether something is good or bad, positive or negative, skillful or unskillful, pleasant or unpleasant, distressing or comforting, beautiful or ugly, appetizing or disgusting, successful or unsuccessful, or effective or ineffective. Evaluative variables concern the degree to which the target was valuable; measuring them involves judgments of value to or by some person. They do not describe specific behaviors but rather whether the respondent valued it or thought someone else valued it. I suggest that evaluative psychotherapy process variables reflect the therapist's and/or client's appropriate responsiveness, that is, the extent to which the therapist or client did the right thing.

Evaluative variables can be contrasted with descriptive variables, which concern characteristics that, at least in principle, could be observed by anyone in the right place at the right time with the right skills and equipment. Descriptive variables include the use of the sort of techniques cited earlier as generally uncorrelated with outcome, such as interpretations, Socratic questions, self-disclosures, and assigning homework. The descriptions of these are the same whether or not the behaviors were the right thing to do under the circumstances.

All or almost all of the psychotherapy process variables that consistently predict outcome are evaluative variables. Arguably all of the generally "effective elements of therapy relationships" assembled by Norcross (2002, 2011; Norcross & Lambert, 2019) are substantially evaluative. Examples include alliance, group cohesion, empathy, goal consensus and collaboration, and positive regard. Descriptively, a strong alliance, for example, is not the same across occasions or people. Exhibiting a strong alliance involves different words and actions on different occasions. What is the same is the way the respondents value it. Even variables that at first sound descriptive have modifiers that make them evaluative, for example, "*Repairing* Alliance Ruptures" (Norcross, 2011, p. xv, italics added) and "*Managing* Countertransference" (Norcross, 2011, p. xv, italics added). These measures do not concern whether or not ruptures or countertransference occurred but whether or not the work on them was judged to be successful, that is, whether or not the participants did the right thing.

To put it another way, evaluative measures describe achievements, not actions (Stiles & Wolfe, 2006). To achieve a strong alliance, for example, the therapist must do the right thing over a period of time. The therapist cannot arbitrarily choose to have a strong alliance in the same sense that the therapist can choose to ask a question.

Attempts to Measure Appropriate Responsiveness Descriptively Turn Out Evaluative

Conversely, explicit attempts to assess appropriate responsiveness descriptively seem to yield evaluative measures. In my opinion, Elkin et al. (2014) made the most concerted attempt. Using data drawn from the National Institute of Mental Health collaborative trial for depression (Elkin et al., 1989), "four researchers, . . . all with considerable clinical experience, spent 7 months, meeting bi-weekly, to view and rate videotapes, check discrepancies, and assess reliability" (Elkin et al., 2014, p. 56). They developed a three-part instrument intended to measure therapist responsiveness. Part I, the main focus of their work, consisted of 11 descriptive items that seemed responsive, such as *makes eye contact, uses minimal encouragers,* and *focuses on and demonstrates interest in the patient,* rated at 5-minute intervals. Part II, added late in the process to assess the global atmosphere, consisted of evaluative items based on viewing the entire session, such as *compatible level of discourse* and *appropriate level of emotional quality/intensity.* Part III was a one-item rating of therapist responsiveness in the session. Indexes based on these ratings were compared with measures of patient engagement in therapy, such as early termination. Results showed that factors based on the descriptive features of responsiveness in Part I did not predict engagement (but see the next paragraph); however, the global evaluative items from Part II and the single item responsiveness rating did predict engagement.

The logic of responsiveness suggests the descriptive features failed because more is not always better. As noted earlier, for most descriptive process components, an appropriately responsive therapist approximates an optimum level, which is different for different clients and occasions. This holds for common facilitative behaviors like saying "mm-hm" or making eye contact, as well as for treatment-specific interventions such as assigning homework, two-chair dialogue, or reflection of feeling. This reasoning does not apply when more is always better, as in the case of evaluative variables (Stiles, 1996). Neither does it apply when more is always worse. Elkin et al. (2014) found that a factor consisting of negative descriptive items, such as *disrupts flow, lectures,* and *critical/judgmental,* predicted early termination. If the appropriately responsive level for negative therapist behaviors is none (e.g., Anderson et al., 2012), then more is always worse.

In another explicit effort to measure appropriate, or "attuned," responsiveness, Snyder and Silberschatz (2017) developed the Patient's Experience of Attunement and Responsiveness (PEAR) Scale, which consists of such items as, "My therapist had accurate empathy for my needs and feelings today." It has parallel patient and therapist versions. Exploratory factor analyses distinguished three patient factors and two therapist factors. All of them sound much like other evaluative process scales: *perceived helpfulness, felt empathy,* and *sensed accomplishments* in the patient version; *therapist helpfulness* and *safe-accepted* in the therapist version. In an initial test, the factors showed modest correlations with measures of treatment outcome.

Evaluative Measures Don't Describe Good Process

Here's the rub: Evaluative process measures label and assess whether the process was good or bad, but they don't show what was good or bad about it. Studies using ratings of alliance, empathy, group cohesion, and so forth show that good process predicts good outcome[1] (Norcross, 2002, 2011; Norcross & Lambert, 2019), which is reassuring and publishable. But such studies don't explain what good process is. Different therapist behaviors may yield high ratings on evaluative measures in different cases and at different times, depending on what the client required. Sometimes the right (appropriately responsive) intervention is a question and sometimes an interpretation. Sometimes it may be to assign homework, prescribe a drug, or propose a two-chair exercise. Sometimes the right thing to do is to nod or smile or do nothing.

The right thing is likely to vary depending on, for example, the client's diagnosis, intelligence, education, personality, social situation, stage of life, values, and personal history. The right thing to do is also likely to vary with the therapist's theoretical approach, skills, personality, and demographic characteristics. The right response for a psychoanalytic therapist, for example, is often different from the right response for a cognitive therapist. The right response for a young male therapist may be different from the right response for an old female therapist. The right thing is also likely to differ depending on the stage of therapy, the history of this particular therapeutic relationship, the immediately preceding events, the circumstances of the session, and so forth (see Norcross & Wampold, 2019, for some reviews). The right thing may not be the polite thing or what the client wants at the moment. In some approaches, appropriate therapist responsiveness may entail interventions that cause the client short-term discomfort—not answering a question, confronting an avoided topic, or prescribing exposure to distressing situations—in service of long-term goals.

This is not to say that all evaluative concepts are the same. Sensible conceptual distinctions can be made among them (e.g., see Hatcher, 2015), they can be rated reliably (see next section), and they are associated with widely sought outcomes (but see Footnote 1). A consequence, I think, is a sort of stagnation in psychotherapy process–outcome research, with an ever-increasing array of

---

[1] Most outcome measures, including participant or observer ratings of improvement, effectiveness, or reduced distress, are also evaluative and have related problems. Hans Strupp (1963) put it this way: "As long as one relies on global clinical judgments, like outcome, one substitutes something for real information" (p. 5).

evaluative measures with different names that correlate with outcomes but lack the behavioral specificity needed for detailed theory building.

People Recognize Quality: The Pirsig Phenomenon

Remarkably, considering the complexity, psychotherapy participants and observers can often make reliable ratings of evaluative variables as illustrated by psychometric acceptability of the evaluative measures (reviewed in Norcross, 2002, 2011). Clients, therapists, and, sometimes, experienced judges can distinguish when the process is good or bad—whether an alliance is strong or weak, whether the therapist is being empathic, whether the group is cohesive, and so forth. They can take the circumstances into account and assess how well an intervention responded to the requirements of the moment. In retrospect, judges can even say what was positive or negative about it. However, they cannot specify the right behaviors in advance. I call this the "Pirsig phenomenon," after Robert Pirsig (1974), who argued that people seem able to judge quality in many things, but they cannot specify in general what quality consists of. Perhaps this ability involves what Rogers (1959) called the "organismic valuing process" and what Zajonc (1980) meant in saying "preferences need no inferences" (p. 151). It is as if people have evolved to recognize what is valuable, taking circumstances into account.

WAYS FOLLOWED AND WAYS FORWARD

Responsiveness in various guises has been addressed by researchers for a long time. For example, investigators in child development studied the importance of mothers' appropriate responsiveness to their infants, noting, for example, how infants are upset when their mothers look at them with an unexpressive "still face" (Mesman et al., 2009; Tronick et al., 1978). Research on control-mastery theory focused on clients' unarticulated plans for treatment and the ways therapists respond to the implicit tests clients set (Silberschatz et al., 1986; Weiss, 1993).

Norcross (2002, 2011; Norcross & Wampold, 2019) used the term *responsiveness* in the subtitles of his influential volumes on relationship variables. Caspar and Grosse-Holtforth (2009) noted the problem of responsiveness and argued that a motive-oriented therapeutic relationship offers a way to address responsiveness directly. Hatcher (2015; see also Chapter 2 by Hatcher in this volume) conceptualized responsiveness in therapy and training. Other authors in this book also have accounts of how they became aware of and formulated responsiveness. More pervasively, if research that used evaluative measures is included, then most psychotherapy research has concerned responsiveness.

Engaging With the Responsiveness Problem

In a review of conceptual and empirical work on responsiveness, Kramer and Stiles (2015) distinguished six ways that psychotherapy researchers have engaged with the responsiveness problem: (a) demonstrating effects of responsiveness empirically; (b) measuring responsiveness quantitatively; (c) describing responsiveness qualitatively; (d) using evaluative measures, which incorporate responsiveness; (e) developing clinical interventions that are explicitly responsive; and (f) extending responsiveness concepts to other, related domains (p. 281).

Work on point (b), measuring responsiveness quantitatively, and point (d), using evaluative measures, was discussed extensively in the preceding major sections. Work on the other points has included the following.

Demonstrating Responsiveness

Much of the work in this category involved studying contingencies: how therapists responded differently depending on characteristics of the client or circumstances. For example, in a study suggesting mutual responsiveness, Connolly Gibbons et al. (2003) reported, "therapists used more clarifications and restatements with patients who rated the therapeutic empathy higher, more clarifications and questions with patients who rated higher on depression, and more learning statements with patients who provided more complete interpersonal narratives" (p. 169). Most therapy approaches specify contingencies or markers—indicators of when particular techniques should be used or considered, such as "don't interpret too early" or "use two-chair work for self-evaluative splits." Such effects are sometimes called aptitude-treatment interactions (Snow, 1991). Also placed in this category are naturalistic studies in which therapy participants adjust the duration of treatment to client requirements (e.g., Baldwin et al., 2009; Stiles, Barkham, & Wheeler, 2015).

Qualitative Approaches

Qualitative research takes advantage of the rich observations afforded by case studies and interviews. It is unrestricted by the limits on the number of variables that can be dealt with in statistical models. If each verbal descriptor is considered as a variable, then qualitative research is hugely multivariate, able to simultaneously examine as many variables as there are descriptors in the language. This affords qualitative approaches a more realistically nuanced characterization of responsive human interaction.

Case studies offer great scope for qualitative study of responsiveness (Stiles, 2017). Werbart et al. (2019) contrasted successful and unsuccessful cases of three different therapists and showed how the successful cases were distinguished by the therapists adjusting their way of working to their patients' needs, whereas in the unsuccessful cases the therapists failed to adjust. The research strategy of task analysis (Greenberg, 2007) selects instances of some therapeutic task, such as dealing with unexpressed anger with a parent or overcoming a withdrawal rupture in the therapeutic relationship. The instances are then examined to distinguish and refine a common series of steps required to complete the task.

The discipline of conversational analysis takes moment-by-moment responsiveness as its central topic, examining such phenomena as turn-taking, preferred sequences, silences, conversational rupture, and repair (Labov & Fanshel, 1977; Peräkylä et al., 2008; Smoliak & Strong, 2018). As an illustration, Gaete et al. (2018) described how both power relationships and negotiation about therapeutic interpretations are enacted by what they called "reflexive questions." These utterances are grammatically questions but may also indirectly advance a therapeutic interpretation or advice, for example, "If you did raise these worries with her, do you think she would take it as a lack of trust? . . . As an intrusion into her privacy? . . . Or as an indication of your caring as a parent?" (p. 120). By using the therapist's frame of reference, this intervention redirects the client's understanding and thus exercises the therapist's power. On the other hand, the question form is less presumptuous than a bald interpretation or directive would be, so it allows more leeway for negotiation.

Responsive Treatment Approaches

Some treatment approaches have used responsiveness as an organizing concept. In various ways they describe how each client should receive an individually tailored therapy. Examples include control-mastery theory (Silberschatz, 2005; Weiss, 1993), plan analysis (Caspar, 1995, 2007), and the marker-guided interventions of emotion-focused therapy (Elliott, Watson, et al., 2004; Greenberg, 2002). Pluralistic psychotherapy (Cooper & McLeod, 2007, 2011) suggests that therapists negotiate with their clients about which theoretical approach might best address the client's needs and preferences. Specificity theory (Bacal & Carlton, 2010) argues that each client should and does get an individualized treatment. Smedslund (2012, 2016) proposed that a therapist should be a bricoleur, a jack-of-all-trades who individualizes treatment by drawing on knowledge people share by virtue of being human, understandings acquired though language and culture, and personal familiarity with this particular client rather than using a specific theoretical approach or evidence from formal research.

Some responsive processes seem common across approaches. Examples of research lines that address these include facilitative skills (Anderson, Crowley, et al., 2016; Anderson, Ogles, & Weis, 1999) and alliance rupture repair (Safran & Muran, 1996; Safran et al., 2011; see also Chapter 4 by Eubanks et al. in this volume). Session-level monitoring and feedback (Lambert, 2010) is an increasingly common, explicitly responsive practice. See the other chapters in Part II of this book for accounts of how responsiveness is discussed and implemented within each of a variety of treatment approaches.

Extensions to Other Domains

Responsiveness is ubiquitous. Kramer and Stiles (2015) reviewed a few studies that had explicitly made the link between responsiveness in psychotherapy and responsiveness in related areas, such as clinical supervision and interaction in organizations. For example, Friedlander (2012) suggested that supervisors' appropriate responsiveness may foster appropriate responsiveness by the therapists they supervise. Osatuke et al. (2009) argued that interventions intended to foster interpersonal respect in the workplace must be implemented responsively, taking into account the workers' moment-by-moment requirements.

Suggestions for Further Research

I would like to add three suggestions for further research: unpack evaluative measures, focus on immediate effects, and build an explanatory theory.

Unpack Evaluative Measures

Even though evaluative measures are unspecific, they show what is at stake. They focus researchers' attention on what is valuable in psychotherapy. Unpacking could involve describing (perhaps qualitatively) what exactly happened as dyads achieved their alliance, empathy, group cohesion, and so forth. What led particular clients or therapists to change their response on each item of their alliance rating scale? How did clients and therapists repair ruptures in their relationships (see Chapter 4 by Eubanks et al. in this volume)? Such unpacking would test the limits of the Pirsig phenomenon. It must stay mindful that evaluative measures encompass many different specific events and experiences. The consistencies will not be simple.

Focus on the Immediate Effects

The study of therapists' appropriate responsiveness encompasses responsiveness *to* (e.g., client characteristics, process markers); the approaches, interventions, and responsiveness *with* (e.g., interventions, techniques); and responsiveness *for* (e.g., reduced anxiety, deepening experience, insight). Perhaps the last of these deserves more attention.

Perceptual control theory (Carey et al., 2012; Powers, 2005) suggests that behavior can be best understood as continual adjustments intended to achieve particular effects. To illustrate, the accelerator and brake pedals and steering wheel are continually adjusted to keep a car moving down the road. It would be virtually impossible to describe how to drive by specifying how much to press on the pedals and turn the steering wheel or by specifying eye movements and muscle movements in the arms and legs. Instead, the activity is understood in terms of responding to speed and signs and traffic and keeping the car on the road. Behavior is guided by anticipated perceptions.

Guiding psychotherapy interventions using relevant feedback is the principle underlying monitoring symptom intensity ratings (cf. Lambert, 2010). This can be extended to keeping the therapeutic process on course at a finer-grained level using knowledge of what that course is. And this, in turn, depends on understanding the sequence of changes clients go through on their way to psychological improvement. If therapists know what should come next and can recognize when the process is on or off course, they will be better able to facilitate progress. There are theoretical accounts of this sequence (e.g., Egan, 2002; Hill, 2014; Norcross et al., 2011; Rogers, 1961; Stiles, 2011). Working within such developmental or stage models, research can examine how therapists advance or retard progress through the sequence (e.g., Caro Gabalda et al., 2016; Ribeiro et al., 2016).

Build an Explanatory Theory
Observations on responsive processes are devilishly complex. Any hope of comprehending how psychotherapy works will depend on systematic conceptual work to organize therapeutic responsiveness.

In discussing psychotherapy theory and research, I find it helpful to distinguish explanatory theories from treatment theories because they are evaluated by very different kinds of research. *Explanatory theories* describe what things are and how they are related to each other. In general, scientific theories are explanatory theories. Explanatory theories are evaluated by comparing observations with details of or derivations from the theory. I call this "theory-building research." *Treatment theories* are the concepts that guide clinicians in conducting therapy. Treatment theories are evaluated by testing whether or not the treatments are effective (e.g., clinical trials). I call this "product-testing research" (Stiles, Hill, & Elliott, 2015).

Treatment theories must respect responsiveness, as responsiveness is integral to conducting psychotherapy. However, their purpose is practical, and they may be much less detailed and precise than explanatory accounts. Treatment theories resist change because product-testing research conducted to evaluate them does not address the details of the theory but only the overall efficacy of complex and fluid treatment packages. Even if efficacy differences appear (the Dodo to the contrary), the results of clinical trials do not address the explanation or mechanism.

Some treatment theories are based on explanatory theories, and some familiar theories aspire to be both (see later chapters). The explanatory versions, as well as dedicated explanatory psychotherapy theories, such as attachment theory (see Chapter 3 by Wiseman and Egozi in this volume) and assimilation theory (Stiles, 2011), can be examined in theory building research. Theory-building research studies the details. Some observations confirm expectations, which increases confidence in the theory, and some are unexpected, which may point to *abductions*, that is, to modifications, elaborations, or extensions of the theory (Stiles, 2017). The process is thus self-correcting, and theory is cumulative. It does not directly address the "which is best" question, but it offers a way forward.

CODA

In this chapter, I've tried to explain just a few main points. First, responsiveness is ubiquitous and central to psychotherapy practice, but it poses problems for many of the usual approaches to psychotherapy research. Human interaction is intricately interactive in ways and on time scales that most descriptive variables used in statistical hypothesis testing fail to represent adequately. Second, appropriate responsiveness—doing the right thing—is regularly assessed with evaluative measures. These helpfully quantify the amount or intensity of appropriate responsiveness, but they offer limited understanding of its nature or of how it is achieved. Third, many approaches to practicing and investigating responsiveness have been tried and proposed. The puzzles that responsiveness pose offer many opportunities for careful thought and creativity, as illustrated in this book's other chapters.

REFERENCES

Anderson, T., Crowley, M. E., Himawan, L., Holmberg, J. K., & Uhlin, B. D. (2016). Therapist facilitative interpersonal skills and training status: A randomized clinical trial on alliance and outcome. *Psychotherapy Research*, *26*(5), 511–529. https://doi.org/10.1080/10503307.2015.1049671

Anderson, T., Knobloch-Fedders, L. M., Stiles, W. B., Ordoñez, T., & Heckman, B. D. (2012). The power of subtle interpersonal hostility in psychodynamic psychotherapy: A speech acts analysis. *Psychotherapy Research*, *22*(3), 348–362. https://doi.org/10.1080/10503307.2012.658097

Anderson, T., Ogles, B. M., & Weis, A. (1999). Creative use of interpersonal skills in building a therapeutic alliance. *Journal of Constructivist Psychology, 12*(4), 313–330. https://doi.org/10.1080/107205399266037

Bacal, H. A., & Carlton, L. (2010). *The power of specificity in psychotherapy: When therapy works—and when it doesn't.* Jason Aronson.

Baldwin, S. A., Berkeljon, A., Atkins, D. C., Olsen, J. A., & Nielsen, S. L. (2009). Rates of change in naturalistic psychotherapy: Contrasting dose-effect and good-enough level models of change. *Journal of Consulting and Clinical Psychology, 77*(2), 203–211. https://doi.org/10.1037/a0015235

Barkham, M., Connell, J., Stiles, W. B., Miles, J. N. V., Margison, F., Evans, C., & Mellor-Clark, J. (2006). Dose-effect relations and responsive regulation of treatment duration: The good enough level. *Journal of Consulting and Clinical Psychology, 74*(1), 160–167. https://doi.org/10.1037/0022-006X.74.1.160

Barkham, M., Rees, A., Stiles, W. B., Shapiro, D. A., Hardy, G. E., & Reynolds, S. (1996). Dose-effect relations in time-limited psychotherapy for depression. *Journal of Consulting and Clinical Psychology, 64*(5), 927–935. https://doi.org/10.1037/0022-006X.64.5.927

Carey, T. A., Kelly, R. E., Mansell, W., & Tai, S. J. (2012). What's therapeutic about the therapeutic relationship? A hypothesis for practice informed by Perceptual Control Theory. *The Cognitive Behaviour Therapist, 5*(2–3), 47–59. https://doi.org/10.1017/S1754470X12000037

Caro Gabalda, I., Stiles, W. B., & Pérez Ruiz, S. (2016). Therapist activities preceding setbacks in the assimilation process. *Psychotherapy Research, 26*(6), 653–664. https://doi.org/10.1080/10503307.2015.1104422

Carroll, L. (1865). *Alice's adventures in wonderland.* Macmillan & Co.

Caspar, F. (1995). *Plan Analysis. Towards optimizing psychotherapy.* Hogrefe.

Caspar, F. (2007). Plan Analysis. In T. D. Eells (Ed.), *Handbook of psychotherapy case formulations* (2nd ed., pp. 251–289). Guilford Press.

Caspar, F., & Grosse-Holtforth, M. (2009). Responsiveness—Eine entscheidende Prozessvariable in der Psychotherapie [Responsiveness—A crucial process variable in psychotherapy]. *Zeitschrift für Klinische Psychologie und Psychotherapie, 38*(1), 61–69. https://doi.org/10.1026/1616-3443.38.1.61

Connolly Gibbons, M. B., Crits-Christoph, P., Levinson, J., & Barber, J. (2003). Flexibility in manual-based psychotherapies: Predictors of therapist interventions in interpersonal and cognitive-behavioral therapy. *Psychotherapy Research, 13*(2), 169–185. https://doi.org/10.1093/ptr/kpg017

Cooper, M., & McLeod, J. (2007). A pluralistic framework for counselling and psychotherapy: Implications for research. *Counselling & Psychotherapy Research, 7*(3), 135–143. https://doi.org/10.1080/14733140701566282

Cooper, M., & McLeod, J. (2011). *Pluralistic counselling and psychotherapy.* Sage.

Cox, A., Holbrook, D., & Rutter, M. (1981). Psychiatric interviewing techniques. VI. Experimental study: Eliciting feelings. *The British Journal of Psychiatry, 139*(2), 144–152. https://doi.org/10.1192/bjp.139.2.144

Cox, A., Rutter, M., & Holbrook, D. (1981). Psychiatric interviewing techniques V. Experimental study: Eliciting factual information. *The British Journal of Psychiatry, 139*(1), 29–37. https://doi.org/10.1192/bjp.139.1.29

Egan, G. (2002). *The skilled helper: A problem management approach to helping* (7th ed.). Brooks Cole.

Elkin, I., Falconnier, L., Smith, Y., Canada, K. E., Henderson, E., Brown, E. R., & McKay, B. M. (2014). Therapist responsiveness and patient engagement in therapy. *Psychotherapy Research, 24*(1), 52–66. https://doi.org/10.1080/10503307.2013.820855

Elkin, I., Shea, M. T., Watkins, J. T., Imber, S. D., Sotsky, S. M., Collins, J. F., Glass, D. R., Pilkonis, P. A., Leber, W. R., Docherty, J. P., Fiester, S. J., & Parloff, M. B. (1989). National Institute of Mental Health Treatment of Depression Collaborative Research Program. General effectiveness of treatments. *Archives of General Psychiatry, 46*(11), 971–982. https://doi.org/10.1001/archpsyc.1989.01810110013002

Elliott, R., Hill, C. E., Stiles, W. B., Friedlander, M. L., Mahrer, A. R., & Margison, F. R. (1987). Primary therapist response modes: Comparison of six rating systems. *Journal of Consulting and Clinical Psychology, 55*(2), 218–223. https://doi.org/10.1037/0022-006X.55.2.218

Elliott, R., Watson, J. C., Goldman, R. N., & Greenberg, L. S. (2004). *Learning emotion-focused therapy: The process experiential approach to change.* American Psychological Association. https://doi.org/10.1037/10725-000

Friedlander, M. L. (2012). Therapist responsiveness: Mirrored in supervisor responsiveness. *The Clinical Supervisor, 31*(1), 103–119. https://doi.org/10.1080/07325223.2012.675199

Gaete, J., Smoliak, O., & Couture, S. (2018). Reflexive questions as constructive interventions: A discursive perspective. In O. Smoliak & T. Strong (Eds.), *Therapy as discourse: The language of mental health* (pp. 117–140). Palgrave Macmillan. https://doi.org/10.1007/978-3-319-93067-1_6

Greenberg, L. S. (2002). *Emotion-focused therapy: Coaching clients to work through their feelings.* American Psychological Association. https://doi.org/10.1037/10447-000

Greenberg, L. S. (2007). A guide to conducting a task analysis of psycho-therapeutic change. *Psychotherapy Research, 17*(1), 15–30. https://doi.org/10.1080/10503300600720390

Greenberg, L. S., & Pinsof, W. M. (Eds.). (1986). *The psychotherapeutic process: A research handbook.* Guilford Press.

Hatcher, R. L. (2015). Interpersonal competencies: Responsiveness, technique, and training in psychotherapy. *American Psychologist, 70*(8), 747–757. https://doi.org/10.1037/a0039803

Hill, C. E. (2014). *Helping skills: Facilitating exploration, insight, and action* (4th ed.). American Psychological Association. https://doi.org/10.1037/14345-000

Howard, K. I., Kopta, S. M., Krause, M. S., & Orlinsky, D. E. (1986). The dose-effect relationship in psychotherapy. *American Psychologist, 41*(2), 159–164. https://doi.org/10.1037/0003-066X.41.2.159

Kiesler, D. J. (1973). *The process of psychotherapy: Empirical foundations and systems of analysis.* Aldine.

Kramer, U., & Stiles, W. B. (2015). The responsiveness problem in psychotherapy: A review of proposed solutions. *Clinical Psychology: Science and Practice, 22*(3), 277–295. https://doi.org/10.1111/cpsp.12107

Labov, W., & Fanshel, D. (1977). *Therapeutic discourse: Psychotherapy as conversation.* Academic Press.

Lambert, M. J. (2010). *Prevention of treatment failure: The use of measuring, monitoring, and feedback in clinical practice.* American Psychological Association. https://doi.org/10.1037/12141-000

Luborsky, L., Singer, B., & Luborsky, L. (1975). Comparative studies of psychotherapies: Is it true that "Everyone has won and all must have prizes"? *Archives of General Psychiatry, 32*(8), 995–1008. https://doi.org/10.1001/archpsyc.1975.01760260059004

McDaniel, S. H., Stiles, W. B., & McGaughey, K. J. (1981). Correlations of male college students' verbal response mode use in psychotherapy with measures of psychological disturbance and psychotherapy outcome. *Journal of Consulting and Clinical Psychology, 49*(4), 571–582. https://doi.org/10.1037/0022-006X.49.4.571

Mesman, J., van IJzendoorn, M. H., & Bakermans-Kranenburg, M. J. (2009). The many faces of the Still-Face Paradigm: A review and meta-analysis. *Developmental Review, 29*(2), 120–162. https://doi.org/10.1016/j.dr.2009.02.001

Norcross, J. C. (Ed.). (2002). *Psychotherapy relationships that work: Therapist contributions and responsiveness to patient need.* Oxford University Press.

Norcross, J. C. (Ed.). (2011). *Psychotherapy relationships that work: Evidence-based responsiveness* (2nd ed.). Oxford University Press. https://doi.org/10.1093/acprof:oso/9780199737208.001.0001

Norcross, J. C., Krebs, P. M., & Prochaska, J. O. (2011). Stages of change. In J. C. Norcross (Ed.), *Psychotherapy relationships that work* (2nd ed., pp. 279–300). Oxford University Press. https://doi.org/10.1093/acprof:oso/9780199737208.003.0014

Norcross, J. C., & Lambert, M. J. (Eds.). (2019). *Psychotherapy relationships that work: Vol. 1. Evidence-based therapist contributions.* Oxford University Press.

Norcross, J. C., & Wampold, B. E. (Eds.). (2019). *Psychotherapy relationships that work: Vol. 2. Evidence-based therapist responsiveness.* Oxford University Press. https://doi.org/10.1093/med-psych/9780190843960.001.0001

Orlinsky, D. E., Grawe, K., & Parks, B. K. (1994). Process and outcome in psychotherapy—Noch einmal. In A. E. Bergin & S. L. Garfield (Eds.), *Handbook of psychotherapy and behavior change* (4th ed., pp. 270–376). Wiley.

Orlinsky, D. E., & Howard, K. I. (1978). The relation of process to outcome in psychotherapy. In S. L. Garfield & A. E. Bergin (Eds.), *Handbook of psychotherapy and behavior change* (2nd ed., pp. 283–329). Wiley.

Orlinsky, D. E., & Howard, K. I. (1986). Process and outcome in psychotherapy. In S. L. Garfield & A. E. Bergin (Eds.), *Handbook of psychotherapy and behavior change* (3rd ed., pp. 311–381). Wiley.

Orlinsky, D. E., Rønnestad, M. H., & Willutzki, U. (2003). Fifty years of process–outcome research: Continuity and change. In M. J. Lambert (Ed.), *Bergin and Garfield's handbook of psychotherapy and behavior change* (5th ed., pp. 307–390). Wiley.

Osatuke, K., Moore, S. C., Ward, C., Dyrenforth, S. R., & Belton, L. (2009). Civility, respect, engagement in the workforce (CREW). Nationwide Organization Development Intervention at Veterans Health Administration. *The Journal of Applied Behavioral Science, 45*(3), 384–410. https://doi.org/10.1177/0021886309335067

Peräkylä, A., Antaki, C., Vehviläinen, S., & Leudar, I. (Eds.). (2008). *Conversation analysis and psychotherapy.* Cambridge University Press.

Pirsig, R. M. (1974). *Zen and the art of motorcycle maintenance.* William Morrow.

Powers, W. T. (2005). *Behavior: The control of perception* (2nd ed.). Benchmark.

Reynolds, S., Stiles, W. B., Barkham, M., Shapiro, D. A., Hardy, G. E., & Rees, A. (1996). Acceleration of changes in session impact during contrasting time-limited psychotherapies. *Journal of Consulting and Clinical Psychology, 64*(3), 577–586. https://doi.org/10.1037/0022-006X.64.3.577

Ribeiro, E., Cunha, C., Teixeira, A. S., Stiles, W. B., Pires, N., Santos, B., Basto, I., & Salgado, J. (2016). Therapeutic collaboration and the assimilation of problematic experiences in emotion-focused therapy for depression: Comparison of two cases. *Psychotherapy Research*, *26*(6), 665–680. https://doi.org/10.1080/10503307.2016.1208853

Robinson, L., Delgadillo, J., & Kellett, S. (2020). The dose-response effect in routinely delivered psychological therapies: A systematic review. *Psychotherapy Research*, *30*(1), 79–96. https://doi.org/10.1080/10503307.2019.1566676

Rogers, C. R. (1959). A theory of therapy, personality, and interpersonal relationships as developed by the client-centered framework. In S. Koch (Ed.), *Psychology: A study of a science: Volume III. Formulations of a person and the social context* (pp. 184–256). McGraw-Hill.

Rogers, C. R. (1961). *On becoming a person*. Houghton-Mifflin.

Rosenzweig, S. (1936). Some implicit common factors in diverse methods of psychotherapy. *American Journal of Orthopsychiatry*, *6*(3), 412–415. https://doi.org/10.1111/j.1939-0025.1936.tb05248.x

Russell, R. L., & Stiles, W. B. (1979). Categories for classifying language in psychotherapy. *Psychological Bulletin*, *86*(2), 404–419. https://doi.org/10.1037/0033-2909.86.2.404

Safran, J. D., & Muran, J. C. (1996). The resolution of ruptures in the therapeutic alliance. *Journal of Consulting and Clinical Psychology*, *64*(3), 447–458. https://doi.org/10.1037/0022-006X.64.3.447

Safran, J. D., Muran, J. C., & Eubanks-Carter, C. (2011). Repairing alliance ruptures. *Psychotherapy*, *48*, 80–87. https://doi.org/10.1093/acprof:oso/9780199737208.003.0011

Shapiro, D. A., Barkham, M., Rees, A., Hardy, G. E., Reynolds, S., & Startup, M. (1994). Effects of treatment duration and severity of depression on the effectiveness of cognitive-behavioral and psychodynamic-interpersonal psychotherapy. *Journal of Consulting and Clinical Psychology*, *62*(3), 522–534. https://doi.org/10.1037/0022-006X.62.3.522

Silberschatz, G. (2005). *Transformative relationships: The control-mastery theory psychotherapy*. Routledge.

Silberschatz, G., Fretter, P. B., & Curtis, J. T. (1986). How do interpretations influence the process of psychotherapy? *Journal of Consulting and Clinical Psychology*, *54*(5), 646–652. https://doi.org/10.1037/0022-006X.54.5.646

Sloane, R. G., Staples, F. R., Cristol, A. H., Yorkston, N. J., & Whipple, K. (1975). *Psychotherapy versus behavior therapy*. Harvard University Press. https://doi.org/10.4159/harvard.9780674365063

Smedslund, J. (2012). The bricoleur model of psychological practice. *Theory & Psychology*, *22*(5), 643–657. https://doi.org/10.1177/0959354312441277

Smedslund, J. (2016). Practicing psychology without an empirical evidence-base: The bricoleur model. *New Ideas in Psychology*, *43*, 50–56. https://doi.org/10.1016/j.newideapsych.2016.06.001

Smoliak, O., & Strong, T. (Eds.). (2018). *Therapy as discourse: Practice and research*. Palgrave Macmillan. https://doi.org/10.1007/978-3-319-93067-1

Snow, R. E. (1991). Aptitude-treatment interaction as a framework for research on individual differences in psychotherapy. *Journal of Consulting and Clinical Psychology*, *59*(2), 205–216. https://doi.org/10.1037/0022-006X.59.2.205

Snyder, J., & Silberschatz, G. (2017). The patient's experience of attunement and responsiveness scale. *Psychotherapy Research, 27*(5), 608–619. https://doi.org/10.1080/10503307.2016.1147658

Stiles, W. B. (1987). "I have to talk to somebody." A fever model of disclosure. In V. J. Derlega & J. H. Berg (Eds.), *Self-disclosure: Theory, research, and therapy* (pp. 257–282). Plenum Press. https://doi.org/10.1007/978-1-4899-3523-6_12

Stiles, W. B. (1988). Psychotherapy process–outcome correlations may be misleading. *Psychotherapy: Theory, Research, & Practice, 25*(1), 27–35. https://doi.org/10.1037/h0085320

Stiles, W. B. (1996). When more of a good thing is better: Reply to Hayes et al. (1996). *Journal of Consulting and Clinical Psychology, 64*(5), 915–918. https://doi.org/10.1037/0022-006X.64.5.915

Stiles, W. B. (2009). Responsiveness as an obstacle for psychotherapy outcome research: It's worse than you think. *Clinical Psychology: Science and Practice, 16*(1), 86–91. https://doi.org/10.1111/j.1468-2850.2009.01148.x

Stiles, W. B. (2011). Coming to terms. *Psychotherapy Research, 21*(4), 367–384. https://doi.org/10.1080/10503307.2011.582186

Stiles, W. B. (2013). The variables problem and progress in psychotherapy research. *Psychotherapy, 50*(1), 33–41. https://doi.org/10.1037/a0030569

Stiles, W. B. (2017). Theory-building case studies. In D. Murphy (Ed.), *Counselling psychology: A textbook for study and practice* (pp. 439–452). Wiley.

Stiles, W. B. (2020). Bricoleurs and theory-building qualitative research: Responses to responsiveness. In T. G. Lindstad, E. Stänicke, & J. Valsiner (Eds.), *Respect for thought: Jan Smedslund's legacy for psychology* (pp. 343–359). Springer. https://doi.org/10.1007/978-3-030-43066-5_20

Stiles, W. B., Barkham, M., & Wheeler, S. (2015). Duration of psychological therapy: Relation to recovery and improvement rates in UK routine practice. [corrected]. *The British Journal of Psychiatry, 207*(2), 115–122. https://doi.org/10.1192/bjp.bp.114.145565

Stiles, W. B., Hill, C. E., & Elliott, R. (2015). Looking both ways. *Psychotherapy Research, 25*(3), 282–293. https://doi.org/10.1080/10503307.2014.981681

Stiles, W. B., Honos-Webb, L., & Surko, M. (1998). Responsiveness in psychotherapy. *Clinical Psychology: Science and Practice, 5*(4), 439–458. https://doi.org/10.1111/j.1468-2850.1998.tb00166.x

Stiles, W. B., & Horvath, A. O. (2017). Appropriate responsiveness as a contribution to therapist effects. In L. Castonguay & C. E. Hill (Eds.), *How and why are some therapists better than others? Understanding therapist effects* (pp. 71–84). American Psychological Association. https://doi.org/10.1037/0000034-005

Stiles, W. B., McDaniel, S. H., & McGaughey, K. (1979). Verbal response mode correlates of experiencing. *Journal of Consulting and Clinical Psychology, 47*(4), 795–797. https://doi.org/10.1037/0022-006X.47.4.795

Stiles, W. B., & Shapiro, D. A. (1994). Disabuse of the drug metaphor: Psychotherapy process–outcome correlations. *Journal of Consulting and Clinical Psychology, 62*(5), 942–948. https://doi.org/10.1037/0022-006X.62.5.942

Stiles, W. B., Shapiro, D. A., & Elliott, R. (1986). Are all psychotherapies equivalent? *American Psychologist, 41*(2), 165–180. https://doi.org/10.1037/0003-066X.41.2.165

Stiles, W. B., & Wolfe, B. E. (2006). Relationship factors in treating anxiety disorders. In L. G. Castonguay & L. E. Beutler (Eds.), *Principles of therapeutic change that work* (pp. 155–165). Oxford University Press.

Strupp, H. H. (1963). The outcome problem in psychotherapy revisited. *Psychotherapy: Theory, Research, & Practice, 1*(1), 1–13.

Tronick, E., Als, H., Adamson, L., Wise, S., & Brazelton, T. B. (1978). The infant's response to entrapment between contradictory messages in face-to-face interaction. *Journal of the American Academy of Child & Adolescent Psychiatry, 17*(1), 1–13.

Wampold, B. E., & Imel, Z. E. (2015). *The great psychotherapy debate: The evidence for what makes psychotherapy work* (2nd ed.). Taylor & Francis.

Weiss, J. (1993). *How psychotherapy works*. Guilford Press.

Werbart, A., Annevall, A., & Hillblom, J. (2019). Successful and less successful psychotherapies compared: Three therapists and their six contrasting cases. *Frontiers in Psychology, 10*(816), 816. https://www.frontiersin.org/articles/10.3389/fpsyg.2019.00816/full

Zajonc, R. B. (1980). Feeling and thinking: Preferences need no inferences. *American Psychologist, 35*(2), 151–175.

2

RESPONSIVENESS, THE RELATIONSHIP, AND THE WORKING ALLIANCE IN PSYCHOTHERAPY

ROBERT L. HATCHER

The responsiveness concept is encompassing and complex. This chapter explores and critiques this concept as it has been applied to psychotherapy and psychotherapy research, and it considers how contributions from relationship science and psychoanalysis can bring useful aspects of the responsiveness concept into focus for thinking about psychotherapy and the therapeutic working alliance. This line of inquiry may prove a useful complement to our field's efforts to focus on improving our treatment methods.

Although this volume brings us to the responsiveness concept via its application by Stiles and colleagues to some key results of psychotherapy research (Kramer & Stiles, 2015; Stiles, 2009, 2013; Stiles et al., 1998; Stiles & Horvath, 2017), related versions of the idea have been introduced in the study of close relationships (Reis, 2014; Reis & Clark, 2013; Reis & Gable, 2015) and in psychoanalysis (Bacal, 1985, 1998; Bacal & Carlton, 2011). These contributions share a common viewpoint: Relationships are characterized by ongoing, mutual influence, such that each person's motives, goals, affects, attitudes, and behaviors are affected by those of the other, with each person more or less responsive to the emerging context of the relationship. As a result, the relationship itself has properties not fully predictable from what is known

https://doi.org/10.1037/0000240-003
The Responsive Psychotherapist: Attuning to Clients in the Moment, J. C. Watson and H. Wiseman (Editors)

about its members. In the course of this chapter, I discuss how these different approaches relate to one another and how they shed light on psychotherapy process.

Stiles, Honos-Webb, and Surko introduced the concept of responsiveness to the field of psychotherapy research in 1998 as a general principle of interpersonal interaction:

> We use the term *responsiveness* to describe behavior that is affected by emerging context, including perceptions of others' characteristics and behavior. Insofar as therapist and client respond to each other, responsiveness implies a dynamic relationship between variables, involving bidirectional causation and feedback loops. (p. 439)

This formulation straddles two conceptual domains. It describes two people interacting, each more or less sensitive to and affected by who the other person is and what they are doing, and it describes a world of variables, with complex, bidirectional statistical relationships that can be explained by the variables' links to the nature of the interdependent interaction between the two people. Stiles and colleagues' focus is on the disruptive effect that the nature of interpersonal relationships has on the simple causal and statistical assumptions commonly made in psychotherapy research. For example, if interpretation is seen by clinicians as a key agent of change, why doesn't its use correlate with outcome in psychodynamic therapy? Stiles and colleagues proposed that therapists use techniques responsively—that they use an intervention as much as needed to help the client achieve desired results, and that this amount will vary in a statistically random way across clients, resulting in a net zero correlation with outcome. Stiles and colleagues described the simple assumption that more of an action would lead to more change as "ballistic," because it is based on the idea that it has a direct, unmoderated effect on outcome, with no course correction, as if shot from a cannon. Instead, therapists use techniques to help achieve treatment goals, and they tend to use as much of any given technique as is required, given the state of the treatment, the interaction, and the client. They showed that this reasoning applies to treatment assignment, treatment strategies and tactics, and to moment-to-moment adjustments made by the therapist to the client's reactions to the therapist's intervention.

SPECIFYING THE NATURE AND SCOPE OF THE RESPONSIVENESS CONCEPT

As a concept, responsiveness is extraordinarily broad. Any object or process in nature is responsive to emerging conditions to one degree or another; light, for example, bends in response to the gravity of stars, although it is not pursuing any goal or intention. Many other processes in nature involve bidirectional causality and feedback loops, as in the gravitational interaction among the moon, the earth, and ocean tides. A subset of these interactions involves partners, each pursuing goals that are themselves modified by the interaction with the other, and this is the domain that Stiles and colleagues operate in when they apply the responsiveness concept to the goal-oriented interactions of clients and therapists. This goal-oriented kind of responsiveness distinguishes interaction between people from the responsiveness that is a general principle for all phenomena in nature.

Stiles and colleagues have discussed some key features of this goal-oriented responsiveness. As a general property of interaction among people, they noted that this responsiveness occurs in multiple timeframes—"on time scales that range from months to milliseconds" (Stiles et al., 1998, p. 440)—with the implication that people are responsive to tiny shifts and indications, such as tone of voice or gesture, as well as to major, enduring features, such as cultural background or the organization in which the encounter is taking place. Further, each instance of responsive action may respond to many levels at once: A single response may simultaneously address and be affected by the client's tone of voice, shift of subject, emergence of feeling, reference to the therapist, and new symptoms; actions described by the client; the previous session's content; racial, ethnic, gender, economic, cultural, and other differences; and the institutional context of the treatment—overall, by the wide range of contexts in which therapy occurs. And reciprocally, the same holds for the client.

For each of these features, multiple motives may be involved, serially or simultaneously, beyond the therapist's overall motivation to optimize the client's positive growth. Negative as well as positive motivations (goals), helpful as well as harmful, play varying roles in the interaction (Castonguay et al., 2010). The client's tone of voice may feel critical to the therapist and evoke a defensive or hostile response in turn (Wolf et al., 2017); the client's self-pity may evoke disgust as well as compassion; the client's race or ethnicity (Hayes et al., 2016), racial attitudes, moral choices, and religious preferences—really, anything about the client—may evoke motives and feelings in the therapist, which affect subsequent responses, motives, and feelings that may assist or detract from the overall aim to promote the client's optimal growth. And these responses, in turn, affect the participants' subsequent, equally complex responses.

Further, goal-directed responsiveness involves each party not only seeking ways to reach goals in the context of the other's responses but also changing the goals themselves in response to emerging context (Fitzsimons et al., 2015). Another way to say this is that people look for opportunities to pursue their various goals in their interactions with others and make continual adjust-ments to their goals in light of emerging context.

Goal-directed responsiveness as a property of the therapy dyad has direct links to the concept of the alliance in therapy, and particularly to Bordin's (1979) concept of the working alliance. Bordin proposed that the working alliance is a collaboration between client and therapist using agreed-upon tasks to work toward agreed-upon goals, supported by a sufficiently strong and resilient mutual bond (Hatcher & Barends, 2006). To establish and main-tain a satisfactory working alliance, there must be sufficient responsiveness on the part of both therapist and client—each must be able to recognize the goals of the other, and each to identify and pursue a way that they can work together toward the client's goals as articulated in a responsive exchange with the therapist. I discuss the links between responsiveness and the working alliance more fully later.

The implications of responsiveness for research, however, are problematic. The upshot is that what may look like a straightforward variable—a tech-nique (e.g., cognitive restructuring, interpretation, an empathic response) or a treatment method (e.g., cognitive behavioral therapy [CBT] for anxiety)—itself varies complexly, depending on the emerging context between the client and the therapist. As Kramer and Stiles (2015) put it, "The responsiveness critique is that a psychotherapeutic intervention (the 'what') is not a coherent entity but a fluid, adaptive process that stands in the way of the straight-forward answers everyone would like" (p. 289). Stiles and colleagues argue that research must honor this complexity in order to address the nature of psychotherapy.

However, this responsiveness concept and framework has such broad and complex implications that it quickly becomes difficult to manage. There are so many moving parts—multiple, overlapping, and interacting timeframes, motives, and goals for each participant. Stiles and colleagues faced a chal-lenge in shaping a manageable version of the responsiveness concept that could be serviceable in explaining the variables problem in psychotherapy research.

APPROPRIATE RESPONSIVENESS

Stiles and colleagues' original use of the responsiveness concept was to help explain unexpected findings in psychotherapy research (see also Chapter 1 by Stiles in this volume). In doing so, they introduce a more focused version of the concept, centered primarily on the role of the therapist. In addi-tion, rather than dealing with the range of therapists' positive and negative motivations, they propose an overall positive, helpful trend for all therapists to act so as to yield desired outcomes for their clients, generally doing what's best for their clients. They called this "appropriate responsiveness": "doing what is required to produce some desired outcome such as reduction in symptoms or improvement in life functioning, or to meet some standard, such as acting consistently within some conceptual system (e.g., psychoanalytic or cognitive-behavioral theory)" (Stiles et al., 1998, p. 440). They described appropriate responsiveness as "the essence of good practice," "a core operating principle for clinicians," and "part of being an expert who intuitively discriminates seemingly similar situations and decides how to intervene differentially across time" (Kramer & Stiles, 2015, p. 279).

Summarized by Stiles and Horvath (2017) as "do the right thing," the utility of this way of thinking about responsiveness for explaining the variables problem in psychotherapy research is evident. Across different treatment approaches, therapists share the same overall goal of helping clients toward good outcomes, and to get there, they all tend to "do the right thing" within the framework of their particular treatment approach. This helps explain why so many studies end up showing more or less equivalent outcomes across a variety of treatments for the same issues, the "Dodo Bird verdict" (Stiles et al., 1998). Thus, there are various ways to "do the right thing." Therapists use their techniques responsively, their judgment informed by subsequent events (e.g., the client's response to an intervention) that help them decide whether to continue with more of the technique (e.g., interpretation, cognitive restructuring, explaining the cognitive model), to combine the technique with other techniques (e.g., adding more warmth to a comment), or to switch to another technique. This fact works against the desire of researchers and to some extent of clinicians to measure the use of a technique as a variable—generally with the idea that more of it would be better.

The choice of the term "appropriate responsiveness" is a good match for Stiles and colleagues' (1998) model that includes the idea that responsiveness may refer to "doing what is required to . . . meet some standard, such as acting consistently within some conceptual system (e.g., psychoanalytic or cognitive-behavioral theory)" (p. 440). This idea is presented alongside the idea of doing what is required to produce a desired outcome, and they are combined in their more recent formulation: Therapists tend to "do the right thing at the right time, considering the client, the context, and their therapeutic approach" (Kramer & Stiles, 2015, p. 279). This formulation seems particularly fitting in the context of psychotherapy research, which generally requires adherence to a treatment manual. Under these conditions, therapists have special incentives to consider the requirements of their treatment approach, and to behave appropriately as expected. This imperative extends to the broad effort to encourage or require practitioners to adhere to an empirically supported treatment (EST; e.g., Watts et al., 2014). Although Stiles and colleagues' 1998 formulation of "meeting some standard or acting consistently within some conceptual system" (p. 440) seems to put allegiance to the theory above responsiveness to the client, they likely intend it to indicate the responsive use of a set of theory-based techniques, directed toward goals as framed within the approach in use.

Nevertheless, this aspect of appropriate responsiveness rests somewhat uneasily in Stiles and colleagues' work when they extend their consideration to the practicing therapist in general. In this context they noted, for example, that "therapists may respond to emerging indications of client requirements by changing their strategy and even their theoretical approach to treatment" (Stiles et al., 1998, p. 441). Perhaps this is an indication of the additional questions and perspectives that arise when the broader responsiveness paradigm is to look outside the domain of psychotherapy research to the world of clinical practice, where therapists, sensitive to the needs and current states of their clients, look for the most effective way to help them in the present moment. Exploring this possibility can start with the role of the treatment model.

CONSIDERING THE ISSUE OF RESPONSIVENESS IN SPECIFIED TREATMENT APPROACHES

The field's wide commitment to ESTs has drawn attention to therapists' adherence to treatment manuals and protocols, and to the relationship of adherence to outcome. This is the domain of responsiveness as "doing what is required . . . to meet some standard, such as acting consistently within some conceptual system" (Stiles et al., 1998, p. 440). A fair amount of work has been done to assess both the consistent use of theory-based techniques under the rubric of adherence and the skillful, appropriate use of these techniques, understood as competence. A number of research reports indicate that therapists can remain generally adherent while at the same time accommodating their use of approved techniques to particular client needs (e.g., Connolly Gibbons et al., 2003; Hardy et al., 1998; Kendall & Frank, 2018; Marques et al., 2019) and remaining appropriately responsive within the theoretical framework of their approach.

However, contrary to expectations, research that tests the relationship between adherent and competent delivery of specified treatments and client outcome has not produced clear or compelling findings, as reported in Webb et al.'s (2010) meta-analysis of 36 relevant studies. Overall, the ability of these factors to predict outcome has varied widely across studies, such that

Webb and colleagues' meta-analysis shows a net zero effect for both (see also Baldwin & Imel, 2013). Collyer et al. (2020) found a similar result in their meta-analysis for treatment of children and adolescents. In a study examining levels of adherence and competence in a group of community settings as compared with research settings, McLeod and colleagues (2019) found significantly lower rates on both dimensions in the community settings but no differences in outcomes for the clients. These results suggest that adherence and competence in a given treatment method have more complex relationships with outcome than might be expected, and a number of important questions follow: What are therapists doing when they are not adherent? What leads therapists to be nonadherent? Can nonadherence actually improve outcomes? What changes in treatment methods could be made to optimize outcomes?

An approach to these questions can be helped by recent findings that, although there are demonstrable differences between therapists in their levels of adherence, there are also sizeable differences within each therapist's caseload, as reported by Baldwin and Imel (2013), Boswell et al. (2013), Imel et al. (2011), and Maiwald et al. (2019), for example. As these researchers have noted, the fact that therapists tend to vary in adherence across clients points to the mutual, interactive influence of the dyad on the therapist's choice of interventions, as the responsiveness model predicts.

The responsiveness model takes into consideration that therapists encounter a wide range of challenges and opportunities in their interaction with clients. When their treatment approach offers a range of techniques that can be drawn upon to meet these challenges, things can go well. This effect was recognized by researchers demonstrating varying use of adherent techniques within the manual's framework, depending on client characteristics (Connolly Gibbons et al., 2003; Falkenström et al., 2013; Hardy et al., 1998; Marques et al., 2019; Zilcha-Mano, 2018).

When therapists encounter a challenge from their client that is not well matched to techniques provided by their treatment approach, they look for ways to deal with the challenge. Therapists may "do the right thing," finding techniques in their personal or professional repertoires that meet the demands of the situation and making good use of nonadherent techniques to optimize outcome. For example, Aviram et al. (2016) showed that CBT therapists treating clients with generalized anxiety disorder varied in their responses to client resistance early in treatment. Clients had better success when their therapists, though untrained in motivational interviewing (W. R. Miller & Rollnick, 2002), incorporated techniques compatible with this approach. Similarly, Katz and colleagues (2019) showed that adherent, psychodynamically trained therapists who nevertheless used small amounts of CBT-compatible techniques produced enhanced treatment outcomes with clients who were depressed.

On the other hand, sometimes therapists double down on the very same adherent techniques that aggravated the problem in the first place. For example, in a 1996 study, Castonguay et al. found that some CBT therapists attempted to resolve strains in the alliance by pointing out the distortions in the client's thinking about the therapist. Not surprisingly, these instances led to poorer outcomes, as the lack of suitable technical options led to unresponsive use of sanctioned techniques. Barber et al. (2003) reported similar doubling down for some highly skilled CBT therapists as they struggled to accommodate the special motivational challenges of cocaine addicts.

Unsatisfactory therapist responses are more studied in the literature and generally involve the activation of aggressive, hostile, and/or critical responses by their clients' behaviors in session. These client behaviors include anger, hostility, and aggression (Baldwin & Imel, 2013; Boswell et al., 2013); resistance, including rejection of the treatment model, belittling the therapist, reluctance to stay on track, evasion, and complaining about the therapist and the therapy (Zickgraf et al., 2016); and disengagement (Snippe et al., 2019). These client responses tend to pull therapists off track (although they may result from therapist behaviors that provoke negativity), leading therapists to lose their bearings, becoming "deskilled" (Boswell et al., 2013).

APPROPRIATE RESPONSIVENESS VERSUS OPTIMAL RESPONSIVENESS

Bacal (1985, 1998), a practicing psychoanalyst, took a somewhat different, more fully process-oriented approach to responsiveness, which he called "optimal" responsiveness. Bacal noted that a treatment model, as a system of prescribed and proscribed interventions, is indispensable for any therapist. However, he stressed that any given approach risks failing to recognize that what is therapeutic for a particular client is highly variable and cannot be known on the basis of theory alone (Bacal & Carlton, 2011). Theory and research can help the therapist identify potentially helpful behaviors, but optimal responsiveness does not limit the range of possible interventions, given the constraints of ethical practice; it involves taking advantage of opportunities that emerge in the ongoing process to engage and help the client. Thus, Bacal (1985) defined *optimal responsiveness* as "the responsivity of the analyst that is therapeutically most relevant at any particular moment in the context of a particular patient and his illness" (p. 202). Because of the unique and complex features of any therapist–client dyad, optimal responsiveness "denote[s] that therapeutic efficacy necessarily embraces diverse and differential responsivity to individual therapeutic need" (Bacal, 1998, p. 151).

Optimal responsiveness describes an ideal, in which the therapist seeks a response that best assists the client toward treatment goals. The thrust of the studies discussed previously is that therapists, while guided in many respects by their treatment approaches, will tend to use other, "nonadherent" responses when presented with challenges or opportunities by the client for which an adherent response is unspecified or for some reason seems less satisfactory. Although Stiles and colleagues' assumption that therapists are guided by positive, helpful motives is likely generally true, therapists are especially challenged to find positive opportunities when clients express negativity, and a number of studies note the need to develop techniques to address these events so as to foster good outcomes (e.g., Boswell et al., 2013; Zickgraf et al., 2016).

This perspective points to the disruptive features of the responsiveness concept for any established treatment model. If optimal responsiveness can potentially mean that the therapist should do whatever is necessary to help the client (within professional and ethical bounds), and if responsive therapists to some extent move outside their treatment models to use unsanctioned interventions to assist their work toward client goals, what are the implications for the role of the treatment model in our work?

THE POSITIVE ROLE OF TREATMENT MODELS

Treatment models help therapists maintain a framework of positive, goal-directed motivations and actions, and help sustain their ethical and professional position, further supporting the therapist in maintaining consistently positive, helpful clinical motivations. The fact that therapists can be pulled into negative interactions poses a challenge to these treatment models (e.g., Boswell et al., 2013; Zickgraf et al., 2016), but as these problematic interactions are identified, methods can be devised to address them and even to turn them to positive use. On the other hand, acknowledging that therapists tend to look for opportunities beyond the prescribed scope of the treatment model—and that such steps can be beneficial to client progress—would help maintain the flexibility needed to provide optimal care.

Further, having a clear, coherent technical and theoretical approach may itself be responsive to the needs of many, if not most, clients. This is Wampold and colleagues' argument in their contextual model of psychotherapy (e.g., Wampold & Imel, 2015). On the one hand, optimal responsiveness may not imply or require maximum theoretical and technical flexibility. On the other hand, it follows that a given treatment model may be responsive to the needs of some clients but not others, as suggested by dropout rates across treatment approaches around 20% (Swift & Greenberg, 2012), by non-improvement rates ranging from 30% to 65% (Lambert, 2017), and by studies demonstrating the positive role of client choice of treatment in successful outcome (e.g., Lindhiem et al., 2016). This is why Stiles and colleagues have noted that therapists may change to a different treatment approach when the one in use does not meet the client's needs. Overall, it seems important to distinguish the requirement for a clearly specified set of interventions necessary for researching the efficacy of a treatment—that is, adherence—from the flexibility needed for responsive practice by a given therapist with a given client—that is, optimal responsiveness. Ultimately, the implication is that responsive therapists in practice, unless otherwise constrained, adhere to treatment methods insofar as they believe and experience the method to be responsive to the client's treatment needs, and not for the sake of the method itself. To the extent that the therapist honors the treatment method, it is not for the method's sake but with the conviction that the method and its techniques are as optimal as the therapist can be in response to the client's needs.

While exploring how this model of responsiveness applies to psychotherapy, I have lingered on the topic of treatment method because it is a significant factor in the therapeutic relationship between client and therapist. Along the way, I have noted the role of negative therapist motivations and behaviors, which may be responsive in the broad sense of being induced by client behaviors (e.g., Wolf et al., 2017) but detract from optimal responsiveness. As much as we therapists may like to think that our clients are primarily influenced by our special techniques—including interpretation, cognitive restructuring, behavioral experiments, and empathic reflection—the responsiveness framework asks us to consider and make good use of the fact that the client responds to the full range of our behaviors, needs, attitudes, likes and dislikes, feelings, and so on as they are manifested in the treatment relationship, and that may be experienced as helpful, harmful, or neutral by the client. And the client's responses, in turn, may be equally complex.

I have considered responsiveness at two different levels. The first is the overall level of the fuller responsiveness model, encompassing the entire mutually influential, evolving relationship. The second level focuses on the therapist as a goal-directed, responsive agent, dedicated to enhancing the client's well-being and operating within a relationship thoroughly characterized by mutual influence, reciprocal causation, and feedback loops. Stepping back to view the treatment relationship from the broader responsiveness perspective opens up far more areas of inquiry than can be addressed in a single chapter. Because the relationship is between human beings, and because every therapist has had decades of experience in personal relationships, the needs, desires, expectations, and attitudes that have been shaped in these relationships will be available in the treatment relationship and will potentially influence it (Caspar, 2017; Hatcher, 2015). Additionally, in my emphasis on the therapist's responsiveness, I have not focused on the client's responsiveness and its role in treatment, nor have I addressed the other features that are present in all relationships, including therapeutic relationships, that affect the nature and quality of the therapist's (and client's) responsiveness. Let us turn to some of these points now.

SUPPORTIVE RESPONSIVENESS IN CLOSE RELATIONSHIPS

The study of close relationships—"relationship science"—is a strong research field with an extensive body of theory that dates back to Kelley's (1979) work on interpersonal relationships. In their overview of core theoretical principles, Finkel et al. (2017) identified a concept of close relationships widely shared over the years and across theories: "Partners are dependent on one another to obtain good outcomes and facilitate the pursuit of their most important needs and goals" (p. 388). Further, these needs and goals, as they emerge in the relationship, are themselves shaped and modified by the relationship with the partner (Fitzsimons et al., 2015). These broad definitions indicate that relationship studies operate in the same conceptual frame of responsiveness as described by Stiles and colleagues in 1998.

The concept of partner responsiveness is a major topic in relationship studies. Reis and colleagues have done extensive theoretical and research work in this area, based on the idea that "responsiveness consists of partners interacting in ways such that they understand, value, and support each other in fulfilling important personal needs and goals" (Reis & Clark, 2013, p. 400). Reis (2014) identified responsiveness as a central feature across many different theoretical models of close relationships:

> Embedded within each of these specific theories is the general idea that when partners are felt to be responding supportively to important needs, goals, values, or preferences in the self-concept, emotional well-being is enhanced and effective emotional self-regulation is facilitated. On the other hand, when partners are seen to be responding critically or when their response is perceived to be controlling or contingent, emotional well-being suffers and emotional self-regulation is impaired. I refer to these phenomena as perceived partner responsiveness and unresponsiveness. (p. 257)

Responding supportively consists of not only warmth and encouragement but also any kind of response that furthers the needs and goals of the other

(Reis & Clark, 2013). In this way, responsiveness as defined by Reis and colleagues corresponds closely to appropriate and especially to optimal responsiveness as discussed previously. Several features of this approach to responsiveness are notable. Similar to Stiles and colleagues, this is a specialized version of the broader responsiveness concept, focused on positive assistance for the partner's goals. In addition, responsiveness as conceptualized and studied by Reis and others is not structured around a set of techniques or treatment principles as is typically found in work on psychotherapy. Instead, it focuses on the partner's subjective experience of the other's supportive responsiveness, an experience that is more or less influenced by the actual behavior of the partner (as rated by independent judges; Lemay & Clark, 2015; Pollmann & Finkenauer, 2009). This approach then is focused on a more general level than the treatment model through which the therapist attempts to be responsive to the client in psychotherapy, and highlights the positive effects on the partner of optimal responsiveness per se. Reis (2014) identified three aspects of the partner's behavior that are likely to be beneficial and experienced as responsive in this sense. If the person experiences the partner's understanding of himself or herself as accurate and true, the person's sense of authenticity is enhanced. Believing that one's self is valued and appreciated yields a feeling of validation, the sense that the partner likes, appreciates, and accepts oneself, resulting in enhanced feelings of belongingness and security. In addition, responsiveness may convey a sense that the other is concerned for one's well-being and will provide help when needed. These effects are associated with overall well-being, health, and other positive outcomes (Reis, 2012; Selcuk & Ong, 2013). The benefits of responsiveness extend to self-regulation, the control of one's "thoughts, feelings, and behavior in order to . . . make progress toward valued goals" (Reis, 2014, p. 259). As Reis (2014) put it,

> Perceived partner responsiveness is central to all of these mechanisms. Knowing that a partner has one's back—in other words, that he or she will be available if needed and is willing to provide nurturance or assistance, even if it were to be costly—gives people the emotional wherewithal to deal with challenges and the security to interact with others confidently and nondefensively. (p. 259)

RELATIONAL RESPONSIVENESS AND THE WORKING ALLIANCE

These features overlap substantially with ideas about the working alliance in therapy (Bordin, 1979; Hatcher & Barends, 2006), particularly with the idea of the alliance bond's role. Relationship research emphasizes the key importance of the subjective experience of the other's responsiveness, as Reis summarized earlier. Bordin sought to emphasize the importance of agreement on the goals and tasks of therapy, separating these aspects of the working alliance from the bond of liking, respect, and appreciation. His interest in this regard was to look at the working component of therapy, at how the therapist and client develop a shared engagement in the tasks of treatment, based on a shared understanding of treatment goals. To reach and sustain this agreement, a sufficient bond is needed, with stronger, deeper bonds for therapeutic work that is more intensely personal (Bordin, 1979; Hatcher & Barends, 2006). Appropriate responsiveness, as described by Stiles and colleagues, involves the therapist's sensitive, context-aware use of technique (Bordin's "tasks") to help the client reach treatment goals. However, what relationship science research suggests is that the act of responding appropriately or optimally with techniques to help the client reach treatment goals also promotes the bond with the client. Thus, the distinctions commonly drawn between goal and task consensus and the bond in alliance discussions are likely drawn too sharply. Responsive use of technique promotes the bond; the strengthened subjective bond is itself a good outcome that promotes other good outcomes (e.g., feeling more authentic and valuable as a person); these in turn help the client face difficulties and engage more fully in treatment tasks, making it easier for the therapist to be effectively responsive. Here, also, is a good example of reciprocal causation and feedback loops, and an example of Kramer and Stiles's (2015) observation that "the responsiveness critique is that a psychotherapeutic intervention (the 'what') is not a coherent entity but a fluid, adaptive process that stands in the way of the straightforward answers everyone would like" (p. 289). This link between the subjective bond and therapist responsiveness is implicit in Stiles and colleagues' work, particularly in their assertion that measures of alliance in psychotherapy tap the client's subjective, evaluative sense of the therapist's responsiveness, more than they assess the specific features of goal and task agreement (Kramer & Stiles, 2015; Stiles & Goldsmith, 2010). Of course, this leaves alliance measurement with considerable challenges.

The features of responsiveness identified in relationship research also overlap considerably with Carl Rogers's concept of therapist-offered conditions (1957) as they point to the positive value of the act of responsiveness for clients. Rogers's ideas were adopted and enriched by emotion-focused therapy, where the therapist's responsiveness plays a fundamental role (Watson, 2018). In this regard, Kramer and Stiles (2015) emphasized that responsiveness is not a common factor in psychotherapy, unlike Rogers's conditions, and this is true for the broad concept involving mutual influence and feedback loops. But once the conceptual ground is shifted to the therapist's appropriate or optimal responsiveness, we can see that as relationship research suggests, these features have general, common effects across treatment types.

CLIENT RESPONSIVENESS

Within relationship science, psychotherapy would be considered an asymmetrical communal relationship, in which one person holds responsibility for the welfare of the other (Clark & Aragón, 2013). This means that it is the therapist's responsibility to offer responsiveness to the client. Psychotherapists generally have different expectations when it comes to client responsiveness to the therapist. Clients often present with difficulties in affective, supportive engagement with others. Nevertheless, it is probably fair to say that therapists hope clients will respond positively, with interest and engagement, to their methods, their ideas about treatment goals, their technical interventions, and their genuine interest in the client and his or her welfare. We have an idea of what "the right thing" would be by way of the client's responding, and the therapist's responsiveness is shaped to enhance and maximize the likelihood that the client will respond in this way. Some treatment methods make client responsiveness a key focus of treatment, with the idea of enhancing the client's capacity to respond positively to the therapist (e.g., McCullough, 2000). Others work with the client's difficulties in responsiveness to the therapist as an indicator of more general difficulties with others, as in interpersonal therapy (Weissman et al., 2000) and the analysis of transference. Still others focus more on difficulties in engaging with the therapeutic tasks as pathways to identifying underlying conflicts or habitual thought patterns (e.g., automatic thoughts and schemas in CBT).

From this perspective, the overall goal of evidence-based practice and empirically supported treatment is to identify and use treatment approaches to which, on average, clients are demonstrably responsive. Often a further goal is to show that clients are more responsive to a given approach than to others. From a responsiveness point of view, these are the core arguments for ESTs that have received reliable research support. If the average client is responsive to this treatment, the challenge then becomes how to apply this general finding to a given individual. This must be done responsively, requiring attention to the specifics of the individual client and all of the other factors that the general responsiveness framework points us to. Thoughtful consideration of these issues has grown within the EST domain, including how to maintain fidelity to the underlying principles of a given approach, while introducing congruent modifications to fit individual circumstances (e.g., Asnaani et al., 2018; Kendall & Frank, 2018; Wiltsey Stirman et al., 2017).

DEVELOPING AND ENHANCING THERAPIST RESPONSIVENESS

Appropriate or optimal responsiveness—finding the best way to help the client reach treatment goals—is the "essence of good practice" (cf. Kramer & Stiles, 2015, p. 279), so enhancing one's responsiveness is important to psychotherapists. Some therapists already seem to have this ability in abundance. A few studies indicate that there is a small group of therapists who help virtually everyone they see. These are "supershrinks" (S. D. Miller et al., 2008; Okiishi et al., 2003; see also Baldwin & Imel, 2013). Little is understood about what makes them exceptional. They tend to be attuned to and wholly engaged in helping their clients. They seem to use quite varying approaches, from a warm, engaging empathy to a vigorous, instructive direction. It appears that they have each somehow developed something close to optimal responsiveness across clients. How did they do this, and what, specifically, do they do? The answer, to date, is unknown, pointing to the frontiers of our understanding of responsiveness. But even supershrinks would want to better help their clients.

Our field has developed two general approaches to enhancing therapists' appropriate or optimal responsiveness. The first is through giving therapists feedback on their work with clients, including engaging in deliberate practice. There is an extensive literature on this topic, not reviewed here (e.g., Rousmaniere et al., 2017). Therapists enter training already benefiting from years of feedback received during interpersonal interactions with family, peers, romantic partners, and others. Professional training seeks to help trainees shape their abilities into a responsive, professional helping framework through didactic experiences and supervision, now increasingly with the benefit of video recordings and supplemented by routine monitoring of treatment processes such as alliance and outcome (Caspar, 2017; Hatcher, 2015; Hill & Knox, 2013).

The second general approach is to develop new and enhanced treatment methods. Considered from a responsiveness perspective, each of the myriad treatment approaches could be seen as an effort to refine and enhance therapists' responsiveness to their clients. Arguably, advances in technique grow out of the obstacles therapists encounter, or from new opportunities that they recognize, some involving opportunities seen in obstacles. Many of these advances are not anticipated by the theories that are in use and may in fact modify them. A widely known example is Aaron Beck's clinical observation that his clients' experiences of depressive affect—sadness, frustration, and immobility—were preceded by negative, distorted thoughts of which they were only dimly aware. Beck (2006) reported that this observation, along with his failed (psychoanalytic) theory-guided search for evidence of enhanced hostility in depressed clients' dreams, led him to alter his technique and theory. This is a strong example of nonadherent responsiveness! Much of the evolution of Freud's psychoanalysis was precipitated by limits in his theory and technique that were manifested in client resistance to treatment. In fact, the concept of resistance grew out of Freud's thwarted attempts to help clients recover troubling memories, and the concept of transference arose when the treatment process was interrupted by the client's thoughts and feelings about Freud that, he felt, better fit a childhood figure than himself (e.g., Freud, 1905). Cognitive therapy, developed to address problems that clinicians felt were not effectively dealt with by psychoanalysis, has in subsequent years rediscovered transference and resistance in the course of practice. These developments can all be seen as examples of therapist responsiveness to client behaviors, and they were all intended to enhance the work toward treatment goals. As Beck's account of the origins of cognitive therapy suggests, the responsiveness concept can speak to the motivation behind the development of new treatment approaches. These grow out of some sort of dissatisfaction with an existing treatment method, or a new idea of how to help clients in a better way. The list of these new treatment approaches is long and constantly growing. Of considerable interest is whether the new approaches are an improvement on previous methods and should replace them, or simply offer alternative ways of dealing with problems, but perhaps ways that may be more acceptable or helpful to some clients, thus expanding the overall capacity of the field for responsive care. This question, though not framed in responsiveness terms, is the focus of considerable controversy in the field. Some (e.g., Cuijpers & van Straten, 2011; Wampold & Imel, 2015) argue for equivalence between different treatment approaches, while others dispute this claim (e.g., Wiltsey Stirman et al., 2010).

To deal with this problem, systematic efforts to identify variations in treatment approaches that best help given types of clients, or better yet, a given client, are an important development in the field (Hofmann & Hayes, 2019; Zilcha-Mano, 2018). Under the rubric of personalized approaches to treatment, there are two main streams of work (Zilcha-Mano, 2018). New approaches have been developed to identify multiple client characteristics that in combination help produce a more nuanced treatment recommendation. For example, Cohen and DeRubeis (2018) developed the Personalized Advantage Index for use with clients with depression. Hofmann and Hayes (2019) advocated for a focus on "process-based" therapies that identify evidence-based, modifiable issues and associated interventions for individual clients.

Another approach pinpoints moments of emerging context that call for specific attention in order to optimize therapeutic work. These studies identify markers of key moments in therapy that can help therapists enhance their responsiveness with useful techniques. Westra and Norouzian (2018), for example, showed the value of motivational interviewing techniques when markers of resistance or ambivalence show up in cognitive behavioral therapy. Safran and Muran have conducted extensive work (e.g., 2000) on the use of metacommunication and related techniques to address a subset of resistance markers involving client withdrawal or anger (which they call "alliance ruptures"). Constantino and colleagues (2013) proposed a general framework for identifying markers and responsive interventions that they called "context-responsive psychotherapy" (see also Chapter 7 by Constantino et al. in this volume), using client characteristics and in-session behaviors as markers for differential use of techniques. They used generalized anxiety disorder treatment to illustrate this approach, which focuses on evidence-based modules— that is, bundles of techniques designed to address an emerging problem in treatment. This line of research covers a range of these issues, such as the client's treatment expectations and beliefs (e.g., Coyne et al., 2019), and involves demonstrating the utility of these modules for treatment outcomes (making them "evidence based").

As much as these new research- and evidence-based approaches to training and treatment selection may help enhance client outcomes, the clinicians involved must apply every one of them responsively.

CONCLUSION

Responsiveness is a useful guide to help keep psychotherapists open to new information and opportunities. It is a counterweight to our wish to pin things down, to be certain about what to do, and to master our situation and environment. Its inclusive, encompassing scope warns us not to settle for what we think is certain—to be alert to changing conditions, new threats and opportunities, and limits to what we know and can do. The quest for optimal responsiveness, and to know what it is, may be as complex and challenging as the interactions it describes.

REFERENCES

Asnaani, A., Gallagher, T., & Foa, E. B. (2018). Evidence-based protocols: Merits, drawbacks, and potential solutions. *Clinical Psychology: Science and Practice*, *25*(4), e12266–e12270. https://doi.org/10.1111/cpsp.12266

Aviram, A., Westra, H. A., Constantino, M. J., & Antony, M. M. (2016). Responsive management of early resistance in cognitive–behavioral therapy for generalized anxiety disorder. *Journal of Consulting and Clinical Psychology*, *84*(9), 783–794. https://doi.org/10.1037/ccp0000100

Bacal, H. A. (1985). Optimal responsiveness and the therapeutic process. In A. Goldberg (Ed.), *Progress in self psychology* (Vol. 1, pp. 202–227). Guilford Press.

Bacal, H. A. (Ed.). (1998). *Optimal responsiveness: How therapists heal their patients.* Jason Aronson.

Bacal, H. A., & Carlton, L. (2011). *The power of specificity in psychotherapy: When therapy works—and when it doesn't.* Jason Aronson.

Baldwin, S. A., & Imel, Z. E. (2013). Therapist effects: Findings and methods. In M. J. Lambert (Ed.), *Bergin and Garfield's handbook of psychotherapy and behavior change* (5th ed., pp. 258–297). Wiley.

Barber, J. P., Liese, B. S., & Abrams, M. J. (2003). Development of the Cognitive Therapy Adherence and Competence Scale. *Psychotherapy Research, 13*(2), 205–221. https://www.tandfonline.com/doi/abs/10.1093/ptr/kpg019

Beck, A. T. (2006). How an anomalous finding led to a new system of psychotherapy. *Nature Medicine, 12*(10), 1139–1141. https://doi.org/10.1038/nm1006-1139

Bordin, E. S. (1979). The generalizability of the psychoanalytic concept of the working alliance. *Psychotherapy: Theory, Research & Practice, 16*(3), 252–260. https://doi.org/10.1037/h0085885

Boswell, J. F., Gallagher, M. W., Sauer-Zavala, S. E., Bullis, J., Gorman, J. M., Shear, M. K., Woods, S., & Barlow, D. H. (2013). Patient characteristics and variability in adherence and competence in cognitive-behavioral therapy for panic disorder. *Journal of Consulting and Clinical Psychology, 81*(3), 443–454. https://doi.org/10.1037/a0031437

Caspar, F. (2017). Professional expertise in psychotherapy. In L. G. Castonguay & C. E. Hill (Eds.), *How and why are some therapists better than others? Understanding therapist effects* (pp. 193–214). American Psychological Association. https://doi.org/10.1037/0000034-012

Castonguay, L. G., Boswell, J. F., Constantino, M. J., Goldfried, M. R., & Hill, C. E. (2010). Training implications of harmful effects of psychological treatments. *American Psychologist, 65*(1), 34–49. https://doi.org/10.1037/a0017330

Castonguay, L. G., Goldfried, M. R., Wiser, S., Raue, P. J., & Hayes, A. M. (1996). Predicting the effect of cognitive therapy for depression: A study of unique and common factors. *Journal of Consulting and Clinical Psychology, 64*(3), 497–504. https://doi.org/10.1037/0022-006X.64.3.497

Clark, M. S., & Aragón, O. R. (2013). Communal (and other) relationships: History, theory development, recent findings, and future directions. In J. A. Simpson & L. Campbell (Eds.), *The Oxford handbook of close relationships* (pp. 255–280). Oxford University Press.

Cohen, Z. D., & DeRubeis, R. J. (2018). Treatment selection in depression. *Annual Review of Clinical Psychology, 14*(1), 209–236. https://doi.org/10.1146/annurev-clinpsy-050817-084746

Collyer, H., Eisler, I., & Woolgar, M. (2020). Systematic literature review and meta-analysis of the relationship between adherence, competence and outcome in psychotherapy for children and adolescents. *European Child & Adolescent Psychiatry, 29*, 417–431. https://doi.org/10.1007/s00787-018-1265-2

Connolly Gibbons, M. B., Crits-Christoph, P., Levinson, J., & Barber, J. (2003). Flexibility in manual-based psychotherapies: Predictors of therapist interventions in interpersonal and cognitive-behavioral therapy. *Psychotherapy Research, 13*(2), 169–185. http://www.tandfonline.com/doi/abs/10.1093/ptr/kpg017

Constantino, M. J., Boswell, J. F., Bernecker, S. L., & Castonguay, L. G. (2013). Context-responsive psychotherapy integration as framework for a unified clinical science: Conceptual and empirical considerations. *Journal of Unified Psychotherapy and Clinical Science*, *2*(1). https://www.researchgate.net/publication/235745350

Coyne, A. E., Constantino, M. J., & Muir, H. J. (2019). Therapist responsivity to patients' early treatment beliefs and psychotherapy process. *Psychotherapy*, *56*(1), 11–15. https://doi.org/10.1037/pst0000200

Cuijpers, P., & van Straten, A. (2011). New psychotherapies for mood and anxiety disorders: Necessary innovation or waste of resources? *Canadian Journal of Psychiatry*, *56*(4), 251. https://doi.org/10.1177/070674371105600413

Falkenström, F., Granström, F., & Holmqvist, R. (2013). Therapeutic alliance predicts symptomatic improvement session by session. *Journal of Counseling Psychology*, *60*(3), 317–328. https://doi.org/10.1037/a0032258

Finkel, E. J., Simpson, J. A., & Eastwick, P. W. (2017). The psychology of close relationships: Fourteen core principles. *Annual Review of Psychology*, *68*(1), 383–411. https://doi.org/10.1146/annurev-psych-010416-044038

Fitzsimons, G. M., Finkel, E. J., & vanDellen, M. R. (2015). Transactive goal dynamics. *Psychological Review*, *122*(4), 648–673. https://doi.org/10.1037/a0039654

Freud, S. (1905). On psychotherapy (1905 [1904]). In *The standard edition of the complete psychological works of Sigmund Freud: Vol. 7 (1901–1905). A case of hysteria: Three essays on sexuality and other works* (pp. 255–268). Hogarth Press.

Hardy, G. E., Shapiro, D. A., Stiles, W. B., & Barkham, M. (1998). When and why does cognitive-behavioral treatment appear more effective than psychodynamic-interpersonal treatment? Discussion of the findings from the Second Sheffield Psychotherapy Project. *Journal of Mental Health*, *7*(2), 179–190. https://doi.org/10.1080/09638239818229

Hatcher, R. L. (2015). Interpersonal competencies: Responsiveness, technique, and training in psychotherapy. *American Psychologist*, *70*(8), 747–757. https://doi.org/10.1037/a0039803

Hatcher, R. L., & Barends, A. W. (2006). How a return to theory could help alliance research. *Psychotherapy*, *43*(3), 292–299. https://doi.org/10.1037/0033-3204.43.3.292

Hayes, J. A., McAleavey, A. A., Castonguay, L. G., & Locke, B. D. (2016). Psychotherapists' outcomes with White and racial/ethnic minority clients: First, the good news. *Journal of Counseling Psychology*, *63*(3), 261–268. https://doi.org/10.1037/cou0000098

Hill, C. E., & Knox, S. (2013). Training and supervision in psychotherapy: Evidence for effective practice. In M. J. Lambert (Ed.), *Handbook of psychotherapy and behavior change* (6th ed., pp. 775–811). Wiley.

Hofmann, S. G., & Hayes, S. C. (2019). The future of intervention science: Process-based therapy. *Clinical Psychological Science*, *7*(1), 37–50. https://doi.org/10.1177/2167702618772296

Imel, Z. E., Baer, J. S., Martino, S., Ball, S. A., & Carroll, K. M. (2011). Mutual influence in therapist competence and adherence to motivational enhancement therapy. *Drug and Alcohol Dependence*, *115*(3), 229–236. https://doi.org/10.1016/j.drugalcdep.2010.11.010

Katz, M., Hilsenroth, M. J., Gold, J. R., Moore, M., Pitman, S. R., Levy, S. R., & Owen, J. (2019). Adherence, flexibility, and outcome in psychodynamic treatment of depression. *Journal of Counseling Psychology, 66*(1), 94–103. https://doi.org/10.1037/cou0000299

Kelley, H. H. (1979). *Personal relationships: Their structures and processes.* Erlbaum.

Kendall, P. C., & Frank, H. E. (2018). Implementing evidence-based treatment protocols: Flexibility within fidelity. *Clinical Psychology: Science and Practice, 25*(4), 1–12. https://doi.org/10.1111/cpsp.12271

Kramer, U., & Stiles, W. B. (2015). The responsiveness problem in psychotherapy: A review of proposed solutions. *Clinical Psychology: Science and Practice, 22*(3), 277–295. https://doi.org/10.1111/cpsp.12107

Lambert, M. J. (2017). Maximizing psychotherapy outcome beyond evidence-based medicine. *Psychotherapy and Psychosomatics, 86*(2), 80–89. https://doi.org/10.1159/000455170

Lemay, E. P., & Clark, M. S. (2015). Motivated cognition in relationships. *Current Opinion in Psychology, 1,* 72–75. https://doi.org/10.1016/j.copsyc.2014.11.002

Lindhiem, O., Bennett, C. B., Orimoto, T. E., & Kolko, D. J. (2016). A meta-analysis of personalized treatment goals in psychotherapy: A preliminary report and call for more studies. *Clinical Psychology: Science and Practice, 23*(2), 165–176. https://doi.org/10.1111/cpsp.12153

Maiwald, L. M., Junga, Y. M., Lang, T., Montini, R., Witthöft, M., Heider, J., Schröder, A., & Weck, F. (2019). The role of therapist and patient in-session behavior for treatment outcome in exposure-based cognitive behavioral therapy for panic disorder with agoraphobia. *Journal of Clinical Psychology, 75*(4), 614–626. https://onlinelibrary.wiley.com/doi/abs/10.1002/jclp.22738

Marques, L., Valentine, S. E., Kaysen, D., Mackintosh, M.-A., Dixon De Silva, L. E., Ahles, E. M., Youn, S. J., Shtasel, D. L., Simon, N. M., & Wiltsey Stirman, S. (2019). Provider fidelity and modifications to cognitive processing therapy in a diverse community health clinic: Associations with clinical change. *Journal of Consulting and Clinical Psychology, 87*(4), 357–369. https://doi.org/10.1037/ccp0000384

McCullough, J. P., Jr. (2000). *Treatment for chronic depression: Cognitive Behavioral Analysis System of Psychotherapy (CBASP).* Guilford Press.

McLeod, B. D., Southam-Gerow, M. A., Jensen-Doss, A., Hogue, A., Kendall, P. C., & Weisz, J. R. (2019). Benchmarking treatment adherence and therapist competence in individual cognitive-behavioral treatment for youth anxiety disorders. *Journal of Clinical Child and Adolescent Psychology, 48*(Suppl. 1), S234–S246. https://doi.org/10.1080/15374416.2017.1381914

Miller, S. D., Hubble, M., & Duncan, B. (2008). Supershrinks: What is the secret of their success? *Psychotherapy in Australia, 14*(4), 14–22.

Miller, W. R., & Rollnick, S. (2002). *Motivational interviewing: Preparing people for change* (2nd ed.). Guilford Press.

Okiishi, J., Lambert, M. J., Nielsen, S. L., & Ogles, B. M. (2003). Waiting for supershrink: An empirical analysis of therapist effects. *Clinical Psychology & Psychotherapy, 10*(6), 361–373. https://doi.org/10.1002/cpp.383

Pollmann, M. M. H., & Finkenauer, C. (2009). Investigating the role of two types of understanding in relationship well-being: Understanding is more important than knowledge. *Personality and Social Psychology Bulletin, 35*(11), 1512–1527. https://doi.org/10.1177/0146167209342754

Reis, H. T. (2012). Perceived partner responsiveness as an organizing theme for the study of relationships and well-being. In L. Campbell & T. J. Loving (Eds.), *Interdisciplinary research on close relationships: The case for integration* (pp. 27–52). American Psychological Association. https://doi.org/10.1037/13486-002

Reis, H. T. (2014). Responsiveness: Affective interdependence in close relationships. In M. Mikulincer & P. R. Shaver (Eds.), *Mechanisms of social connection: From brain to group* (pp. 255–271). American Psychological Association. https://doi.org/10.1037/14250-015

Reis, H. T., & Clark, M. S. (2013). Responsiveness. In J. A. Simpson & L. Campbell (Eds.), *The Oxford handbook of close relationships* (pp. 400–423). Oxford University Press.

Reis, H. T., & Gable, S. L. (2015). Responsiveness. *Current Opinion in Psychology, 1,* 67–71. https://doi.org/10.1016/j.copsyc.2015.01.001

Rogers, C. R. (1957). The necessary and sufficient conditions of therapeutic personality change. *Journal of Consulting Psychology, 21*(2), 95–103. https://doi.org/10.1037/h0045357

Rousmaniere, T., Goodyear, R. K., Miller, S. D., & Wampold, B. E. (Eds.). (2017). *The cycle of excellence: Using deliberate practice to improve supervision and training.* Wiley-Blackwell. https://doi.org/10.1002/9781119165590

Safran, J. D., & Muran, J. C. (2000). *Negotiating the therapeutic alliance: A relational treatment guide.* Guilford Press.

Selcuk, E., & Ong, A. D. (2013). Perceived partner responsiveness moderates the association between received emotional support and all-cause mortality. *Health Psychology, 32*(2), 231–235. https://doi.org/10.1037/a0028276

Snippe, E., Schroevers, M. J., Tovote, K. A., Sanderman, R., Emmelkamp, P. M. G., & Fleer, J. (2019). Explaining variability in therapist adherence and patient depressive symptom improvement: The role of therapist interpersonal skills and patient engagement. *Clinical Psychology & Psychotherapy, 26*(1), 84–93. https://doi.org/10.1002/cpp.2332

Stiles, W. B. (2009). Responsiveness as an obstacle for psychotherapy outcome research: It's worse than you think. *Clinical Psychology: Science and Practice, 16*(1), 86–91. https://doi.org/10.1111/j.1468-2850.2009.01148.x

Stiles, W. B. (2013). The variables problem and progress in psychotherapy research. *Psychotherapy, 50*(1), 33–41. https://doi.org/10.1037/a0030569

Stiles, W. B., & Goldsmith, J. Z. (2010). The alliance over time. In J. C. Muran & J. P. Barber (Eds.), *The therapeutic alliance: An evidence-based guide to practice* (pp. 44–62). Guilford Press.

Stiles, W. B., Honos-Webb, L., & Surko, M. (1998). Responsiveness in psychotherapy. *Clinical Psychology: Science and Practice, 5*(4), 439–458. https://doi.org/10.1111/j.1468-2850.1998.tb00166.x

Stiles, W. B., & Horvath, A. O. (2017). Appropriate responsiveness as a contribution to therapist effects. In L. G. Castonguay & C. E. Hill (Eds.), *How and why are some therapists better than others? Understanding therapist effects* (pp. 71–84). American Psychological Association. https://doi.org/10.1037/0000034-005

Swift, J. K., & Greenberg, R. P. (2012). Premature discontinuation in adult psychotherapy: A meta-analysis. *Journal of Consulting and Clinical Psychology, 80*(4), 547–559. https://doi.org/10.1037/a0028226

Wampold, B. E., & Imel, Z. E. (2015). *The great psychotherapy debate: The research evidence for what works in psychotherapy* (2nd ed.). Routledge. https://doi.org/10.4324/9780203582015

Watson, J. C. (2018). Empathy and responsiveness in emotion-focused therapy. In O. Tishby & H. Wiseman (Eds.), *Developing the therapeutic relationship: Integrating case studies, research, and practice* (pp. 235–255). American Psychological Association. https://doi.org/10.1037/0000093-011

Watts, B. V., Shiner, B., Zubkoff, L., Carpenter-Song, E., Ronconi, J. M., & Coldwell, C. M. (2014). Implementation of evidence-based psychotherapies for posttraumatic stress disorder in VA specialty clinics. *Psychiatric Services, 65*(5), 648–653. https://doi.org/10.1176/appi.ps.201300176

Webb, C. A., DeRubeis, R. J., & Barber, J. P. (2010). Therapist adherence/competence and treatment outcome: A meta-analytic review. *Journal of Consulting and Clinical Psychology, 78*(2), 200–211. https://doi.org/10.1037/a0018912

Weissman, M. M., Markowitz, J. C., & Klerman, G. L. (2000). *Comprehensive guide to interpersonal psychotherapy*. Basic Books.

Westra, H. A., & Norouzian, N. (2018). Using motivational interviewing to manage process markers of ambivalence and resistance in cognitive behavioral therapy. *Cognitive Therapy and Research, 42*(2), 193–203. https://doi.org/10.1007/s10608-017-9857-6

Wiltsey Stirman, S., Gamarra, J. M., Bartlett, B. A., Calloway, A., & Gutner, C. A. (2017). Empirical examinations of modifications and adaptations to evidence-based psychotherapies: Methodologies, impact, and future directions. *Clinical Psychology: Science and Practice, 24*(4), 396–420. https://doi.org/10.1111/cpsp.12218

Wiltsey Stirman, S., Toder, K., & Crits-Christoph, P. (2010). New psychotherapies for mood and anxiety disorders. *Canadian Journal of Psychiatry, 55*(4), 193–201. https://doi.org/10.1177/070674371005500402

Wolf, A. W., Goldfried, M. R., & Muran, J. C. (2017). Therapist negative reactions: How to transform toxic experiences. In L. G. Castonguay & C. E. Hill (Eds.), *How and why are some therapists better than others? Understanding therapist effects* (pp. 175–192). American Psychological Association. https://doi.org/10.1037/0000034-011

Zickgraf, H. F., Chambless, D. L., McCarthy, K. S., Gallop, R., Sharpless, B. A., Milrod, B. L., & Barber, J. P. (2016). Interpersonal factors are associated with lower therapist adherence in cognitive–behavioural therapy for panic disorder. *Clinical Psychology & Psychotherapy, 23*(3), 272–284. https://doi.org/10.1002/cpp.1955

Zilcha-Mano, S. (2018). Major developments in methods addressing for whom psychotherapy may work and why. *Psychotherapy Research, 29*(6), 693–708. https://doi.org/10.1080/10503307.2018.1429691

3

ATTACHMENT THEORY AS A FRAMEWORK FOR RESPONSIVENESS IN PSYCHOTHERAPY

HADAS WISEMAN AND SHARON EGOZI

Bowlby and Ainsworth's attachment theory (Ainsworth et al., 1978; Bowlby, 1969/1982, 1973, 1980, 1988) appears to offer an especially solid framework for conceptualizing therapist responsiveness and attunement to clients' relational needs in psychotherapy. In the quest for "pathways of connections and integration" between different domains in psychology and psychotherapy (Castonguay, 2011), attachment theory and research in many ways provide "a royal road" for building connections between the science of relationships and psychotherapy relationships (Wiseman, 2017). Among attachment theory's unique points of strength that make it suitable for exploring the concepts of responsiveness and attunement in psychotherapy are (a) it has an exceptionally strong empirical base, providing a bridge between clinical thinking and empirical research (Eagle, 2013; Fonagy, 2001; Mikulincer & Shaver, 2007); (b) it offers a strong foundation for integration between diverse psychotherapy orientations (Connors, 2011; Gold, 2011); (c) it encompasses a developmental lifespan approach, "from the cradle to the grave" (Bowlby, 1969/1982); (d) it is a theory of affect regulation and defensive processes (Connors, 2011) with

https://doi.org/10.1037/0000240-004
The Responsive Psychotherapist: Attuning to Clients in the Moment, J. C. Watson and H. Wiseman (Editors)

implications for psychopathology and psychotherapy (Mallinckrodt, 2010; Mikulincer et al., 2013); and (e) it provides potentially powerful means for connecting psychotherapy researchers and clinicians (Eagle & Wolitzky, 2009; Farber & Metzger, 2009; Slade, 2016).

In this chapter, we use attachment theory as a framework to begin the pathway to conceptualization of therapists' responsiveness to their clients by considering the responsiveness of parents to their infants. Research in developmental psychology on mother–infant attachment flourished following Ainsworth et al.'s (1978) groundbreaking strange situation paradigm. First, we touch on the nature of early infant–parent interaction to highlight the centrality of responsiveness in infant–parent bonds. Second, we consider key concepts in attachment theory that are applicable to responsiveness in psychotherapy: the provision of a secure base by parents and by therapists and internal working models and relationship representations. We then turn to consider attachment dynamics in psychotherapy, focusing on therapist responsiveness to client attachment needs through regulating therapeutic distance. We provide narrative illustrations (derived from interviews with clients about their experiences with their therapists) that depict lack of responsiveness and appropriate responsiveness, as well as misattunement and attunement. Finally, we present relevant assessment tools for attachment processes and research.

RESPONSIVENESS IN THE ATTACHMENT PATHWAY

Considering conceptualizations of responsiveness by diverse theoretical approaches in relationship science, Reis (2013) viewed attachment theory as featuring caregiver responsiveness to infants' expressions of need or distress as accounting for socioemotional development. As Bowlby (1969/1982) first theorized and Ainsworth et al.'s (1978) subsequent research confirmed, infants with caregivers who respond sensitively and supportively to them learn to be confident about their caregivers' availability and responsiveness. This sense of confidence, or felt security, is internalized and generalized to other caregivers, providing a foundation for the development of secure internal working models that serve the individual throughout life. Thus, attunement and appropriate parent responsiveness to infants' needs are the hallmark of secure attachment. In relation to the findings of prospective studies on the association between infant attachment and maternal responsive behavior, Holmes (1993) stated, "Mothers of secure one-year-olds are *responsive to their babies*, mothers of insecure-avoidants are *unresponsive*, and mothers of insecure-ambivalents are *inconsistently responsive*" (p. 107).

Some Evidence From Infant-Parent Interaction Research

Babies and the adults who care for them are built to bond with one another. There is a growing body of evidence that shows that infants and the adults who care for them possess reciprocal, coevolved characteristics designed to ensure that strong emotional bonds form between them (Zeifman, 2013). The term "coregulation" (Hofer, 1995) in infant–caregiver emotional bonds reflects the process of mutual reliance of relationship partners used to regulate personal physiological states. Research has shown that infants possess an inborn sensitivity to subtle cues and emotional feedback of the parent in face-to-face interaction, being highly attuned to signs of their parent's emotional availability and contingent responsiveness. Zeifman (2013) reviewed evidence from experiments that tested the reactions of infants to experimentally induced disturbance in the rhythmic, turn-taking exchanges of infants and caregivers. For example, after infants (6–9 weeks old) and mothers established free-flowing positive communication, the researcher played back to the infants a time-lagged video (a segment of the mother's behavior to the infant as it had been a minute prior, rather than as it was occurring in real time), which lacked the contingent responsiveness of the normal mother–infant interaction in the previous part of the experiment. Although the video preserved the quality of the mother's behavior in every other way, the infants became unsettled and upset in response to the noncontingent feedback of the mother and reacted by turning away, frowning, touching their own bodies and clothing, and often crying (Murray & Trevarthen, 1986).

Tronick's still-face procedure (Tronick et al., 1978) is a well-recognized procedure in infant research that demonstrates young infants' sensitivity to contingent feedback and responsiveness from the caregiver. In this procedure, following a period of normal face-to-face interaction, the mother is instructed by the experimenter to assume a neutral, nonresponsive facial expression for several minutes. Experiments applying the procedure have been conducted with newborn infants only hours after birth, infants 2 to 3 months of age, and infants 6 months and older. Newborns, although they have no experience-based expectations for the caregiver's contingent feedback and responsiveness, display discontent during the still-face portion of the interaction by averting their gaze, closing their eyes, and grimacing at higher rates (Nagy, 2008). At age 2 to 3 months, infants react to the mother's lack of responsiveness with even more obvious displeasure by turning their faces away, arching their backs, frowning, and often crying and, by age 6 months, by turning their faces (Tronick et al., 1978). By 6 months of age, they not only show measurable signs of physiological deregulation (e.g., increases in heart rate) but also "go to great lengths to behaviorally re-engage their frozen-conversation partners" (e.g., by waving their hands, screaming, and protesting; Zeifman, 2013, p. 54). As Zeifman (2013) concluded, "Collectively, these experiments demonstrate that from the earliest age infants are attentive to caregiver cues of availability and responsiveness" (p. 54).

Tronick and his colleagues have studied mutual regulatory processes between mothers and infants during face-to-face interactions using measures of behavior and affect (see Tronick, 2007, for a review of 3 decades of this work). They found that mothers and infants engage in self-directed and other-directed actions during face-to-face interaction in an effort to maintain optimal levels of self- and dyadic arousal and engagement. According to the mutual regulation model (Tronick, 1989), infants play a major agentic role in regulating the interaction and modulating its intensity and their own internal state. Caregivers vary in the degree to which they apprehend and learn their infants' messages and thus vary in how much they help (or hinder) the infants' regulation. Temporal features of the interaction reveal contingencies of signaling, synchrony, and attunement, and both caregivers and infants use nonverbal forms of communication that convey meaning. O'Brien and colleagues (2013) reviewed the ways that the mutual regulation model has been connected to the understanding of therapeutic relational processes. They suggested that early work on mutual regulation and that of many other developmental and psychological researchers (e.g., Beebe & Lachmann, 2002; Fonagy, 2002; Tronick et al., 1998) have had a profound impact on the conceptualization of therapeutic processes in contemporary relational psychotherapies (Safran & Muran, 2000; see also Chapter 4 by Eubanks et al. in this volume).

Provision of a Secure Base by Parents

Ainsworth introduced the concept of secure base in her seminal work on infant–mother/caretaker attachment (Ainsworth et al., 1978). Bowlby (1988) formulated the concept of *A Secure Base* (the title of his last book) as a central feature of his model of parenting:

> the provision by both parents of a secure base from which a child or an adolescent can make sorties into the outside world and to which he can return knowing for sure that he will be welcomed when he gets there, nourished physically and emotionally, comforted if distressed, reassured if frightened. (p. 11)

Bowlby explained that he used the term "base" to connote that the parents' role is similar to the officer commanding a military base, with the base serving as the home from which the expeditionary force sets out and to which it can retreat in the case of setback. Although much of the time the role of the base is that of waiting, it is vital, for only when there is confidence that the base is secure can the force dare press forward and take risks. A parent ensures the provision of a secure base by being available and responsive when called upon and ready to intervene actively only when clearly necessary, thereby encouraging autonomy (appropriate to the child's developmental capabilities and state of mind). Provided the child experiences the parent as available and responsive when called upon, the child feels secure enough to explore (Ainsworth, 1967) and feels they have a home base to return to when in difficulty (Bowlby, 1988).

Internal Working Models and Relationship Representations

Bowlby posited that on the basis of early attachment experiences with caregivers, individuals develop mental representations of self and others that he called "internal working models" (IWMs; Bowlby, 1969/1982, 1973, 1980). IWMs of self and other in attachment relationships help individuals anticipate, interpret, and guide interactions with partners, such as in parent–child or intimate relationships (Bretherton & Munholland, 2008). According to Bowlby, the IWMs a child develops are largely a reflection of actual events rather than fantasy: "The particular form that a person's working model takes is a fair reflection of the types of experiences he has had in his relationships with attachment figures" (Bowlby, 1973, p. 297). Eagle (2013) drew attention to this as a major point of contention between Bowlby's attachment theory and the strong emphasis in psychoanalysis on fantasy and psychic reality (for a historical view on Bowlby the psychoanalyst and the psychoanalytic community, see Berman, 2016, and Eagle, 2013).

Given that IWMs are the product of the particular repeated experiences children have with their caregivers that form their internalized expectations and beliefs of self and the attachment figure, it follows that there are individual differences in IWMs. Variations in working models, and hence in attachment system functioning, depend on the availability, sensitivity, and responsiveness of attachment figures in time of need. Security of attachment, an outgrowth of the child's experiencing attachment figures as available, sensitive, and responsive during times of emotional distress, leads the child to develop a generally positive model of others (i.e., expecting others to be available and responsive). Out of those same experiences, the child develops a complementary positive model of the self as worthy of assistance, affection, and love (Bowlby, 1962/1982). In contrast, insecure attachment is the outgrowth of the child's experience of attachment figures as responding insensitively and in a noncontingent manner by either not responding or being intrusive. Thus, children learn that they cannot feel confident they can rely on their caregivers' availability and responsiveness, which fosters insecure working models of attachment in later childhood and adulthood (Kobak & Madsen, 2008). It is in this respect that Reis (2013) viewed the centrality of caregiver responsiveness in attachment theory as key in considering the various theoretical conceptualizations of responsiveness in relationship science.

THE THERAPIST'S ROLE: FIVE THERAPEUTIC TASKS

Applying attachment theory to the therapeutic process, Bowlby (1988) viewed the therapist's role as providing

> the conditions in which his patient can explore his representational models of himself and his attachment figures with a view to reappraising and restructuring them in light of the new understanding he acquires and the new experiences he has in the therapeutic relationship. (p. 138)

Toward this end, Bowlby (1988, pp. 138–139) outlined five interrelated therapeutic tasks:

1. The therapist provides the client a secure base for exploration of their thoughts and feelings, analogous to the mother providing her child a secure base from which to explore the world, by being a trusted companion who enables the exploration of painful aspects of the client's life.

2. The therapist assists in the exploration of expectations and unconscious biases in forming relationships with others.

3. The therapist encourages examination of how the client's early parenting experiences are related to the relationship that develops between the two of them.

4. The therapist helps the client see the past for what it is and conceive healthier alternative ways of thinking and acting.

5. The therapist assists in examining the client's relationship with the therapist in the here and now of the sessions in relation to the client's working models of self and other as they play out in the therapeutic relationship.

ATTACHMENT DYNAMICS IN THE THERAPEUTIC RELATIONSHIP

An attachment-informed approach to conceptualizing the therapeutic relationship between client and therapist postulates that this relationship is likely to reactivate clients' long-standing expectations about the availability and responsiveness of others (Bowlby, 1988; Eagle & Wolitzky, 2009; Farber &

Metzger, 2009; Mallinckrodt, 2010; Wiseman & Tishby, 2014). Given that clients' working models dictate their expectations from their therapist, individual differences in attachment style will lead to different manifestations and dynamics in the development of the therapeutic relationship (Wiseman & Atzil-Slonim, 2018). An individual's location in the two-dimensional space defined by attachment avoidance and attachment anxiety reflects both the person's sense of attachment security and the ways in which the person deals with threats and distress. Individuals who score low on these dimensions are generally secure and tend to use constructive and effective affect regulation strategies. Those who score high on either the anxiety or the avoidant dimension (or both) suffer from attachment insecurities and tend to rely on secondary attachment strategies.

In order to cope with threats individuals experience when they feel that their efforts to meet their emotional needs through a secure relationship have failed, they shift to one of two secondary attachment strategies. Individuals who rely on *hyperactivating strategies* intensify dependency needs and closeness in their relations with attachment figures, whereas those who rely on *deactivating strategies* increase distance so as not to get hurt (Mikulincer & Shaver, 2007). Hyperactivation of attachment behaviors is attributed to people with high attachment anxiety. These people seek greater proximity to the attachment figure, exhibit maximal amplification of attachment behaviors, and show hypersensitivity to any sign of rejection. Deactivation of attachment behaviors is attributed to people with high attachment avoidance who expend a great deal of cognitive effort in diverting attention from distressing situations or from recognizing or expressing thoughts and emotions ascribed to attachment (Mikulincer & Shaver, 2019). These diverse attachment strategies call upon therapists to consider how to work with clients with hyperactivating versus deactivating strategies in order to work through their insecurities and establish a secure relationship with the therapist and to build a working alliance that enables collaboration in therapy (Mallinckrodt, 2010; Mikulincer et al., 2013).

THERAPIST RESPONSIVENESS TO CLIENTS' ATTACHMENT NEEDS: REGULATING THERAPEUTIC DISTANCE

A principal implication of attachment theory regarding the question of how therapists can enhance their appropriate responsiveness involves tailoring the therapeutic relationship to clients' attachment needs. Consider the situation in which an adult meets a (normative) young child for the first time. A sensitive response would require giving the child some time to become familiar with the adult's new presence in the room and monitoring the distance that feels comfortable for the child. Indeed, the strange situation procedure includes episodes of being left with a stranger with and without the presence of the attachment figure in the room (Ainsworth et al., 1978). Regulating interpersonal distance in everyday interactions with strangers, teachers, and peers is a sign of social competence. In forming new romantic relationships, regulating distance is often an issue and plays out in "dancing too close" versus "dancing too far." Particularly in times of distress, the appropriate distance for one person is different from that of another and is influenced by each person's attachment history. Clients meeting their therapist for the first session bring into the psychotherapy room their tendency to feel comfort, or more often discomfort, with closeness versus distance. This tendency is closely tied to their attachment history with attachment figures and their current attachment patterns. Hence, being attuned and responsive to clients' attachment needs (internal working models of self and other) requires the therapist to regulate the appropriate therapeutic distance in the therapeutic relationship.

Taking an attachment approach to the psychotherapy relationship, Mallinckrodt (2010) developed the concept he termed "therapeutic distance," defined as "the level of transparency and disclosure in the psychotherapy relationship from both client and therapist, together with the immediacy, intimacy, and emotional intensity of a session" (Daly & Mallinckrodt, 2009, p. 559). Interviews with experienced interpersonal therapists suggest that in order to foster a secure attachment in the relationship, they attempt to regulate the therapeutic distance between themselves and the client while tailoring this distance to meet the specific client's attachment needs (Daly & Mallinckrodt, 2009; Mallinckrodt et al., 2015). Mallinckrodt's (2010) model, therapeutic gratification, relief, anxiety, or frustration (T-GRAF), assumes that for therapists to adopt a therapeutic distance that will provide their clients a corrective emotional experience, they must take into account both the client's attachment strategy and the changing phases of therapy. During the initial engagement phase, therapists largely need to accede to the client's desired (but ultimately maladaptive) level of therapeutic distance. Later, during the working phase, therapists gradually attempt to steer the relationship toward a more optimal level of therapeutic distance. The therapeutic distance optimal for each phase is regulated by the therapist depending on the client's hyperactivating versus deactivating strategies.

Hyperactivating clients (high in attachment anxiety) tend to feel that their therapist is too distant (cold, remote, not helpful enough). To establish a secure base during the initial engagement phase with these clients, therapists should attempt to be responsive to these clients' need for closeness by minimizing the therapeutic distance as much as possible. Only during more advanced phases of therapy, once the relationship is established, should therapists attempt to gradually increase the therapeutic distance in a manner that allows their clients to experience autonomy and independence. By encouraging self-reliance and supporting independent decisions at this more advanced phase, therapists offer hyperactivating clients the needed corrective emotional experience.

In contrast, deactivating clients (high in attachment avoidance) sense that their therapist is too close (pushing for too much disclosure and emotional proximity). To establish a secure base, during the initial engagement phase of therapy therapists should attempt to be responsive to these clients' need for distance by respecting it and allowing a great deal of distance. Only during more advanced phases of therapy, once the relationship is established, should therapists attempt to begin to challenge these needs by establishing a closer, more engaged and caring relationship. Once these clients are engaged and feel more secure, they more freely disclose upsetting topics to the therapist, which is the corrective emotional experience needed for deactivating clients (Mallinckrodt et al., 2015).

MARKERS OF CLOSENESS AND DISTANCE DYNAMICS IN CLIENT-THERAPIST RELATIONAL NARRATIVES

In previous research, we examined how clients and their therapists experienced the relational dance between them at various phases of psychodynamic psychotherapy (Schattner & Tishby, 2018; Wiseman, 2017; Wiseman & Tishby, 2017) through client–therapist relational narratives collected through relationship anecdotes paradigm (RAP) interviews (Luborsky & Crits-Christoph, 1998; Wiseman & Tishby, 2017). Applying the core conflictual relationship theme (CCRT) method to these narratives, we assigned Response of Other (RO) and Response of Self (RS) ratings to enable observation of representations of others and representations of self that correspond to internal working models (Atzil-Slonim et al., 2016). In the sections that follow, we focus on responsiveness and attunement experiences as revealed in narratives regarding closeness and distance dynamics in the client–therapist dyad. We first consider markers of lack of responsiveness and misattunement and then illustrate responsiveness and attunement as experienced by both client and therapist. These illustrations are drawn from clients' narratives about meaningful interactions with their therapist recounted in the RAP interviews during ongoing psychodynamic psychotherapy.[1]

---

[1]The identities of all clients in this chapter's narratives have been disguised to protect client confidentiality.

Therapist Lack of Responsiveness: Too Distant

Client narratives in which clients experience the therapist as too distant depict the therapist as being inattentive, uninvolved, and unresponsive.

"As If He Forgot About It": Experiencing the Therapist as Inattentive and Detached

The client in the following narrative felt that the therapist was detached and uninvolved (too distant) because he did not hold on to what she had told him in the previous session:

> In the last session, the whole session we talked about my brother who lives abroad coming for a visit, and I was really excited because he was scheduled to arrive home exactly when I would be returning home after my therapy session—same day, same hour. So, we talked about it the entire session. He [the therapist] asked if my brother and I are close friends and how I feel about him coming, and this and that. And then in the next session, the first thing I expected him to say was, "OK, your brother arrived; let's talk about it." And he didn't say anything about it, like, didn't ask me anything, didn't talk about it at all, didn't mention it, as if he forgot about it. . . . And I felt that maybe he isn't a good therapist. That he . . . I don't know, that he doesn't know what he is doing . . . like, it didn't make sense to me, like . . . I was sure that he would ask me about it. I thought, "What, isn't he caring, isn't he interested, doesn't he remember, doesn't he even have a memory?"

The client expected the therapist to ask her about her brother's visit and perceived his not bringing it up as a lack of responsiveness (to the material from the previous session). In narrating this experience to the RAP interviewer (at the early stage of therapy, Session 5), she questioned the therapist's competence and caring for her and suspected that the therapist failed to hold her in his mind between sessions (Schröder et al., 2009).

"We Did Not Talk for 10 Minutes, and She Looks at Me and Doesn't Say a Word": Experiencing Therapist Silence as Unresponsiveness

The client in the narrative that follows expected the therapist to help her talk and experienced the therapist's letting her remain silent as being inattentive to her needs:

> We have a lot of silent moments because I do not volunteer information; I prefer to be asked. My previous therapist (a social worker) used to ask questions like a TV interviewer. And that was very comfortable for me. But here I can't come in with something that upsets me and just pour it out. I must get her guidance. One time we didn't talk for 10 minutes, and she looks at me and does not say a word. It annoyed me, so I asked her to ask me questions, so she answered, "What do you want me to ask you?" So it is a question, but a stupid one. . . . I felt like she was not attentive to my needs. . . . I have no idea what she feels

about the therapy, about me, about the things I say. Does she identify with them? Does she feel empathy? . . . Maybe she understood what I meant, but she didn't take it a step further.

This client experienced the therapist not breaking the silence in the session (at the early stage of therapy, Session 5) as the therapist being distant and inaccessible and lacking true interest in what the client needed from her. Of course, silence in itself does not entail failure to be responsive because the therapist being present in silence can be experienced as attuning in the moment to the clients' needs. Silence can be helpful ("silence is golden") depending on client factors, therapist factors, and relationship factors (Hill et al., 2018).

Therapist Misattunement: Too Close

Client narratives in which clients experienced the therapist as too close depict the therapist as being overinvolved and misattuned to the way the client feels about the significance of the therapist and therapy in their life.

"I Do Not See the Therapy as a Relationship": Experiencing the Therapist as Overly Intimate

The client in the following narrative seemed troubled by what she perceived as her therapist's overinvolvement in her life (too close). In a session at the advanced stage of therapy (Session 28), she had discussed with her therapist a relatively new romantic relationship, and she recalled his response:

> Then he [the therapist] came in and said, "Now you have two relationships in your life," that both relationships started about at the same time. I said to him, "I do not see it as two relationships. I see my relationship with my romantic partner as a couple relationship, and I do not see the therapy as a relationship." That word "relationship" frightened me, because it means a commitment. These are the little things that make me feel uncomfortable [with the therapist]. (adapted from Wiseman & Tishby, 2017, p. 289)

"It Does Not Affect the Relationship": Experiencing the Therapist as Assuming Too Much Emotional Connection

In a session with the client, the therapist announced she was pregnant and would take maternity leave; in the narrative that follows, the client (at the advanced stage of therapy, Session 28) seemed to feel uncomfortable about her own indifference to this announcement:

> Not long ago the therapist told me that she is pregnant, and she wanted us to talk about it. I told her I had already noticed, but hadn't said anything because I didn't want to embarrass her. I said that I was happy for her, and she asked

what I think about our relationship and if it [the pregnancy] will affect it, that she will have to go on maternity leave and whether I am angry. But the truth is, I didn't have anything to say except, "Congratulations." . . . These questions were strange for me; I didn't think about it, and didn't feel that way. I thought it was natural that there would be a break, but she looked very worried, as if it would bother me or be difficult for me. She thought it would affect the relationship and she wanted me to tell her how, and I didn't know how it would affect it, and I also thought it does *not* affect it. It's something that happens, and it's natural and OK; I'm not a child. [Interviewer: What did you feel?] I feel nothing about that issue. I guess I'm not experiencing the therapy as something emotional, or maybe I don't let myself feel. And I wouldn't like it to be any other way, because it's not a place to feel envy or emotional. I mean, if there are two sides—the first total dependency on the therapist and the other not being dependent at all—then I'm closer to the second.

In these two illustrations of misattunement, both therapists failed to regulate the appropriate distance from their client, assuming that the client wished closeness with them. Both therapists' responses seem incongruent and misattuned to the way their clients felt about the importance of the relationship with the therapist in their lives. The first therapist assumed that the relationship with him was as important as the client's new romantic relationship. The second assumed that the client felt affected by the therapist's maternity leave and must have been angry with her about the anticipated break. However, the client appeared to guard herself from developing dependence and, in response to the therapist's announcement, did not express any feelings of protest or sense of abandonment.

Therapist Appropriate Responsiveness and Attunement

Appropriate responsiveness and attunement are depicted by a client–therapist dyad who independently recounted their experiences in the following narratives. The client, from her perspective, experienced her therapist as fully attuned and responding authentically to what she needed in the moment; the therapist, from his perspective, felt that he was being responsive to her in an appropriate and authentic relational manner.

Client's Narrative: "I Want an Authentic Reaction"
The client in the following narrative told the interviewer that one of her great dilemmas was whether to wear a short dress because that would mean showing her legs, which she felt would reveal a big weakness, "as if I were wearing my wounds on my legs, or scars, more exactly." She felt that for her this would be "a very big exposure, very much like nakedness." Two weeks

before, she had gone into a store, saw a short dress she loved, tried it on, and decided it looked very nice on her. She bought it knowing that it would just hang in her closet. She talked to her therapist about it:

> We talked about it in the session, and he really encouraged me to wear it. Yesterday I came to the session wearing the dress, and when I came into the room, he looked at my dress and said, "You are wearing the dress." I said "Yes, I did it," and he understands exactly what that means for me, that it is awfully sensitive. We talked about what reaction I would like to get from those around me. So I told him that anybody who tells me that they don't notice it at all is biased. If my girlfriends tell me, "Oh, it's nothing, nobody can see it," then they are pretending, and the saleswoman in the shop will obviously say that nobody sees it, because she wants to sell me the dress [laughs]. We reached the conclusion that I want some sort of authentic reaction. I want somebody to come and tell me, "You look nice in the dress" or "You don't look good in the dress." And then, before I left, he said, "You look nice in the dress." I said, "Thank you, but you're not objective" [giggles]. Then he said, "True." I left smiling.
>
> It goes back to the subject of nakedness, I think that it's scary, I mean. You open up so much to a person [her voice becomes weepy]. It is kind of scary because, like, what will happen afterwards. It's clear that it has to end; I am not developing some sort of dependency here or anything like that . . . but it makes you wonder if I'll manage to create something real like this. Something so nonjudgmental, so accepting, so supportive—he is very understanding. He doesn't get scared. He helps me understand myself, understand the monster, helps me dig deeper into those feelings. I feel a kind of great appreciation. Gratitude.

Therapist's Narrative: "I Was Really Free, I Was Authentic"
The therapist in the following narrative also referred to the time the client talked with him about her "dress dilemma." He recounted the interaction between them in the session in which she began to disclose to him why she would not feel comfortable wearing the short dress:

> A few sessions ago, she told me that she'd gone to buy a dress, and at a certain point she said it was very embarrassing because she wasn't feeling comfortable in the dress, because she didn't want people to see . . . and I didn't understand what she meant, and I asked her what it was that she didn't want people to see. Then there was silence, and she started crying really bitterly. It was heartbreaking. I was terribly embarrassed because I thought I'd asked her something that I shouldn't have, I really had no clue; we were talking about a dress, but I understood it embarrassed her. I asked if something in my questions was inappropriate, or hurtful. And she shook her head, and then she told me that she had some scars on her legs, and that she hadn't told almost anyone about them, but she told me.

I think that it was a very special moment because it was as if she laid herself bare in the dress. She told me about the scars, as if she were showing them to me. I also felt a kind of gratitude. There was something very intense in that moment, a sense of intimacy. I feel she could expose one of her deepest fears and survive it. It says that she's taken another very big step. And it says that she trusts that I will survive this exposure. As a person, I really feel that what she talked about, I mean the ability to lay herself bare in front of someone else, it's a terribly scary moment. I really felt that it didn't scare me. I saw her there in her beauty, and not in her scars. I felt she didn't only show me something, but also gave me something human. As a therapist, looking back, it was great. We were able to get to something new that she hadn't thought about and I hadn't thought about. I was really free, I was authentic, and that also helped. I felt it was for the client's sake, and that it made me feel good.

Attunement and appropriate responsiveness in this dyad were apparent in the congruence between the experiences of the client and therapist. The meeting between their relational needs was expressed by their use of the same words in narrating their experience (they were interviewed independently by different interviewers): "exposure," "scary," "authentic," and "gratitude." At this advanced stage of therapy (Session 28), the matching between the attachment patterns of the therapist and client and the therapist's appropriate distance regulation provided the kind of corrective experience that this insecurely attached client needed in order to revise her working models of self and other.

IN-SESSION ATTACHMENT PROCESSES: MEASURES AND RESEARCH

In-session measures that have been developed to shed light on responsiveness with an attachment framework include the assessment of therapeutic distance and the study of communication patterns and attunement.

Assessment of Therapeutic Distance

On the basis of Mallinckrodt's theoretical therapeutic distance model, Mallinckrodt et al. (2015) developed the Therapeutic Distance Scale (TDS) to assess how clients experience the process of their therapist's attempts to regulate therapeutic distance. The TDS is a client self-report questionnaire composed of four subscales: (a) Too Distant and (b) Too Close (referring to clients' experience of therapeutic distance) and (c) Growing Autonomy and (d) Growing Engagement (referring to the expansion of their internal working model). Their preliminary findings showed significant associations between clients' therapeutic distance experience assessed by the TDS and attachment characteristics (anxiety and avoidance) assessed using the Experiences in Close Relationships Scale (ECR; Brennan et al., 1998). Specifically, at the outset of therapy, significant correlations were found between clients' attachment anxiety and their sense that their therapists were too distant, and between clients' attachment avoidance and their sense that their therapists were too close. They also tested the associations at a more advanced phase of therapy for a subsample of clients ($n = 17$) who established secure attachment to their therapist (measured with the Client Attachment to Therapist Scale; see Mallinckrodt et al., 1995; Mallinckrodt & Jeong, 2015). The findings indicated that for these clients, as predicted, pretherapy ECR Avoidance was positively correlated with TDS Growing Engagement; however, contrary to expectations, no correlation was found between ECR Anxiety and TDS Growing Autonomy (Mallinckrodt et al., 2015).

Taking a relational perspective that highlights the mutual aspects of the encounter between client and therapist (Aron, 1996; Muran, 2019; Safran & Muran, 2000; see also Chapter 5 by Tishby in this volume), we developed the Therapeutic Distance Scale Observer version (TDS–O; Egozi et al., 2020) to assess the therapeutic distance as experienced by each partner in the dyad. The TDS–O includes a version for the client and one for the therapist. Like the self-report TDS, the Observer versions also comprise four scales: Too Distant (the partner is perceived as distant and inaccessible), Too Close (the partner is perceived as intrusive and forcing closeness), Growing Autonomy (therapy encourages clients to make independent decisions and to take the initiative, from either the client's or the therapist's view), and Growing Engagement (clients' ability to discuss sensitive issues and relinquish concerns regarding the need to reveal themselves, from either the client's or the therapist's view; Egozi et al., 2020).

In a recent study (Egozi et al., 2021), we tested the associations of client attachment and therapist attachment with the TDS–O applied to relational narratives that clients and their therapists narrated about meaningful moments between them at the beginning and advanced stages of long-term psychodynamic therapy (after Sessions 5, 15, and 28). Contrary to expectations, client attachment anxiety did not relate to their perception of the therapist as too distant at the beginning of therapy (Session 5); however, as expected, it did relate to less autonomy among clients in therapy as reported in therapists' narratives at the beginning stage and as reported in clients' narratives at the advanced stage (Session 28). Client attachment avoidance was related to their feeling that the therapist was too close at the beginning stage and the middle stage (Session 15) and to less engagement at the beginning stage. These correlations appeared only in clients' narratives and disappeared at the advanced stage, as expected from the T-GRAF model. Therapist attachment anxiety predicted therapist granting of less autonomy in beginning therapy and more therapist engagement in the advanced stages of therapy only in therapists' narratives. Their clients, however, perceived them as more distant at the middle stage. Therapist avoidance in the beginning stage predicted clients' perception of the therapist as too close and granting less autonomy but did not predict the therapist's experience. Therapist attachment avoidance predicted therapist perception of the client as too distant in early therapy, whereas their clients perceived them as both too distant and too close at the same stage. In advanced therapy, however, therapist attachment avoidance positively predicted therapist perception of the client as both too distant and less too close, whereas clients' narratives did not reveal any unique characteristics (Egozi et al., 2021).

These findings support the assumption that client attachment dimensions relate to diverse emotional needs in the therapeutic relationship at different phases. Moreover, in order to be responsive to clients' emotional needs and enable a secure base and corrective emotional experience, therapists need to be aware of their own attachment characteristics (for a review on therapist attachment, see Strauss & Petrowski, 2017).

Assessment of Communication Patterns and Attunement

Talia et al. (2014) suggested that language, as a social behavior, inevitably affects relationships and that people use language subconsciously to convey the type of response they ask from their partner. They originated the Patient Attachment Coding System (PACS), which assesses language and communication patterns in order to examine whether clients with different attachment classifications reveal distinct patterns in their use of language to regulate closeness and connection with their listener (Talia et al., 2017). Applying the PACS to single-session transcripts, they found that different Adult Attachment Interview (AAI; George et al., 1996) attachment classifications (coded independently) related to different ways of communication (Talia et al., 2014):

- *Secure clients* convey their present experience openly. They disclose their emotions in the here and now (e.g., "I feel frustrated," "I am happy") and share vivid narratives of past experiences that clearly convey their feelings in the present. Secure clients also communicate needs in the therapeutic relationship and share their present intentions, autonomous reflections, and positive experiences. These speech acts, rated on the PACS Proximity Seeking, Contact Maintaining, and Exploring scales, allow the therapist to take part in the client's experience, reflect or elaborate by asking questions, and get close.

- *Avoidant clients* tend to decline requests to express their feelings or are reluctant to describe their experiences in sufficient detail; they tend to downplay recent experiences (positive or negative) or convey unwillingness to do something about the situation. These types of communication, rated by the PACS Avoidance and Downplaying scales, preempt any kind of support and connection by shifting the listener's attention from the speaker's internal state.

- *Preoccupied clients* share their experience in a one-sided, exaggerated, or confusing way that leaves little room for the therapist to respond. For example, they may persuade the therapist to join their point of view alone (involving markers) or convey their experience in an impersonal, difficult-to-understand way (merging markers). These patterns tend to limit the extent to which the therapist is able to make meaning of clients' experience, leaving no room for contradiction, challenge, or elaboration, and these clients actually disregard the therapist's interventions.

Studies using the PACS with different samples in a range of therapeutic modalities have confirmed that AAI classifications predict marked differences in clients' in-session communication and that by analyzing such differences in a single session, one can predict clients' AAI classification (Talia et al., 2017). These patterns also appeared in posttreatment interviews conducted by an unfamiliar interviewer (Talia, Miller-Bottome, Wyner, et al., 2019). Specifically, the PACS Exploring scale has been shown to be closely associated with clients' independently obtained ratings of mentalizing in the context of the AAI (Talia, Miller-Bottome, Katznelson, et al., 2019). Finally, accumulating evidence shows that the PACS Security scale predicts greater resolution of alliance ruptures (Miller-Bottome et al., 2018, 2019), as well as greater physiological synchronization between client and therapist (Kleinbub et al., 2020).

Recently, Talia et al. (2020) developed the Therapist Attunement Scales (TASc), a transcript-based instrument that assesses ways in which therapists verbally attune to their clients. They suggested that therapists' attachment classifications are associated with their distinct communication about clients' internal states, which they refer to with the term "attunement" (Talia et al., 2020). In the initial validation study of the TASc, significant relationships were found between therapists' AAI classifications and their TASc scores:

- *Secure therapists* made conjectures on the client's internal state, presenting them as questions in sessions (leaving the client room to explore); they also used empathic validation and joining of client's experience by disclosing the impact that the client had on them.

- *Avoidant therapists* used clarifications that minimized the affect implicit in the client's disclosures (e.g., "So, you are feeling a bit sad right now"), and when they offered a validation of the client's self-states, they did so on the basis of an external fact or reason.

- *Preoccupied therapists* used coercing intervention in which they offered their insight on the internal states of another person without presenting it as their personal view (objective stance; e.g., "Your teacher is just trying to help you, obviously") or quoted a purported past occurrence of the client talking to themselves (e.g., "So you were thinking, 'I'm here, and I don't know what to do'").

Overall, the findings of Talia and colleagues (2020) regarding the PACS and the TASc underscore the effects of both client and therapist attachment classification on the communication patterns in the dyad. In terms of therapist attunement and responsiveness, secure communication patterns contribute to enhancing attunement and responsiveness, whereas avoidant and preoccupied communication patterns may result in misattunement and nonresponsiveness.

CONCLUSION

Responsiveness has been described as "behavior that is affected by emerging context, including perceptions of others' characteristics and behavior. Insofar as therapist and client respond to each other, responsiveness implies a dynamic relationship between variables, involving bidirectional causation and feedback loops" (Stiles et al., 1998, p. 439). Outlining the contributions of attachment concepts to the understanding of the therapeutic relationship, Holmes (2009) pointed to McCluskey's (2005) term "goal-corrected empathic attunement," which refers to a continual process of goal correction or mutual adjustment between client and therapist as they attempt to stay on track. In responsiveness terms, such empathic goal correction would involve attuning in the moment and making microadjustments to clients' changing relational needs in light of emerging context. Therapists' empathic attunement has been found to lead to improvement in clients' affect regulation capacities, depression, self-esteem, self-criticism, and neediness, and it is especially crucial in the case of insecurely attached clients (Watson, 2018; Watson et al., 2014). The markers for regulating distance that we described in this chapter call for therapist empathic attunement that is appropriately responsive to clients' attachment needs as they emerge in the client–therapist interaction at various phases of therapy. Clients with different attachment patterns, especially those who are insecurely attached (anxious, avoidant, or both), require different types of therapist responsive behavior. Therapists' awareness of their own attachment patterns, and the way these meet the patterns of their clients, is crucial for the development of a secure base and for facilitating a corrective emotional experience.

Appropriate responsiveness, meaning doing the right thing at the right time, also depends on the history of the particular therapeutic relationship, immediately preceding events, the circumstances of the session, and many other factors (Kramer & Stiles, 2015; Stiles & Horvath, 2017). Although our analysis of regulation of distance was based on relational narratives rather than on session transcripts of actual client–therapist in-session behavior, these recollected accounts depict the subjective experiences of the client and therapist in the therapeutic relationship (Wiseman & Atzil-Slonim, 2018; Wiseman & Tishby, 2017). We suggest that there is much to gain from these narratives because they tell us in essence whether the interaction is experienced as the right thing at the right time. For example, the therapist who responded "What do you want me to ask you?" to the client's request that instead of being silent the therapist ask her questions, is perhaps attempting to adhere to psychodynamic therapy (the training orientation of the therapists in the study), but this response was experienced by the client as an empathic failure (Hatcher, 2015; see also Chapter 2 by Hatcher in this volume). In contrast, in the example of appropriate responsiveness and attunement presented in the client and therapist narratives, the therapist's response "You look nice in the dress" does not seem to adhere to psychodynamic therapy, or perhaps to any other specific psychotherapy orientation, but for this client it did appear to be the right thing at the right time. We see this kind of therapist response as appropriate responsiveness that conveys validation as well as understanding and caring (the three components of perceived responsiveness in adult couple relationships, according to Reis, 2013). For this client, it appeared to be the right thing within this timing and context; however, it no doubt might have been harmful to the same client earlier on in therapy or if it was said in a flirtatious manner.

Future research on responsiveness and attunement from an attachment perspective is needed to make more fine-grained observations on the meeting of client and therapist attachment patterns, in-session attachment communication processes, and their relation to psychotherapy outcome. In training and supervision to enhance responsiveness, therapists can learn to identify attachment needs and attachment-related verbal communication patterns in order to impact in-session change and final outcome.

REFERENCES

Ainsworth, M. D. S. (1967). *Infancy in Uganda: Infant care and the growth of attachment.* John Hopkins Press.

Ainsworth, M. D. S., Blehar, M. C., Waters, E., & Wall, S. (1978). *Patterns of attachment: Psychological study of the strange situation.* Erlbaum.

Aron, L. (1996). *A meeting of minds: Mutuality in psychoanalysis.* The Analytic Press.

Atzil-Slonim, D., Wiseman, H., & Tishby, O. (2016). Relationship representations and change in adolescents and emerging adults during psychodynamic psychotherapy. *Psychotherapy Research, 26*(3), 279–296. https://doi.org/10.1080/10503307.2015.1010627

Beebe, B., & Lachmann, F. (2002). *Infant research and adult treatment: Co-constructing interactions.* The Analytic Press.

Berman, E. (2016). John Bowlby, psychoanalyst. In J. Bowlby, *A secure base: Parent–child attachment and healthy human development* (Hebrew version, pp. 17–28). Am Oved Publishers.

Bowlby, J. (1973). *Attachment and loss: Vol. 2. Separation: Anxiety and anger.* Hogarth Press.

Bowlby, J. (1980). *Attachment and loss: Vol. 3. Loss: Sadness and depression.* Basic Books.

Bowlby, J. (1982). *Attachment and loss: Vol. 1. Attachment* (2nd ed.). Basic Books. Original work published 1969

Bowlby, J. (1988). *A secure base: Clinical applications of attachment theory.* Routledge.

Brennan, K. A., Clark, C. L., & Shaver, P. R. (1998). Self-report measurement of adult attachment: An integrative overview. In J. A. Simpson & W. S. Rholes (Eds.), *Attachment theory and close relationships* (pp. 46–76). Guilford Press.

Bretherton, I., & Munholland, K. A. (2008). Internal working models in attachment relationships: Elaborating a central construct in attachment theory. In J. Cassidy & P. R. Shaver (Eds.), *Handbook of attachment: Theory, research, and clinical applications* (pp. 102–127). Guilford Press.

Castonguay, L. G. (2011). Psychotherapy, psychopathology, research and practice: Pathways of connections and integration. *Psychotherapy Research, 21*(2), 125–140. https://doi.org/10.1080/10503307.2011.563250

Connors, M. E. (2011). Attachment theory: A "secure base" for psychotherapy integration. *Journal of Psychotherapy Integration, 21*(3), 348–362. https://doi.org/10.1037/a0025460

Daly, K. D., & Mallinckrodt, B. (2009). Experienced therapists' approach to psychotherapy for adults with attachment avoidance or attachment anxiety. *Journal of Counseling Psychology, 56*(4), 549–563. https://doi.org/10.1037/a0016695

Eagle, M. N. (2013). *Attachment and psychoanalysis: Theory, research, and clinical implications.* Guilford Press.

Eagle, M., & Wolitzky, D. L. (2009). Adult psychotherapy from the perspectives of attachment theory and psychoanalysis. In J. H. Obegi & E. Berant (Eds.), *Attachment theory and research in clinical work with adults* (pp. 379–409). Guilford Press.

Egozi, S., Tishby, O., & Wiseman, H. (2020). Changes in clients' and therapists' experiences of therapeutic distance during psychodynamic therapy. *Journal of Clinical Psychology.* Advance online publication. https://doi.org/10.1002/jclp.23077

Egozi, S., Tishby, O., & Wiseman, H. (2021). Therapeutic distance in client–therapist narratives: Client attachment, therapist attachment, and dyadic effects. *Psycho-*

therapy Research. Advance online publication. https://doi.org/10.1080/10503307. 2021.1874069

Farber, B. A., & Metzger, J. A. (2009). The therapist as secure base. In J. H. Obegi & E. Berant (Eds.), *Attachment theory and research in clinical work with adults* (pp. 46–70). Guilford Press.

Fonagy, P. (2001). *Attachment theory and psychoanalysis*. Other Press.

Fonagy, P. (2002). *Affect regulation, mentalization, and the development of the self*. Other Press.

George, C., Kaplan, N., & Main, M. (1996). *Adult Attachment Interview* (3rd ed.). Department of Psychology, University of California, Berkeley.

Gold, J. (2011). Attachment theory and psychotherapy integration: An introduction and review of the literature. *Journal of Psychotherapy Integration, 21*(3), 221–231. https://doi.org/10.1037/a0025490

Hatcher, R. L. (2015). Interpersonal competencies: Responsiveness, technique, and training in psychotherapy. *American Psychologist, 70*(8), 747–757. https://doi.org/ 10.1037/a0039803

Hill, C. E., Kline, K. V., O'Connor, S., Morales, K., Li, X., Kivlighan, D. M., Jr., & Hillman, J. (2018). Silence is golden: A mixed methods investigation of silence in one case of psychodynamic psychotherapy. *Psychotherapy, 56*(4), 577–587. https://doi.org/10.1037/pst0000196

Hofer, M. A. (1995). Hidden regulators: Implications for a new understanding of attachment, separation, and loss. In S. Goldberg, R. Muir, & J. Kerr (Eds.), *Attachment theory: Social, developmental, and clinical perspectives* (pp. 203–230). The Analytic Press.

Holmes, J. (1993). *John Bowlby and attachment theory*. Routledge.

Holmes, J. (2009). From attachment research to clinical practice: Getting it together. In J. H. Obegi & E. Berant (Eds.), *Attachment theory and research in clinical work with adults* (pp. 490–514). Guilford Press.

Kleinbub, J. R., Talia, A., & Palmieri, A. (2020). Physiological synchronization in the clinical process: A research primer. *Journal of Counseling Psychology, 67*(4), 420–437. https://doi.org/10.1037/cou0000383

Kobak, R., & Madsen, S. (2008). Disruptions in attachment bonds: Implications for theory, research, and clinical intervention. In J. Cassidy & P. R. Shaver (Eds.), *Handbook of attachment: Theory, research, and clinical applications* (pp. 23–47). Guilford Press.

Kramer, U., & Stiles, W. B. (2015). The responsiveness problem in psychotherapy: A review of proposed solutions. *Clinical Psychology: Science and Practice, 22*(3), 277–295. https://doi.org/10.1111/cpsp.12107

Luborsky, L., & Crits-Christoph, P. (1998). *Understanding transference: The core conflictual relationship theme method*. American Psychological Association. https:// doi.org/10.1037/10250-000

Mallinckrodt, B. (2010). The psychotherapy relationship as attachment: Evidence and implications. *Journal of Personal and Social Relationships, 27*(2), 262–270. https://doi.org/10.1177/0265407509360905

Mallinckrodt, B., Choi, G., & Daly, K. D. (2015). Pilot test of a measure to assess therapeutic distance and its association with client attachment and corrective experience in therapy. *Psychotherapy Research, 25*(5), 505–517. https://doi.org/10.1080/ 10503307.2014.928755

Mallinckrodt, B., Gantt, D. L., & Coble, H. M. (1995). Attachment patterns in the psychotherapy relationship: Development of the Client Attachment to Therapist Scale. *Journal of Counseling Psychology, 42*(3), 307–317. https://doi.org/10.1037/0022-0167.42.3.307

Mallinckrodt, B., & Jeong, J. (2015). Meta-analysis of client attachment to therapist: Associations with working alliance and client pretherapy attachment. *Psychotherapy, 52*(1), 134–139. https://doi.org/10.1037/a0036890

McCluskey, U. (2005). *To be met as a person: The dynamics of attachment in professional encounters.* Karnac.

Mikulincer, M., & Shaver, P. R. (2007). *Attachment in adulthood: Structure, dynamics, and change.* Guilford Press.

Mikulincer, M., & Shaver, P. R. (2019). Attachment orientations and emotion regulation. *Current Opinion in Psychology, 25*(1), 6–10. https://doi.org/10.1016/j.copsyc.2018.02.006

Mikulincer, M., Shaver, P. R., & Berant, E. (2013). An attachment perspective on therapeutic processes and outcomes. *Journal of Personality, 81*(6), 606–616. https://doi.org/10.1111/j.1467-6494.2012.00806.x

Miller-Bottome, M., Talia, A., Eubanks, C., Safran, J. D., & Muran, J. C. (2019). Secure in-session attachment predicts rupture resolution: Negotiating a secure base. *Psychoanalytic Psychology, 36*(2), 132–138. https://doi.org/10.1037/pap0000232

Miller-Bottome, M., Talia, A., Safran, J. D., & Muran, J. C. (2018). Resolving alliance ruptures from an attachment-informed perspective. *Psychoanalytic Psychology, 35*(2), 175–183. https://doi.org/10.1037/pap0000152

Muran, J. C. (2019). Confessions of a New York rupture researcher: An insider's guide and critique. *Psychotherapy Research, 29*(1), 1–14. https://doi.org/10.1080/10503307.2017.1413261

Murray, L., & Trevarthen, C. (1986). The infant's role in mother–infant communications. *Journal of Child Language, 13*(1), 15–29. https://doi.org/10.1017/S0305000900000271

Nagy, E. (2008). Innate intersubjectivity: Newborns' sensitivity to communication disturbance. *Developmental Psychology, 44*(6), 1779–1784. https://doi.org/10.1037/a0012665

O'Brien, K. M., Afzal, K., & Tronick, E. (2013). Relational psychophysiology and mutual regulation during dyadic therapeutic and developmental relating. In J. H. D. Cornelius-White, R. Motschnig-Pitrik, & M. Lux (Eds.), *Interdisciplinary handbook of the person-centered approach* (pp. 183–197). Springer. https://doi.org/10.1007/978-1-4614-7141-7_13

Reis, H. T. (2013). Relationship well-being: The central role of perceived partner responsiveness. In C. Hazan & M. I. Campa (Eds.), *Human bonding: The science of affectional ties* (pp. 283–307). Guilford Press.

Safran, J. D., & Muran, J. C. (2000). *Negotiating the therapeutic alliance: A relational treatment guide.* Guilford Press.

Schattner, E., & Tishby, O. (2018). Patient and therapist relational patterns: Implicit negotiations. In O. Tishby & H. Wiseman (Eds.), *Developing the therapeutic relationship: Integrating case studies, research, and practice* (pp. 61–80). American Psychological Association. https://doi.org/10.1037/0000093-004

Schröder, T., Wiseman, H., & Orlinsky, D. (2009). "You were always on my mind": Therapists' intersession experiences in relation to their therapeutic practice, professional characteristics, and quality of life. *Psychotherapy Research, 19*(1), 42–53. https://doi.org/10.1080/10503300802326053

Slade, A. (2016). Attachment and adult psychotherapy: Theory, research, and practice. In J. Cassidy & P. R. Shaver (Eds.), *Handbook of attachment: Theory, research, and clinical applications* (3rd ed., pp. 759–779). Guilford Press.

Stiles, W. B., Honos-Webb, L., & Surko, M. (1998). Responsiveness in psychotherapy. *Clinical Psychology: Science and Practice, 5*(4), 439–458. https://doi.org/10.1111/j.1468-2850.1998.tb00166.x

Stiles, W. B., & Horvath, A. O. (2017). Appropriate responsiveness as a contribution to therapist effects. In L. G. Castonguay & C. E. Hill (Eds.), *How and why are some therapists better than others? Understanding therapist effects* (pp. 71–84). American Psychological Association. https://doi.org/10.1037/0000034-005

Strauss, B. M., & Petrowski, K. (2017). The role of the therapist's attachment in the process and outcome of psychotherapy. In L. G. Castonguay & C. E. Hill (Eds.), *How and why are some therapists better than others? Understanding therapist effects* (pp. 117–138). American Psychological Association. https://doi.org/10.1037/0000034-008

Talia, A., Daniel, S. I. F., Miller-Bottome, M., Brambilla, D., Miccoli, D., Safran, J. D., & Lingiardi, V. (2014). AAI predicts patients' in-session interpersonal behavior and discourse: A "move to the level of the relation" for attachment-informed psychotherapy research. *Attachment & Human Development, 16*(2), 192–209. https://doi.org/10.1080/14616734.2013.859161

Talia, A., Miller-Bottome, M., & Daniel, S. I. F. (2017). Assessing attachment in psychotherapy: Validation of the Patient Attachment Coding System (PACS). *Clinical Psychology & Psychotherapy, 24*(1), 149–161. https://doi.org/10.1002/cpp.1990

Talia, A., Miller-Bottome, M., Katznelson, H., Pedersen, S. H., Steele, H., Schröder, P., Origlieri, A., Scharff, F. B., Giovanardi, G., Andersson, M., Lingiardi, V., Safran, J. D., Lunn, S., Poulsen, S., & Taubner, S. (2019). Mentalizing in the presence of another: Measuring reflective functioning and attachment in the therapy process. *Psychotherapy Research, 29*(5), 652–665. https://doi.org/10.1080/10503307.2017.1417651

Talia, A., Miller-Bottome, M., Wyner, R., Lilliengren, P., & Bate, J. (2019). Patients' Adult Attachment Interview classification and their experience of the therapeutic relationship: Are they associated? *Research in Psychotherapy, 22*(2), 175–188. https://doi.org/10.4081/ripppo.2019.361

Talia, A., Muzi, L., Lingiardi, V., & Taubner, S. (2020). How to be a secure base: Therapists' attachment representations and their link to attunement in psychotherapy. *Attachment & Human Development, 22*(2), 189–206. https://doi.org/10.1080/14616734.2018.1534247

Tronick, E. Z. (1989). Emotions and emotional communication in infants. *American Psychologist, 44*(2), 112–119. https://doi.org/10.1037/0003-066X.44.2.112

Tronick, E. Z. (2007). *The neurobehavioral and social–emotional development of infants and children.* Norton.

Tronick, E., Als, H., Adamson, L., Wise, S., & Brazelton, T. B. (1978). The infant's response to entrapment between contradictory messages in face-to-face interaction. *Journal of the American Academy of Child Psychiatry, 17*(1), 1–13. https://doi.org/10.1016/S0002-7138(09)62273-1

Tronick, E. Z., Bruschweiler-Stern, N., Harrison, A. M., Lyons-Ruth, K., Morgan, A. C., Nahum, J. P., Sander, L., & Stern, D. N. (1998). Dyadically expanded states of consciousness and the process of therapeutic change. *Infant Mental Health Journal, 19*(3), 290–299. https://doi.org/10.1002/(SICI)1097-0355(199823)19:3<290::AID-IMHJ4>3.0.CO;2-Q

Watson, J. C. (2018). Empathy and responsiveness in emotion-focused therapy. In O. Tishby & H. Wiseman (Eds.), *Developing the therapeutic relationship: Integrating case studies, research, and practice* (pp. 235–255). American Psychological Association. https://doi.org/10.1037/0000093-011

Watson, J. C., Steckley, P. L., & McMullen, E. J. (2014). The role of empathy in promoting change. *Psychotherapy Research, 24*(3), 286–298. https://doi.org/10.1080/10503307.2013.802823

Wiseman, H. (2017). The quest for connection in interpersonal and therapeutic relationships. *Psychotherapy Research, 27*(4), 469–487. https://doi.org/10.1080/10503307.2015.1119327

Wiseman, H., & Atzil-Slonim, D. (2018). Closeness and distance dynamics in the therapeutic relationship. In O. Tishby & H. Wiseman (Eds.), *Developing the therapeutic relationship: Integrating case studies, research, and practice* (pp. 81–103). American Psychological Association. https://doi.org/10.1037/0000093-005

Wiseman, H., & Tishby, O. (2014). Client attachment, attachment to the therapist and client–therapist attachment match: How do they relate to change in psychodynamic psychotherapy? *Psychotherapy Research, 24*(3), 392–406. https://doi.org/10.1080/10503307.2014.892646

Wiseman, H., & Tishby, O. (2017). Applying relationship anecdotes paradigm interviews to study client–therapist relationship narratives: Core conflictual relationship theme analyses. *Psychotherapy Research, 27*(3), 283–299. https://doi.org/10.1080/10503307.2016.1271958

Zeifman, D. M. (2013). Built to bond: Coevolution, coregulation, and plasticity in parent–infant bonds. In C. Hazan & M. I. Campa (Eds.), *Human bonding: The science of affectional ties* (pp. 41–73). Guilford Press.

4

RESPONSIVENESS TO RUPTURES AND REPAIRS IN PSYCHOTHERAPY

CATHERINE F. EUBANKS, JOEY SERGI, AND
J. CHRISTOPHER MURAN

The *alliance*, often defined as a purposeful collaboration on the tasks and goals of therapy and the presence of an affective bond between patient and therapist (Bordin, 1979; Safran & Muran, 2000), has received extensive empirical support as a predictor of positive outcomes and a key variable in understanding the therapeutic change process (Flückiger et al., 2018). As interest in the alliance has increased, researchers have turned their attention to the inextricable role of therapist responsiveness in the alliance-building process (Stiles & Horvath, 2017). *Therapeutic responsiveness* refers to the mutual influence patient and therapist have on each other throughout treatment, an ongoing ebb and flow of behaviors that are influenced by the emerging context of the therapy relationship (Stiles et al., 1998). The alliance can be understood as coconstructed by both participants in the therapeutic dyad (Safran & Muran, 2000), and due to the mutuality inherent in the construct, responsiveness within the alliance framework should also be examined through a two-person perspective. Stiles and colleagues (Stiles et al., 1998; see also Chapter 1, this volume) coined the term *appropriate responsiveness* to refer to moments in which therapists become aware of a shifting therapeutic

https://doi.org/10.1037/0000240-005
The Responsive Psychotherapist: Attuning to Clients in the Moment, J. C. Watson and H. Wiseman (Editors)

context and adjust their behavior in response to their patient's need. Appropriate responsiveness is beneficial to a treatment at any stage; however, when a rupture occurs in the alliance, it becomes a crucial element for success. In fact, the process of successfully repairing a rupture not only explicitly values responsiveness, it also requires it.

UNDERSTANDING RUPTURES AND REPAIRS

Drawing on Bordin's (1979) conceptualization of the alliance, a *rupture* in the working alliance between the patient and therapist can be characterized as a disagreement on the goals of therapy, a lack of collaboration on therapy tasks, or a strain in the therapeutic dyad's affective bond (Eubanks, Muran, & Safran, 2019). Ruptures can be described in terms of two subtypes: *confrontation* ruptures, in which there is movement *against* the other or the work of therapy, and *withdrawal* ruptures, in which there is movement *away* from the other or the work of therapy (Eubanks, Muran, & Safran, 2019). Repairing a rupture requires responsiveness: Therapists must be attuned and responsive to their patients in order to identify when a rupture has occurred and to determine the best pathway to repair it based on the unique factors of the therapeutic dyad in that moment. Responsiveness to moment-by-moment shifts in the alliance is essential because while the term *rupture* often calls to mind a dramatic breakdown, in practice ruptures are often subtle misattunements that can have a cumulative effect on both the alliance and the therapy outcome.

Responsiveness in Rupture Research

Although a relatively nascent area of research (Muran, 2019), a growing number of studies have found a relationship between rupture repair and positive treatment outcomes, including symptom improvement and less premature dropout (Eubanks, Muran, & Safran, 2019). It is worth noting that elements of responsiveness are intrinsic to the rupture research literature. The majority of studies on alliance rupture and repair have relied on naturalistic observation of these phenomena in psychotherapy via the use of patient and therapist self-reports—either direct self-reports of ruptures and repairs or indirect methods of inferring the presence of ruptures and repairs from fluctuations in patient and therapist alliance ratings (Eubanks, Muran, & Safran, 2019; Eubanks-Carter et al., 2010). Patients and therapists need to possess some degree of attunement to the therapy relationship in order to observe and report that a rupture in the alliance is taking place.

Therapist recognition of ruptures is particularly important because it positions therapists to be optimally responsive in these key clinical moments. A number of studies have found evidence suggesting that therapist recognition of a rupture is related to subsequent improvements in alliance or outcome (e.g., Atzil-Slonim et al., 2015; Chen et al., 2018; Rubel et al., 2018; Zilcha-Mano et al., 2017, 2019). However, evidence indicates that many therapists may struggle with the crucial step of rupture recognition. Research examining different perspectives (patient, therapist, and observer) on the alliance and ruptures suggests that, although therapists generally report more ruptures than patients (Eubanks, Muran, & Safran, 2019), therapists may still miss some ruptures. For example, a study comparing an observer-based method (the Rupture Resolution Rating System, or 3RS) to self-report found that observer ratings of confrontation ruptures predicted patient dropout, while patient and therapist self-report of ruptures did not (Eubanks, Lubitz, et al., 2019). Evidence from qualitative studies points to the difficulties therapists can have identifying ruptures: Therapists can be unaware of their patients' dissatisfaction (Regan & Hill, 1992), and this lack of awareness is associated with clients quitting therapy (Rhodes et al., 1994). Withdrawal ruptures, which are subtler and perhaps less emotionally charged, may be particularly difficult for therapists to recognize (Eubanks et al., 2018).

Rupture Identification: Interpersonal and Intrapersonal Rupture Markers

One way therapists can identify that a rupture is taking place is by closely observing interpersonal rupture markers. Rupture markers can act as contingencies (Stiles & Horvath, 2017) within the responsiveness framework: "moments or markers that indicate when certain interventions are more likely to be appropriate" (p. 73). Much of the rupture literature has described rupture markers in terms of patient behaviors (Eubanks, Lubitz, et al., 2019; Eubanks, Muran, & Safran, 2019; Safran & Muran, 2000), but therapists can also observe rupture markers in their own behaviors in session (Eubanks, 2019; Muran & Eubanks, 2020). The most frequently used observer-based measure of ruptures is the Rupture Resolution Rating System (3RS; Eubanks et al., 2015; see also Muran & Eubanks, 2020). In the following example,[1] we draw on the rupture markers in the 3RS to illustrate interpersonal behaviors that can indicate the presence of a confrontation rupture.

---

[1] The identities of the clients in this chapter's case examples have been disguised to protect client confidentiality.

PATIENT: I'm not making any progress. You aren't helping me.

The patient expresses the confrontation markers of "complaints about progress in therapy" and "complaints about the therapist."

THERAPIST: Therapy takes two people. You haven't been doing your part. You never do the homework I assign.

The therapist responds to the patient's complaints by criticizing the patient.

In the next example, the patient and therapist move away from each other via a series of withdrawal rupture markers.

PATIENT: (*smiling*) It's been so hard since my husband passed away. It's hard to be alone.

The patient's affect is incongruent with the content of her speech—a "content/affect split" withdrawal marker.

THERAPIST: Yes, loneliness can be very difficult.

The therapist starts to move away from the patient's experience by speaking in abstract terms—a withdrawal marker of "abstract communication."

PATIENT: I heard someone refer to it as an epidemic of loneliness. It might be linked to changing demographics and the rise of social media.

The patient joins the therapist in "abstract communication" that also serves to "shift the topic" away from the patient's experience.

THERAPIST: Yes, I just read an interesting article about that. I can send it to you.

The therapist continues with "abstract communication" that further "shifts the topic" away from the patient.

PATIENT: (*with a soft sigh and a tight smile*) Yes, that would be very helpful.

The patient avoids voicing her growing sense that the therapist is not really helping her by being overly "deferential and appeasing," another withdrawal marker.

In addition to closely observing the interpersonal field, therapists should also attend to their internal experience, as their feelings provide clues about what is occurring in the therapeutic relationship (Muran & Eubanks, 2020; Safran & Muran, 2000). The therapist's experience of feeling tense, irritated, or bored may be the first indication that something is amiss in the alliance and can provide a window into the patient's experience. Furthermore, if therapists are unable to fully access their experience, it is more likely that their actions will be motivated by unconscious or dissociated feelings, rendering it difficult to be appropriately responsive to the patient.

Therapist Attitudes for Working With Ruptures

For therapists to address ruptures responsively and effectively, they need to approach rupture resolution with certain attitudes (Muran & Eubanks, 2020). Ruptures are dyadic phenomena, and therapists must be willing to take responsibility for their contribution to difficulties in the alliance. Working with ruptures can evoke feelings in the therapist that are difficult to tolerate; experiences such as confusion, incompetence, guilt, and irritation are not uncommon. It is important for clinicians to develop their abilities to recognize, tolerate, and explore any negative feelings that arise within themselves to ensure that they can do the same for their patients; the hope is that therapists will respond to ruptures in a manner that facilitates emotion coregulation for both patient and therapist (Muran & Eubanks, 2020).

The humility that stems from accepting the dyadic nature of ruptures is important for guarding against the cognitive biases that can impair our ability to accurately gauge the quality of the alliance (e.g., Garb & Boyle, 2015). For example, confirmation bias could lead therapists to attend to information that fits their expectations and disregard information that does not; this could prevent therapists from recognizing that an agreeable patient is employing deference as a form of withdrawal, or that a challenging patient is starting to show signs of vulnerability. Therapists must be able to recognize and track subtle movements to be appropriately responsive to them.

Responsive therapists also need to cultivate compassion. If we address ruptures from a place of anger or frustration, the patient is likely to feel criticized. In addition to maintaining compassion toward the patient, responsive therapists need to be compassionate toward themselves. Shame and self-criticism can become overwhelming and all-consuming; self-compassion enables therapists to acknowledge their mistakes while remaining attuned to the patient.

Responsive therapists should court curiosity. Ruptures can be stressful, and research on cognition and decision making has found that our thinking tends to become more rigid and narrow when we are under stress (Muran & Eubanks, 2020). We can counteract this tendency by developing a deep curiosity about our patients, our own experience, and how they shift from moment to moment.

Responsive therapists can also practice patience. Patience is needed to enter into and explore a difficult moment of rupture, rather than rushing to avoid it or to fix it. The research findings on rupture repair can be a useful point of reference; if rupture repair is associated with good outcome (Eubanks, Muran, & Safran, 2019), then we can view ruptures as opportunities for progress rather than as obstacles or setbacks.

RESPONSIVE RUPTURE RESOLUTION

As Stiles and Horvath (2017) pointed out, a strong alliance is not a "technique"; rather, it is an accomplishment that stems from acting and responding appropriately over a period of time. Implicit in the therapist attitudes described previously is a willingness to engage in a continuous back-and-forth process in which therapists are alternating their attention between their inner experience and the patient's inner experience. Ultimately, identifying the best path toward resolving a rupture will require the therapist to consider the unique factors of the dyad at the moment the rupture occurs. While no step-by-step guide to rupture resolution exists (nor should it), responsive intervention selection can be enhanced and informed by considering the meaning underlying a rupture as well as the contextual factors in which the rupture occurs.

Intersecting Relational Needs

It can be helpful to center the meaning of a rupture within a working conceptualization of interpersonal processes for the patient you are working with. The process of repairing ruptures can provide a corrective experience for the patient by meeting the patient's needs for recognition or validation and challenging the patient's expectations that others will be hostile or neglectful (Christian et al., 2012). In determining which resolution strategy to use, the therapist should consider the patient's relational needs and the kind of relationship that would be corrective for the patient. This is part of the reason it is unlikely that a specific type of rupture would call for a specific type of resolution response, as every rupture must be understood within a relational context that is particular to that patient and that therapist in that moment.

Therapists can draw on their knowledge of the patient's diagnosis, background, and presenting problems to help them identify how they could best meet their patient's relational needs. The therapist can also gain some understanding based on the types of ruptures that emerge in the work. Confrontation and withdrawal markers can be understood as stemming from the tension that arises as patients and therapists navigate opposing needs for agency and relatedness within the therapeutic dyad (Safran & Muran, 2000). Through a series of task-analytic studies, Safran and Muran (e.g., Safran & Muran, 1996) developed a stage-process model that can be helpful in identifying the common fears and needs underlying rupture markers.

When patients exhibit a confrontation marker, they are prioritizing their need for agency over their need for relatedness; they are moving against the other to protect themselves and maintain control. According to Safran and Muran's model, the goal with a confrontation rupture is to help the patient contact their underlying vulnerability. The best way to achieve this aim will depend on the kind of corrective experience that is responsive to the patient's relational needs. If the patient is accustomed to others responding to their hostility with counterhostility, the therapist can foster a corrective experience by validating the patient's concerns and nondefensively acknowledging the therapist's contribution to the rupture. If the patient expects the aggression to drive others away, the therapist can facilitate a corrective experience by actively engaging the patient, setting reasonable limits, and demonstrating that the therapist will not give up on the patient.

Many therapists find it difficult to be on the receiving end of aggression, particularly for a prolonged period of time. It is critical that therapists remain aware of and curious about their internal experience and be willing to acknowledge their own contributions to the interaction as it unfolds. Staying in touch with the vulnerability at the heart of most confrontations can help therapists maintain a compassionate stance. If the therapist is struggling with a response, it can be useful to articulate this struggle; this helps the therapist feel less trapped and freer to maneuver, and it also models reflective emotion regulation for the patient. For example, a therapist might respond to a patient displaying an aggressive confrontation marker by saying, "I'm a little hesitant to respond right now because I don't want to escalate what is happening between us."

Patient withdrawal markers represent a patient striving for relatedness at the cost of agency (Safran & Muran, 2000); because the patient anticipates a negative response from others, the patient concludes that the best way to protect the self and the relationship is to avoid directly expressing their needs. A goal of attending to withdrawal markers is to assist the patient in identifying and expressing the underlying need, and to validate their self-assertion. If a patient who tells avoidant stories or uses abstract, intellectualized language is accustomed to being politely ignored, the therapist might foster a corrective experience by actively engaging and interrupting them with questions that show that the therapist is paying close attention to the patient's communication. If a patient is used to being controlled by others, the therapist might be more cautious about redirecting or cutting off the patient's longwinded narratives.

Being responsive to withdrawal markers can be challenging because they are subtle; therapists may overlook or unwittingly collude with them. For example, a therapist may find themselves laughing as a patient tells a humorous story about a distressing family dynamic. The therapist, noting the content/affect split, might then say, "I see we're both laughing because you're telling this story in a funny way, but I wonder if there is another feeling we're not talking about."

We have presented confrontation markers and withdrawal markers as distinct for ease of explanation, but in reality ruptures often include mixtures of both confrontation and withdrawal, and therapists' efforts to address one rupture can lead to additional ruptures (Safran & Muran, 2000). Therapists need to be able to move nimbly and flexibly with the patient and the process in order to be responsive to what is happening right now.

In thinking about how rupture repair can provide a corrective experience for patients, it is important to note that it is not just the patient's relational needs and fears that are relevant; the therapist's response to the patient is also informed by the therapist's relational patterns, which may complement or clash with the patient's needs in that moment (Eubanks, 2019). For example, in a systematic case study that compared good and poor alliance cases seen by the same therapist (Schattner et al., 2017), the therapist's needs for intimacy and closeness met the patient's needs for recognition and support in the case with a good alliance. In the poor alliance case, however, the patient perceived that same therapist's pursuit of closeness as intrusive. To add to the complexity, the intersecting relational needs of the patient and the therapist are constantly shifting. We have described this complexity in terms of "intersubjective negotiation" (Muran & Eubanks, 2020; see also Pizer, 1998) to highlight the continuous process of how patients' and therapists' needs and desires are negotiated in relation to each other. Therapists have their own underlying needs for self-definition (e.g., "I need you to respect my competence by following my intervention") and relatedness (e.g., "I care about you and want to feel close to you"), and tensions inevitably arise as therapists' needs and desires intersect with those of patients.

Context-Dependent Rupture Resolution Strategies

Rupture resolution strategies can be described in terms of immediate and exploratory strategies. Immediate strategies focus on repairing a rupture quickly to return to the therapeutic work that was underway prior to the rupture. In contrast, exploratory strategies shift the focus of the session to exploring the rupture and the needs or concerns that underlie it.

Immediate Resolution Strategies

Immediate resolution strategies can be direct or indirect. A *direct* strategy involves an explicit acknowledgment that a rupture is occurring, whereas with an *indirect* strategy the rupture is resolved without being explicitly acknowledged. At this point, the rupture research literature has not demonstrated that one approach—direct immediate, indirect immediate, or exploratory—is more effective than the others, as the most effective option likely depends on what is most responsive to that particular therapeutic dyad in that specific moment. The task analyses conducted by Safran and Muran (e.g., 1996), as well as task analyses of rupture repair in interpersonal-psychodynamic therapy with depressed patients (Agnew et al., 1994), cognitive analytic therapy with patients with borderline personality disorder (Bennett et al., 2006; Daly et al., 2010); and emotion-focused therapy with couples (Swank & Wittenborn, 2013) all featured explicit acknowledgment and collaborative exploration of the rupture as the initial steps in the resolution process. However, task analyses of cognitive behavior therapy (CBT) for depression (Aspland et al., 2008) and CBT for borderline personality disorder (Cash et al., 2014) concluded that direct acknowledgment of the rupture was not necessary. In these models, therapists resolved ruptures via an indirect, immediate strategy of responsively changing the therapy task—for example, letting go of the next item on the therapist's agenda to explore the issue that was most salient for the client at that moment.

Exploratory Resolution Strategies

An exploratory approach to rupture resolution involves directly exploring the patient's and the therapist's experience of the rupture with a goal of increasing awareness of what is transpiring between them. As this kind of exploration can be challenging, the patient—and the therapist—may be tempted to move away from the exploration. When a therapist attempts to explore a confrontation rupture, patients are likely to move away either from their expressed aggression or from the vulnerability underlying it. Each form of avoidance results in shifts between self-states; often a patient shifts into a state of anxiety or guilt about an expression of aggression, and then back into an aggressive state when the anxiety and guilt become intolerable. Similarly, patients may come into contact with the vulnerability underlying the confrontation and may shift back into a more familiar aggressive stance (Safran & Muran, 2000). Exploration of a withdrawal rupture may lead to a similar pattern as patients start to express their needs, but then become anxious about how the therapist will respond and return to familiar avoidant behaviors. To successfully navigate these moments, therapists must remain attuned to these shifts and bring the patient's attention to them. If therapists are either distracted by or unaware of their own emotional responses to the patient's aggression or avoidance, it will be difficult to track these shifts. To aid the regulation of their own emotional responses, therapists can invite an exploration of the patient's concerns around the impact of their statements on the therapist or invite collaborative curiosity about the therapist's own withdrawal behaviors.

Resolution Choice Points

When deciding which resolution strategy would be most responsive, therapists also need to consider the goals of treatment, the costs and benefits of pausing the current therapy task to attend to a rupture, and the strength and quality of the bond. Take, for example, the following situation:

THERAPIST: I'd like for you to try writing down the negative thoughts you have throughout the day.

PATIENT: (*nervously laughs*) Um, are you sure this is going to be helpful? It seems a little silly.

This example includes elements of confrontation (a complaint about a therapy task) as well as withdrawal (nervous laughter and hesitation about directly expressing the complaint). A direct, immediate resolution strategy could involve the therapist validating the patient's defensiveness and providing a rationale for the therapy task. Such an approach could be helpful if the therapist believes that engaging the patient with this task will serve the goals of therapy and is responsive to the current strength of the bond and the patient's relational needs. A patient who has had difficulty trusting others might appreciate a transparent, direct approach. Also, on reflection, the therapist might realize that they initially failed to adequately explain the therapy task and that providing a rationale is an appropriate response to the therapist's contribution to the rupture.

However, if the therapist is concerned that at this point in therapy, a direct approach might antagonize the patient or engender too much anxiety and distract from a therapy goal that the therapist believes is important to prioritize right now, the therapist can instead use an indirect immediate strategy, such as responsively shifting the task to something more in line with the patient's comfort level. In this way, there is no discussion or negotiation of the rupture event, but the rupture is resolved in that the patient and therapist are able to resume working collaboratively. For an aggressive patient and an anxious therapist, such a response could constitute an unhelpful capitulation, but for a patient who is accustomed to not being heard or respected, a thoughtful accommodation by the therapist could provide a helpful corrective experience.

Alternatively, the therapist could choose an exploratory approach of discussing the patient's concerns around recording negative thoughts. Particularly given the mixed expression of confrontation and withdrawal, the exploration could take different directions depending on which elements become most salient in the moment. Exploration of the rupture might bring up anxiety about being vulnerable in front of others and lead the therapist to encourage the patient to contact their fears and desires around being seen and understood. Or the exploration might lead the therapist to encourage the patient to more directly assert their concerns about the task and the ways in which it is not meeting the patient's needs in this moment, and this could spur the therapist to validate and empower the patient in their self-assertion. The takeaway message here is that there is not one correct pathway for responsive rupture resolution. An awareness of the needs underlying a rupture should be balanced with the contextual factors of the moment in which it emerges.

Metacommunication

Metacommunication, or communicating about the communication process, is a key strategy underlying all direct rupture resolution. Metacommunication can be an important tool for a responsive therapist as it invites both parties to step back and examine the patient's experience, the therapist's experience, and the interpersonal field. Therapists should keep the focus on the here and now and invite collaborative exploration through direct questions such as "What's going on here between us?" or observations such as "It seemed like your mood shifted, am I reading you right?" A therapist could also initiate a dialogue by disclosing their internal experience.

The practice of metacommunication encourages many elements of responsiveness. Metacommunication has been referred to as "mindfulness in interaction" for its goal of bringing awareness to a dynamic interaction as it unfolds (Muran & Eubanks, 2020; Safran & Muran, 2000). Through metacommunication, the intersecting needs of the patient and the therapist can be brought into relief. As patients and therapists metacommunicate, they put words to feelings, which also promotes emotion regulation. Awareness is the priority initially, not change. Focusing on the concrete, specific details of a therapeutic interaction in the here and now, with respect for the uniqueness of each encounter, will help the patient—and the therapist—develop greater experiential awareness. This awareness helps patients become better observers of their own behavior, which fosters positive change. Responsive therapists will also monitor their own experience and be open to acknowledging their contributions to the dynamic.

Metacommunication, although important, is just the first step of an exploratory rupture repair process (Muran et al., 2010). It is important for therapists to recognize that in their attempts to metacommunicate, it is common to create more ruptures. In the following example, a therapist initiates rupture resolution by metacommunicating. In the process, however, he creates another rupture by focusing on metacommunicating about the relationship while missing the patient's concerns about not being in agreement on tasks and goals of therapy.

PATIENT: It just feels a little . . . I don't know, unclear what we are working on here.

THERAPIST: Hmm, you're feeling unsure what we're doing? Can you say more about that?

PATIENT: (*sighs*) I . . . I don't know.

THERAPIST: You just sighed there; it seems like that was a shift. Am I picking up on that right?

PATIENT: I feel like I said it already.

THERAPIST: You feel like you already told me why you sighed?

PATIENT: No . . . (*uncovers face in frustration*). Just that I already told you how I'm feeling, and you're not getting it.

THERAPIST: So something I am saying is making you feel misunderstood?

PATIENT: I'm not sure, just . . . forget it.

THERAPIST: Well, I think this is important that we talk about this.

PATIENT: (*laughs*) What exactly do you want to talk about?

THERAPIST: This feeling of being misunderstood.

PATIENT: This just . . . feels a little, um, silly. I think you might be trying to address my point, and this is what you think is important to focus on. I'm not sure.

THERAPIST: So when I try to stay focused on your feeling of being misunderstood, what comes up for you?

PATIENT: Just that I'm frustrated, and it feels like we're wasting our session time talking about something that isn't important to me.

THERAPIST: I can see how that would be frustrating. I wonder if . . . something feels especially difficult about discussing our relationship?

PATIENT: No, no, no (*lets out a frustrated chuckle*). I just feel in a bind here . . . this really feels like a waste of time, but you think it's important so, I guess I need to go along.

THERAPIST: Hmm, so discussing what might be happening between us feels like a waste of time?

In this scenario, the therapist relies heavily on metacommunication techniques but is not fully attuned to the process and fails to recognize that the dyad has become embedded in another rupture. Ironically, the therapist re-creates the patient's initial complaint about a lack of agreement on therapy goals and tasks by rigidly adhering to one resolution strategy instead of being responsive to the patient's unfolding experience. The therapist's misattunement leads both members of the dyad to become locked in a cycle; the impact of the therapist's rigidity points to the importance of ongoing responsivity and flexibility within rupture repair.

DIVERSITY CONSIDERATIONS

The ability to be responsive within the rupture-repair process can be especially important when working with clients from diverse backgrounds. Attention to the establishment and maintenance of a positive alliance has been shown to be especially important when working with disempowered populations (Davis et al., 2015). Although it has not been systematically examined, it has been suggested in the rupture literature that ethnocultural and demographic differences between patients and therapists such as gender, race, ethnicity, religion, socioeconomic class, and sexual orientation can contribute to more frequent alliance ruptures (Eubanks, Muran, & Safran, 2019; Muran, 2007). This is indirectly supported by research suggesting that minority clients regularly report weaker alliances than their nonminority counterparts (Koo et al., 2016; Walling et al., 2012).

A cultural rupture can be difficult to define, and one can argue that all ruptures are linked to the differences in power, identity, and experience that lie between the patient and therapist and impact their respective needs for and pursuits of self-definition and relatedness (Muran, 2007; Muran & Eubanks, 2020). We are defining a *cultural rupture* as a strain or incongruence between patient and therapist that stems from a cultural misunderstanding or slight. While the majority of research in this area has focused on therapist-initiated ruptures toward a cultural minority client (e.g., Hook et al., 2017), patient biases can also contribute to a rupture with a therapist from a different cultural background.

Shelton and Delgado-Romero (2011) referred to microaggressions, "communications of prejudice and discrimination expressed through seemingly meaningless and unharmful tactics . . . [that] deliver a hidden denigrating, hostile, or negative message about a person or a group" (p. 10), as a form of cultural rupture. In our experience, microinvalidations, or communications that subtly exclude or nullify the feelings, thoughts, or experiences of a person (Sue & Sue, 2008), are the most commonly committed microaggressions in therapy. An example of a microinvalidation is when a therapist politely asks a gay man if he has a girlfriend or a wife, or when a client asks their gay male therapist the same question.

Beyond being difficult to define, cultural ruptures may also be more difficult to detect. Thus, therapists working with clients from different cultural backgrounds should be especially attuned to the possibility of a cultural misunderstanding leading to a rupture and be aware that cultural ruptures may look and function differently from other types of ruptures. In a study of lesbian, gay, and bisexual individuals who have experienced microaggressions, researchers found that behavioral responses tended to cluster in three categories: passive coping, confrontational coping, and protective coping (Nadal et al., 2011). Both passive and protective coping involved avoidant behaviors, such as changing the topic or not responding, that might align with withdrawal rupture markers. Similarly, confrontational coping behaviors, such as becoming defensive, may align with confrontation rupture markers. Although the study did not directly examine microaggressions within the context of the therapeutic relationship, it provided insight into how clients may respond to microaggressions coming from their therapists.

It is important to acknowledge, however, that clients may respond differently to their therapists than they do to others they encounter in their daily lives. Safran and Muran (2000) highlighted the importance of therapists being aware of the power differential in the therapist–client relationship throughout the rupture-resolution process, and this is particularly salient when therapists from a majority group are working with clients from a minority group. Many members of minority groups often respond to microaggressions in their everyday life with internal questioning and inaction (Nadal et al., 2011), or they employ a strategy of "picking and choosing one's battles" (Lewis et al., 2013) that may result in an individual choosing not to directly address a microaggression directed against them. The power differential between client and therapist may exacerbate clients' reluctance to point out or confront cultural ruptures in therapy. With these factors in mind, it is likely that minority clients more often display withdrawal rupture markers. Therapists should be prepared to proactively address their contribution to the interaction and use direct resolution strategies. When a therapist explicitly and nondefensively accepts responsibility for a cultural rupture, clients will likely feel validated that their reactions were appropriate to the situation. In addition, a respectful exploration of the cultural rupture may provide a corrective experience for clients who feel they cannot be assertive when they experience microaggressions in the outside world (Spengler et al., 2016). Given evidence suggesting that the use of proactive coping strategies in response to microaggressions is linked with lower psychological distress (Sanchez et al., 2018), facilitating patients' self-assertion in the context of cultural ruptures is important.

Therapists may struggle to distinguish between clinical, cultural, and personal issues as causes of ruptures. Gaztambide (2012) suggested that in these situations, it is important that therapists disclose their lack of knowledge and invite the patient to give feedback. This process is not only empowering for the client but also provides the therapist with valuable data to discern how the rupture is related to the client's culturally constructed ways of understanding and relating. Research on microaggressions with racial and ethnic minority clients suggests that the majority of microaggressions go undiscussed: Owen et al. (2014) found that although 53% of racial and ethnic minority clients reported experiencing a microaggression in therapy, only 24% of client and therapist dyads discussed the experience. This may stem from therapist resistance to exploring their biases and clinical errors with their clients (Spengler et al., 2016) or from the fact that cultural ruptures may be harder to detect. Therapists can educate themselves on resolution strategies and common microaggressions for the populations they are working with and be sensitive to both client markers and their own internal experiences. As Altman (2009) noted, if therapists are unable to address their discomfort with cultural difference and confront problematic unconscious interactions in themselves, they will be unable to process these interactions therapeutically as well.

Cultural ruptures can result from good intentions. In the following example, a therapist is working with a woman discussing the challenges and discrimination she felt when she worked on a U.S. military base. In this instance, it is precisely the therapist's attempts at working within an intersectional and culturally competent framework that create a rupture.

PATIENT: It was just a really hard time for me. I felt like I was at everybody's mercy and I had no respect.

THERAPIST: It sounds like it was really rough. I can't imagine what it was like for you as a Middle Eastern woman.

The therapist tries to validate the patient's difficult experience by acknowledging the ways her minority identities intersected to exacerbate the difficulties of her experience. Although this can be an affirming way to work, patients may or may not find this lens helpful depending on their own experience of intersecting identities and minority stress.

PATIENT: *(becomes flushed, raises her voice, and waves her hands in front of her to indicate a "no" motion)* No, no, no, it wasn't even about that. It really had more to do with how big of a gap there was in our educations, I had an advanced degree and these guys, they were . . . they hardly graduated high school. I don't view myself as any ethnicity, I am a global citizen. Anyway, it probably wasn't such a big deal . . .

The patient displays a mix of confrontation and withdrawal markers. Initially, the patient rejects the therapist's interpretation of the event (confrontation). She then quickly moves into withdrawal by denying the importance of an event likely relevant to the therapy and attempting to shift the topic. Her suggestion that this "wasn't such a big deal" functions as an effort to preserve the relationship with the therapist.

THERAPIST: I feel like I might have insulted you just there . . .

The therapist uses the resolution technique of acknowledging her contribution to the rupture. In this moment, the therapist's internal cues of anxiety have signaled that something is amiss. The therapist tolerates the discomfort of addressing the rupture by focusing on the potential value of providing a corrective experience by exploring what is transpiring between them.

PATIENT: *(tone has returned to normal, and patient is speaking in a measured way)* Well, I just don't view my being Middle Eastern as having anything to do with who I am as a person. I really, um, consider myself to be a global citizen and like, my degree was really focused globally so, it was just not, um, the case.

The patient may be withdrawing by engaging in denial. More important, the change in tone and the intellectualized statements suggest that the patient is withdrawing via abstract communication.

THERAPIST: I see what you mean. I think when I made that statement, I was trying to touch upon how it must have been hard to be dropped into a situation where, you know, knowing that you view yourself that way, other people were maybe, um, not so on board with it . . . and were disrespecting you because of those pieces of your identity.

The therapist begins by validating the patient's defensive response and then goes on to clarify the misunderstanding by explaining the intent of the original statement.

PATIENT: I think before I did feel insulted, but now I understand what you mean. (*Patient begins to cry.*)

THERAPIST: What did that bring up for you just then?

By inviting the patient's thoughts and feelings, the therapist facilitates metacommunication about what is transpiring between them.

PATIENT: The way they would treat me, they were just terrible to me and it was so hard to feel like it was, like, not just because I was Middle Eastern, but also because I was a woman. I was so naive and idealistic to think I was an American improving America and then to not be seen that way . . .

THERAPIST: And maybe my comment made it feel like I was seeing you the same way those men were?

PATIENT: I think at first, yeah.

RESEARCH AND TRAINING IMPLICATIONS

Responsiveness and the rupture repair process are inextricably linked; one cannot exist without the other. They are also similar in that each is notoriously difficult to measure and teach, as the "right response" can never be specified before an event occurs. While the "right response" will always vary, therapists can be trained to be more attuned to internal and external markers, to be aware of likely obstacles, and to ask themselves the questions necessary to tailor their interventions to better fit the client and the circumstances. A major benefit of the rupture repair paradigm is that it can be applied to the theoretical orientation or modality therapists are already most comfortable using, enhancing responsiveness across approaches.

There is evidence that therapists vary in their abilities to build and maintain strong alliances (Del Re et al., 2012), but there is also evidence that therapists' abilities to maintain alliances can be increased through training. One example is alliance-focused training (AFT), a supervision approach designed to enhance therapists' abilities to detect and work constructively with alliance ruptures and negative therapeutic process (Eubanks-Carter et al., 2015; Muran et al., 2010). AFT explicitly values responsiveness and has been demonstrated to improve interpersonal process for trainees, even when working with clients typically considered more difficult to treat such as those with comorbid diagnoses or personality disorders (Muran et al., 2018). Training programs hoping to enhance clinician responsiveness can adopt the principles of AFT, such as training therapists to recognize ruptures, to consider the mutuality of all interventions, to monitor what is taking place in the therapeutic relationship on an ongoing basis, and to utilize a nondefensive stance in exploring therapists' internal experiences as they navigate difficult moments in therapy.

In their discussion of the future of responsiveness research, Stiles and Horvath (2017) called for an answer to the question "What kinds of signals are they [therapists] tuned to, and how do they use this information to make the intervention better fit the client and the circumstances?" (p. 80). Continued research in the area of rupture repair, with specific attention to rupture markers (signals), specific resolution strategies (interventions), and the factors that moderate patients' responses to them, can help provide an answer to this question. Although we will never have a step-by-step guide to rupture repair that fits every patient, research such as this will go a long way toward improving appropriate responsiveness to difficult moments across approaches.

REFERENCES

Agnew, R. M., Harper, H., Shapiro, D. A., & Barkham, M. (1994). Resolving a challenge to the therapeutic relationship: A single-case study. *The British Journal of Medical Psychology, 67*(2), 155–170. https://doi.org/10.1111/j.2044-8341.1994.tb01783.x

Altman, N. (2009). *The analyst in the inner city: Race, class, and culture from a psychoanalytic lens*. Analytic Press.

Aspland, H., Llewelyn, S., Hardy, G. E., Barkham, M., & Stiles, W. (2008). Alliance ruptures and rupture resolution in cognitive-behavior therapy: A preliminary task analysis. *Psychotherapy Research, 18*(6), 699–710. https://doi.org/10.1080/10503300802291463

Atzil-Slonim, D., Bar-Kalifa, E., Rafaeli, E., Lutz, W., Rubel, J., Schiefele, A.-K., & Peri, T. (2015). Therapeutic bond judgments: Congruence and incongruence. *Journal of Consulting and Clinical Psychology, 83*(4), 773–784. https://doi.org/10.1037/ccp0000015

Bennett, D., Parry, G., & Ryle, A. (2006). Resolving threats to the therapeutic alliance in cognitive analytic therapy of borderline personality disorder: A task analysis. *Psychology and Psychotherapy: Theory, Research and Practice, 79*(3), 395–418. https://doi.org/10.1348/147608305X58355

Bordin, E. S. (1979). The generalizability of the psychoanalytic concept of the working alliance. *Psychotherapy: Theory, Research, & Practice, 16*(3), 252–260. https://doi.org/10.1037/h0085885

Cash, S. K., Hardy, G. E., Kellett, S., & Parry, G. (2014). Alliance ruptures and resolution during cognitive behaviour therapy with patients with borderline personality disorder. *Psychotherapy Research, 24*(2), 132–145. https://doi.org/10.1080/10503307.2013.838652

Chen, R., Atzil-Slonim, D., Bar-Kalifa, E., Hasson-Ohayon, I., & Refaeli, E. (2018). Therapists' recognition of alliance ruptures as a moderator of change in alliance and symptoms. *Psychotherapy Research, 28*(4), 560–570. https://doi.org/10.1080/10503307.2016.1227104

Christian, C., Safran, J. D., & Muran, J. C. (2012). The corrective emotional experience: A relational perspective and critique. In L. G. Castonguay & C. E. Hill (Eds.), *Transformation in psychotherapy: Corrective experiences across cognitive behavioral, humanistic, and psychodynamic approaches* (pp. 51–67). American Psychological Association. https://doi.org/10.1037/13747-004

Daly, A.-M., Llewelyn, S., McDougall, E., & Chanen, A. M. (2010). Rupture resolution in cognitive analytic therapy for adolescents with borderline personality disorder. *Psychology & Psychotherapy: Theory, Research & Practice, 83*(3), 273–288. https://doi.org/10.1348/147608309X481036

Davis, T. A., Ancis, J. R., & Ashby, J. S. (2015). Therapist effects, working alliance, and African American women substance users. *Cultural Diversity & Ethnic Minority Psychology, 21*(1), 126–135. https://doi.org/10.1037/a0036944

Del Re, A. C., Flückiger, C., Horvath, A. O., Symonds, D., & Wampold, B. E. (2012). Therapist effects in the therapeutic alliance-outcome relationship: A restricted-maximum likelihood meta-analysis. *Clinical Psychology Review, 32*(7), 642–649. https://doi.org/10.1016/j.cpr.2012.07.002

Eubanks, C. F. (2019). Alliance-focused formulation: A work in process. In U. Kramer (Ed.), *Case formulation for personality disorders: Tailoring psychotherapy to the individual client* (pp. 337–354). Elsevier. https://doi.org/10.1016/B978-0-12-813521-1.00017-5

Eubanks, C. F., Burckell, L. A., & Goldfried, M. R. (2018). Clinical consensus strategies to repair ruptures in the therapeutic alliance. *Journal of Psychotherapy Integration, 28*(1), 60–76. https://doi.org/10.1037/int0000097

Eubanks, C. F., Lubitz, J., Muran, J. C., & Safran, J. D. (2019). Rupture Resolution Rating System (3RS): Development and validation. *Psychotherapy Research, 29*(3), 306–319. https://doi.org/10.1080/10503307.2018.1552034

Eubanks, C. F., Muran, J. C., & Safran, J. D. (2015). *Rupture Resolution Rating System (3RS): Manual.* Unpublished manuscript, Mount Sinai-Beth Israel Medical Center, New York.

Eubanks, C. F., Muran, J. C., & Safran, J. D. (2019). Repairing alliance ruptures. In J. C. Norcross & M. J. Lambert (Eds.), *Psychotherapy relationships that work: Evidence-based therapist contributions* (3rd ed., pp. 549–579). Oxford University Press. https://doi.org/10.1093/med-psych/9780190843953.003.0016

Eubanks-Carter, C., Muran, J. C., & Safran, J. D. (2010). Alliance ruptures and resolution. In J. C. Muran & J. P. Barber (Eds.), *The therapeutic alliance: An evidence-based approach to practice and training* (pp. 74–94). Guilford Press.

Eubanks-Carter, C., Muran, J. C., & Safran, J. D. (2015). Alliance-focused training. *Psychotherapy: Theory, Research, & Practice, 52*(2), 169–173. https://doi.org/10.1037/a0037596

Flückiger, C., Del Re, A. C., Wampold, B. E., & Horvath, A. O. (2018). The alliance in adult psychotherapy: A meta-analytic synthesis. *Psychotherapy: Theory, Research, & Practice, 55*(4), 316–340. https://doi.org/10.1037/pst0000172

Garb, H. N., & Boyle, P. A. (2015). Understanding why some clinicians use pseudo-scientific methods: Findings from research on clinical judgment. In S. O. Lilienfeld, S. J. Lynn, & J. M. Lohr (Eds.), *Science and pseudoscience in clinical psychology* (pp. 19–41). Guilford Press.

Gaztambide, D. J. (2012). Addressing cultural impasses with rupture resolution strategies: A proposal and recommendations. *Professional Psychology, Research and Practice, 43*(3), 183–189. https://doi.org/10.1037/a0026911

Hook, J. N., Davis, D., Owen, J., & DeBlaere, C. (2017). *Cultural humility: Engaging diverse identities in therapy*. American Psychological Association. https://doi.org/10.1037/0000037-000

Koo, K. H., Tiet, Q. Q., & Rosen, C. S. (2016). Relationships between racial/ethnic minority status, therapeutic alliance, and treatment expectancies among veterans with PTSD. *Psychological Services, 13*(3), 317–321. https://doi.org/10.1037/ser0000029

Lewis, J. A., Mendenhall, R., Harwood, S. A., & Browne Hunt, M. (2013). Coping with gendered racial microaggressions among Black women college students. *Journal of African American Studies, 17*(1), 51–73. https://doi.org/10.1007/s12111-012-9219-0

Muran, J. C. (2007). A relational turn on thick description. In J. C. Muran (Ed.), *Dialogues on difference: Studies of diversity in the therapeutic relationship* (pp. 257–274). American Psychological Association. https://doi.org/10.1037/11500-029

Muran, J. C. (2019). Confessions of a New York rupture researcher: An insider's guide and critique. *Psychotherapy Research, 29*(1), 1–14. https://doi.org/10.1080/10503307.2017.1413261

Muran, J. C., & Eubanks, C. F. (2020). *Therapist performance under pressure: Negotiating emotion, difference, and rupture*. American Psychological Association. https://doi.org/10.1037/0000182-000

Muran, J. C., Safran, J. D., Eubanks, C. F., & Gorman, B. S. (2018). The effect of alliance-focused training on a cognitive-behavioral therapy for personality disorders. *Journal of Consulting and Clinical Psychology, 86*(4), 384–397. https://doi.org/10.1037/ccp0000284

Muran, J. C., Safran, J. D., & Eubanks-Carter, C. (2010). Developing therapist abilities to negotiate alliance ruptures. *The therapeutic alliance: An evidence-based guide to practice* (pp. 320–340). Guilford Press.

Nadal, K. L., Wong, Y., Issa, M., Meterko, V., Leon, J., & Wideman, M. (2011). Sexual orientation microaggressions: Processes and coping mechanisms for lesbian, gay, and bisexual individuals. *Journal of LGBT Issues in Counseling, 5*(1), 21–46. https://doi.org/10.1080/15538605.2011.554606

Owen, J., Tao, K. W., Imel, Z. E., Wampold, B. E., & Rodolfa, E. (2014). Addressing racial and ethnic microaggressions in therapy. *Professional Psychology, Research and Practice, 45*(4), 283–290. https://doi.org/10.1037/a0037420

Pizer, S. A. (1998). *Building bridges: The negotiation of paradox in psychoanalysis*. Analytic Press.

Regan, A. M., & Hill, C. E. (1992). Investigation of what clients and counselors do not say in brief therapy. *Journal of Counseling Psychology, 39*(2), 168–174. https://doi.org/10.1037/0022-0167.39.2.168

Rhodes, R., Hill, C., Thompson, B., & Elliott, R. (1994). Client retrospective recall of resolved and unresolved misunderstanding events. *The Counseling Psychologist, 41*(4), 473–483. https://doi.org/10.1037/0022-0167.41.4.473

Rubel, J. A., Zilcha-Mano, S., Feils-Klaus, V., & Lutz, W. (2018). Session-to-session effects of alliance ruptures in outpatient CBT: Within- and between-patient associations. *Journal of Consulting and Clinical Psychology*, *86*(4), 354–366. https://doi.org/10.1037/ccp0000286

Safran, J. D., & Muran, J. C. (1996). The resolution of ruptures in the therapeutic alliance. *Journal of Consulting and Clinical Psychology*, *64*(3), 447–458. https://doi.org/10.1037/0022-006X.64.3.447

Safran, J. D., & Muran, J. C. (2000). *Negotiating the therapeutic alliance: A relational treatment guide*. Guilford Press.

Sanchez, D., Adams, W. N., Arango, S. C., & Flannigan, A. E. (2018). Racial-ethnic microaggressions, coping strategies, and mental health in Asian American and Latinx American college students: A mediation model. *Journal of Counseling Psychology*, *65*(2), 214–225. https://doi.org/10.1037/cou0000249

Schattner, E., Tishby, O., & Wiseman, H. (2017). Relational patterns and the development of the alliance: A systematic comparison of two cases. *Clinical Psychology & Psychotherapy*, *24*(2), 555–568. https://doi.org/10.1002/cpp.2019

Shelton, K., & Delgado-Romero, E. A. (2011). Sexual orientation microaggressions: The experience of lesbian, gay, bisexual, and queer clients in psychotherapy. *Journal of Counseling Psychology*, *58*(2), 210–221. https://doi.org/10.1037/a0022251

Spengler, E. S., Miller, D. J., & Spengler, P. M. (2016). Microaggressions: Clinical errors with sexual minority clients. *Psychotherapy: Theory, Research, & Practice*, *53*(3), 360–366. https://doi.org/10.1037/pst0000073

Stiles, W. B., Honos-Webb, L., & Surko, M. (1998). Responsiveness in psychotherapy. *Clinical Psychology: Science and Practice*, *5*(4), 439–458. https://doi.org/10.1111/j.1468-2850.1998.tb00166.x

Stiles, W. B., & Horvath, A. O. (2017). Appropriate responsiveness as a contribution to therapist effects. In L. G. Castonguay & C. E. Hill (Eds.), *How and why are some therapists better than others? Understanding therapist effects* (pp. 71–84). American Psychological Association. https://doi.org/10.1037/0000034-005

Sue, D. W., & Sue, D. (2008). *Counseling the culturally diverse: Theory and practice* (5th ed.). John Wiley & Sons.

Swank, L. E., & Wittenborn, A. K. (2013). Repairing alliance ruptures in emotionally focused couple therapy: A preliminary task analysis. *American Journal of Family Therapy*, *41*(5), 389–402. https://doi.org/10.1080/01926187.2012.726595

Walling, S. M., Suvak, M. K., Howard, J. M., Taft, C. T., & Murphy, C. M. (2012). Race/ethnicity as a predictor of change in working alliance during cognitive behavioral therapy for intimate partner violence perpetrators. *Psychotherapy*, *49*(2), 180–189. https://doi.org/10.1037/a0025751

Zilcha-Mano, S., Eubanks, C. F., & Muran, J. C. (2019). Sudden gains in the alliance in cognitive behavioral therapy versus brief relational therapy. *Journal of Consulting and Clinical Psychology*, *87*(6), 501–509. https://doi.org/10.1037/ccp0000397

Zilcha-Mano, S., Snyder, J., & Silberschatz, G. (2017). The effect of congruence in patient and therapist alliance on patient's symptomatic levels. *Psychotherapy Research*, *27*(3), 371–380. https://doi.org/10.1080/10503307.2015.1126682

PART **II** RESPONSIVENESS
IN DIFFERENT
THERAPEUTIC
APPROACHES

5

RESPONSIVENESS IN PSYCHODYNAMIC RELATIONAL PSYCHOTHERAPY

ORYA TISHBY

The unique feature of psychodynamic relational theory is its focus on therapy as an intersubjective process that occurs on both conscious and unconscious levels. Therapist and client cocreate the meaning and form a unique dyadic relationship. This chapter begins with a presentation of basic concepts in the two-person paradigm, followed by a description of relational events that therapists should be attuned to, such as negotiating the alliance, resolving ruptures in the alliance, attuning to the transference–countertransference matrix, processing enactments, and attuning to dissociated self states. These processes are illustrated by clinical vignettes with commentaries. Research in this area is still quite limited, but a number of recent studies that lend support to relational processes in therapy are presented. The chapter also addresses attunement to diversity and implications for training.

RESPONSIVENESS IN A TWO-PERSON PARADIGM

Relational psychoanalysis focuses on the development of personality in the context of relationships. The relational psychoanalytic approach represents a paradigm shift from one-person psychology, which focuses on the individual

https://doi.org/10.1037/0000240-006
The Responsive Psychotherapist: Attuning to Clients in the Moment, J. C. Watson and H. Wiseman (Editors)

mind and subjective perception of the world, to a two-person psychology, which sees the individual in the context of dyadic interactions with other subjects (Aron, 1996; Curtis & Hirsch, 2011).

From the time a person is born, their mind is constantly interacting with the minds of others, who respond to the person in different ways. In these reciprocal interactions, unique interpersonal patterns develop with different caregivers in a process of mutual regulation and mutual creation (Beebe & Lachmann, 2002; Tronick, 2003). Thus, the self is seen as socially constructed: Early patterns of experience with different people are embedded in the person's mind, creating various self states that continue to develop throughout their life (Bromberg, 1998; Mitchell, 1993). Each self state consists of a relational pattern of self and other, and some self states are conscious, whereas others are less conscious. Together self states function as part of a "healthy illusion of cohesive personal identity—an overarching and experiential state felt as 'me'" (Bromberg, 1998, p. 273).

Relational thinking posits a dissociative model of the mind. In a person with healthy development, there are shifts in self states, with some in the forefront and others temporarily out of awareness. At other moments, the person can shift flexibly to another self state, depending on the context and the interaction. When certain self states are too traumatic to be experienced, they are dissociated from consciousness. If interpreted to the client, or if the client feels a certain emotion from that state, it is experienced as "not me." These dissociated self states reflect not only experiences of abuse and neglect but also experiences of prolonged misattunement to basic needs or rejection of the child's ways of responding to the world. Dissociated self states may manifest themselves in physical symptoms and dreams but also in subtler ways, such as shifts in facial expressions, affect, or body posture. One of the goals of relational therapy is to help clients become aware of these self states so as to increase flexibility and authenticity.

The two-person paradigm has several implications. First, there is no "objective truth," and meaning is coconstructed by both therapist and client. Context plays an important role in understanding clients' subjective experiences: Both the family system and the sociocultural background are important factors in shaping clients' relational patterns and the therapeutic relationship. Therapists should be sensitive to cultural differences between themselves and their clients and discuss these openly (Altman, 2006; Muran, 2007). Second, each therapeutic dyad constitutes the "interactive matrix" (Greenberg, 1995) and creates its own unique process (Tronick, 2003) in which the subjectivities of both therapist and client play a role. Third, the therapeutic relationship does not necessarily represent the client's other relationships.

However, as clients gain insight into some of their interpersonal patterns, they can benefit from reflecting on and processing the therapeutic relationship and how they impact the therapist and other people. This process facilitates the development of mutual recognition, a central concept in the relational literature.

MUTUAL RECOGNITION AND IMPLICIT RELATIONAL KNOWING

Benjamin (1990/1999) coined the term *mutual recognition*, referring to the ability of both partners in a relationship to be attuned to the subjectivity of the other. Being attuned to a significant other requires one to balance the need for recognition and empathy with holding in mind the other person's subjective needs. In moments of high emotional arousal, partners can easily fall into one of two polarities: either (a) submission of one partner to the other and putting aside one's needs to give full recognition to the partner or (b) "destruction," in which one partner dominates the other and claims full recognition at the expense of not being attuned to the other. Benjamin noted that individuals can perceive another person through the lens of need fulfillment (to have their needs recognized) or view the other as a separate subject with their own needs and wishes. In the course of human development, people learn to view the other as a separate subject, and they also learn how to present themselves as subjects in order to get recognition. In adult life, people move flexibly between these two points of view as needed. Thus, responsiveness in this model is the recognition of the client's subjectivity, as different from the therapist's subjectivity, and the recognition of the unique interpersonal pattern that is created with the therapist. Another way in which therapists can be responsive is by helping clients communicate their needs more effectively so that other people can then respond to them. In addition, therapists help clients recognize the needs of others without denying their own.

The Boston Change Process Study Group (2005; Lyons-Ruth et al., 1998) applied models from mother–infant interaction research to learn about microprocess in therapy, which they believed has been insufficiently recognized in the psychoanalytic literature. This group proposed that psychoanalysis and psychodynamic therapy are lacking in terminology to describe the moment-to-moment changes and subtle processes that are core mechanisms of change in psychotherapy. They proposed new terms that describe the relational processes and are relevant to our discussion of responsiveness. One of these terms is *implicit relational knowing*, which describes the process of how client and therapist learn "to be with one another" or "how we do things together." This procedural knowledge, which is different from unconscious representations of the therapist (transference), develops in the context of mutual recognition and coconstruction in the therapeutic process.

WHAT SHOULD RELATIONAL THERAPISTS BE ATTUNED TO? HOW SHOULD THEY MODIFY THEIR INTERVENTIONS?

Relational psychoanalysis focuses on the therapy relationship, attuning to process, alliance ruptures, enactments, and the interplay between transference and countertransference. Therapists are attuned to both verbal and nonverbal client communication on a conscious and unconscious level, paying attention not only to content but also to the moment-to-moment process and to their own spontaneous reactions to the client. This section presents the processes that therapists should be attuned to and ways in which they can become more responsive to their clients in those moments.

Negotiations in the Alliance

Safran and Muran (2000) argued for the value of conceptualizing the work of building the alliance as involving a process of ongoing negotiation between therapist and client. Doran and colleagues (2012) described two dimensions of the alliance that interact with one another: the collaborative dimension (agreement) and the negotiating dimension (disagreement). *Collaboration* takes place when there is agreement between the client and the therapist on tasks and goals and when the client feels trusting of and cared for by the therapist. *Negotiation* describes the ways in which the client and therapist handle strains or disagreements. From the client's perspective, negotiation relates to perceptions of the therapist as willing and able to adjust or modify in response to the client's needs and to be appropriately responsive to the tensions in the bond between them. Negotiation is one way of inviting the client to present their subjective experiences and can relate to minor disagreements, such as disagreement about an interpretation, or more major disagreements, such as what needs are not addressed in therapy.

The session extract that follows is an example of a negotiation on the therapeutic focus in the second session of supportive–expressive psychotherapy (Luborsky, 1984). In this session, the therapist presented the client with the core conflictual relationship theme (CCRT), which was derived from narratives the client had told in the previous session (Luborsky & Crits-Christoph, 1998). The client was a 37-year-old woman with three young children who was in the midst of a marital crisis. She grew up with parents who were very critical and who constantly argued and finally divorced when she was a teenager. She wanted very much to have a family that was different from hers and fantasized about how she would have an "ideal family." In the current situation, she described a strained relationship with her husband, who was rarely at home, blamed her for their problems, and refused to go to couples therapy.[1]

THERAPIST: Following the last session, I went over the narratives and noticed that one theme was repeated in most of them. Let me know what you think of this [presenting the CCRT focus]: "In close relationships, you yearn for closeness and intimacy, wishing that others will 'see you' accurately and have a real interest in you. However, you often feel that people really misperceive you, and what you get is criticism and blaming. You end up feeling very hurt, and then you distance yourself, feeling depressed and frustrated."

CLIENT: Yes, it's true that I seek closeness, but doesn't everybody?

THERAPIST: Yes, we all do, but it seems that this is something that has always been missing for you, so it seems that need is particularly strong.

CLIENT [after thinking for a few minutes]: Yeah, it always has been . . . right. [silence] But I don't think that "distancing" is quite right. I distance sometimes, but what I do most of the times is the opposite: I pursue them with great intensity, and they become stressed out and leave.

THERAPIST: How so? Can you give me an example?

CLIENT: I really need that closeness, as you said, and for them to see me accurately. I often think people are criticizing me even when they are not. . . . I jump on them . . . I try to convince them they are wrong, and when they start distancing, I actually pursue them. I don't understand why I do that. Last week my husband came home, after he had been away for 2 days, and he said he was hungry. I was really mad at him—"You disappear for 2 days and then you want food?" He blamed me for being selfish and left the room, and I ran after him, trying to show him that he was wrong, but he just left, and I let go.

---

[1] The identities of all clients in this chapter's narratives have been disguised to protect client confidentiality.

THERAPIST: I am wondering if you were hurt by his disappearance and felt that he showed up and demanded something from you without noticing how you were feeling at that moment.

CLIENT: Yeah . . . I felt deserted and humiliated, but perhaps I could have been more patient and given him a meal first.

THERAPIST: Would our focus be more accurate if I changed the last part in the following way: "You end up feeling very hurt, and then you try to pursue them in order for them to really see you, but they become stressed, and you end up feeling depressed and frustrated."

CLIENT: Yeah, that's better . . .

In this vignette, the therapist and the client negotiated the focus of treatment so that the client could feel it was a more accurate focus. In this case, being perceived accurately, and allowing her to present herself to the other, was part of this client's CCRT. Thus, the negotiation helped resolve the disagreement about one of the main tasks but was also responsive to one of the client's main needs.

Ruptures in the Alliance and Their Resolution

Safran and colleagues (2011) defined *rupture* as a tension or breakdown in the collaborative relationship between client and therapist. Alliance ruptures vary in intensity from relatively minor tension, of which one or two of the participants may be only vaguely aware, to a more major breakdown. Two broad types of rupture have been identified, withdrawal ruptures and confrontational ruptures, each with its own characteristic patterns and resolution processes (Safran & Kraus, 2014; see Chapter 4 by Eubanks et al. in this volume for further detail on rupture and repair). In the relational approach, in order to be attuned to rupture markers and apply resolution techniques, therapists need to cultivate a stance of ongoing self-awareness of their subjective reactions as a vital source of information and to remain affectively attuned to the subtle interpersonal shifts that occur in the course of treatment. Once they are aware that a rupture has occurred, they can begin to "disembed" from the relational pattern they are caught in. One of the main strategies for disembedding that fits with the relational approach is *metacommunication*, or the process of communicating with the client about how they are communicating in the moment (Safran & Muran, 2000). Metacommunication is grounded in the therapist's immediate experience of some aspect of the therapeutic relationship (either the therapist's own feelings or their experience of some aspect of the client's actions or affect) rather than higher level inferences (Safran & Kraus, 2014). The following narrative provides an example of identifying a rupture and attempting metacommunication:

> Mike has been in therapy throughout college and graduate school. He had always paid a low fee, since his parents were unable to pay, and he earned very little as a student. He was always extremely thankful to me for allowing him to continue paying a low fee and was very much committed to the therapy.
>
> After a few years, Mike got a job in the high-tech industry with a salary that made it possible for him to rent an apartment and upgrade his living. I felt it was time to raise the fee, but I still waited a few months to make sure that he was satisfied with his new job and would remain there for the near future. At the beginning of one of the sessions, he gave me the check for the previous month's sessions. I thanked him and said that since he was now working steadily and earning a higher income, I wanted to discuss raising the fee. He immediately acknowledged that I had been charging him a very low fee and agreed that it was time for an increase. We negotiated and agreed on a higher fee that worked for both of us, and he proceeded to tell me about the events of the week.
>
> After a few minutes, I noticed he was more quiet and remote than usual. I thought I noted a "withdrawal rupture," but I wasn't quite sure. I asked Mike whether something was distracting him, since he seemed unusually distant and preoccupied. He acknowledged that this was so and fell silent. I tried to address some of the questions he raised about his workplace, but I felt I was intellectualizing and not really attuned to him. I commented that our conversation sounded strained, and it seemed that both of us were distancing.
>
> I invited him to tell me what was on his mind, and he responded, slowly, "You clearly deserved a higher fee . . . and you have been very kind to me, but I feel strange. It's like money was not really a part of our relationship up 'til now." He then recalled how he was once injured on a trail while hiking with friends. Someone called the paramedics, and they helped him get up, bandaged his foot, and were extremely nice to him. A week later he received a medical bill in the mail and felt quite angry and cheated. He felt that they didn't really care for him, only for the money, even though he knew this was not true. I asked whether he felt that the discussion of the fee was my way of reminding him that this was a professional relationship, and perhaps he wondered if it was genuine? I offered a transference interpretation: Did he perceive me like the paramedics in his story? like I was really helpful, as he had told me, but I also presented him with the bill (the fee increase)? We discussed this some more, examining our relationship, and the fact that it was genuine and warm, but it also involved a fee (he had brought a check that same session!). I wondered out loud if perhaps he had kept these two aspects of the relationship, the fee and our warm, strong bond, as separate entities in his mind. Thus, I used metacommunication to repair the rupture: observing that our conversation was strained, identifying the rupture, offering a transference interpretation, and examining the interpersonal process.

Attunement to the Transference–Countertransference Matrix and Use of Self-Disclosure

Attuning to transference and countertransference is a core psychodynamic technique; however, relational theory views these phenomena in a two-person paradigm. *Transference* is no longer viewed as mere projection onto a "neutral" therapist, but as the client's conscious and unconscious responses—both cognitive and affective—to the therapist (Maroda, 1991). Clients are sensitive to specific aspects of the therapist's verbal and nonverbal behavior as they reflect on unconscious conflicts or object representations from their inner world. Clients are responding to something real in the therapist but interpreting it in light of their own subjectivity. Similarly, therapists can experience *countertransference,* defined as their conscious and unconscious responses to the client, as a strong affect or a subtle shift in their self state (Bromberg, 1998). These responses are shaped partly by the therapist's unresolved conflicts and partly by the situation in the here and now. Transference and countertransference unfold in conjunction, and the manner in which they are (or are not) addressed by client and therapist leads to an intricate psychological "dance" (Maroda, 1991), called the "transference–countertransference matrix."

Often, the transference–countertransference pattern re-creates the client's central object relations patterns, and gaining insight into this pattern in the here and now is a very powerful emotional experience. Relational theory encourages therapists to participate in recreating the pattern, whereas classical theory advocated resisting the "pull" to reenact the past with the client and sticking to interpretations. The re-creation of conflictual relationship patterns in therapy ultimately leads to new interpersonal experiences as the therapist responds in ways that differ from those of people in the client's life. Maroda (1991) described this process as follows: "All of the above occurs within the context of the patient setting the stage to replay the past, while challenging the therapist to recast his role so that the outcome is different" (p. 70). When the therapist succeeds in navigating the process so that the outcome is really different, the client has a "corrective emotional experience."

One of the interventions used by relational therapists in this process is the therapist's disclosure of countertransference. The disclosure is mostly about the therapist's experience of the session, the therapy, or the relationship, and not about disclosure of personal facts. According to Maroda (2010), focusing on and incorporating the revelation and analysis of the countertransference into psychotherapy technique increases the opportunity for dynamic conflict to be resolved within the therapeutic dyad and enhances the here-and-now relationship. Within the framework of relational theory, self-disclosure increases mutual recognition, and the therapist discloses their subjective experience of the therapy process or the interaction with the client so that the client can "recognize" this experience and how it relates to the client. The therapist also invites the client to respond to this disclosure, thus giving the client recognition as well.

Gorkin (1987) offered three reasons in favor of self-disclosure of countertransference: first, to confirm the client's sense of reality; second, to establish the therapist's honesty or genuineness; and finally, to break through an impasse. Clients who notice that the therapist is tired, hesitant, or perhaps somewhat irritable need confirmation of their perceptions, and not just an interpretation. Further disclosure clarifies to clients how they impact the therapist or other people in similar situations, then breaks through the conflict in the therapeutic dyad that blocks progress. Self-disclosures by the therapist should be handled with caution, taking into account the client's developmental level of functioning, the current state of the therapeutic relationship, and the nature of the transference–countertransference matrix.

Case Example 1: Attuning to Transference and Countertransference and Using Self-Disclosures

The following case example demonstrates attunement to transference and countertransference and the use of self-disclosure as a means of being responsive to the client:

> Ruth, an art teacher in her 40s with persistent depression, considered leaving her high school teaching position in order to develop a project in art education that she had been thinking about for a long time. As she spoke enthusiastically about the project, her whole face lit up and she seemed very excited. I felt that she was looking for a project that would energize her and seem meaningful to her and reflected this back to her. I thought that her plan was a good one and encouraged her to keep on. At the end of the session, she seemed happy and was very thankful.
>
> The following week she was thrilled to tell me that she initiated a meeting with someone in the board of education who promised to support the project and invited her to write up a plan. I thought that I was being responsive to her need for building confidence in choosing her own path. However, in the following session she came in looking crestfallen: There were budget cuts in the board of education, so she was told that the project would have to be postponed. A fellow art teacher who was supposed to be her partner in the project said that she could not commit herself to a full-scale project. Ruth said, "I don't know what got into me. Did I really think I could do this? It seems grandiose now. . . . I feel so ashamed for even thinking that I could develop such a project."
>
> I empathized with her disappointment, and said that these things do take time, but it doesn't mean she has to give up. She responded that I was being "practical" and didn't understand how humiliated she felt. I urged her to tell

me, but she responded, "You and I have a good relationship, but perhaps I shouldn't have started therapy with someone who is a university professor. . . . My mother always wanted me to do a PhD, and she was always disappointed that I didn't." Ruth fell silent for a moment then continued, "I think that if *you* had planned this project, it would have worked." She was very emotional, and in her tone of voice, reference to her mother, and thinking that I could probably pull off her project, I realized that I had not been attuned to her at all.

I reflected a bit and thought to myself that perhaps she was experiencing me like her successful mother, who was always pushing her to stand out, to impress, to excel. Ruth was quite shy as a child, and she sensed her mother's disappointment that she was not more outgoing and vivacious, as the mother was. Listening carefully to her perception of me as "successful" and picking up the sadness in her voice, I thought that this was important transference material that I had overlooked. She was criticizing herself that she had been too ambitious and was incapable of doing what her "mothers" expected her to do.

In line with relational thinking about the transference–countertransference, I also thought about what I may have done or said to trigger these emotions. I wondered if I had expressed too much enthusiasm about the project, quickly "pushing" her rather than simply listening. I asked myself if I was disappointed in her, and realized that although I wasn't, I did jump on the wagon quickly. Perhaps a part of me *did* want to her to "move on" already. She was right that I had been too "practical" and not attuned to her anxiety and ambivalence about her new plan. Perhaps I made it sound too easy (when I said to go ahead), and she was telling me that it may be easy for *me*, but not for her.

All of this went through my mind, and I was trying to process what was happening in the here and now, in the intersubjective space. As these thoughts took on a clearer shape, I asked her in the following session how she experienced my enthusiasm about her project. Ruth responded that she was happy about my initial encouragement, but was also stressed by it. Inquiring about the client's experience of my subjectivity (a relational intervention), I asked whether she felt that I expected her to "spread her wings" and do something special in her life. I also asked if she felt that I was pushing her. Ruth responded that she did not feel pushed, yet my excitement made her stressful, since she thought that I overestimated her abilities.

I made a self-disclosing comment, saying that I really was happy and enthusiastic, and I did not think the project was beyond her capabilities. However, I acknowledged that I had not been attuned to her ambivalence and anxiety about forging ahead with a "grand plan" or her unconscious need to impress me. She responded warmly to my disclosure, saying that her mother never validated her feelings and never admitted to empathic failures, and this was a new experience for her. Thus, attuning to the transference–countertransference matrix and identifying the dance that we were doing opened up new areas of inquiry for us: helping her deal with shame regarding her ambition, ambivalence about success, and need to define to herself whose dreams she was pursuing.

Identifying Enactments and Processing Them

According to relational psychoanalysis, the therapist is a participant observer in the therapy process, rather than an objective observer of the client's inner world. Aron (1996) described the complexity of the analyst's task:

> Analysts must become skillful at participating with patients in an interpersonal interaction, while maintaining some perspective on the analytic field, including their own participation in that field. . . . A balance needs to be maintained between participation and observation, with the recognition that the act of observation is in itself a form of participation, and that the effects of participation must be subject to ongoing examination. (p. 191)

In the course of therapy, clients and therapists are caught in *enactments*, which are unconscious patterns of dyadic interactions to which both the therapist and the client contribute. In an enactment, some aspect of the client's emotional world, which is still nonverbal, is "played out" by both participants. Enactments are unconsciously based, unintended, and unavoidable. At some point, the therapist or client becomes aware of this mutual interaction, which can then be formulated and addressed verbally in the session (Curtis & Hirsch, 2011). Curtis and Hirsch (2011) pointed out the benefits of recognizing and analyzing enactments: "This seemingly unfortunate occurrence may be turned into therapeutic gold when it is recognized and examined" (p. 86).

Case Example 2: Identifying and Processing Enactments With a Client in Debt

The vignette that follows demonstrates an example of an enactment. A therapist in private practice asked to consult a supervisor on one of her clients, a young woman in her 20s diagnosed with borderline personality disorder. She had dropped out of two previous therapies, but the current therapy seemed to be going well, and the relationship was a positive one. The main issues that were discussed were the client's wishes for intimacy and romance, although she constantly felt rejected and very angry at those whom she perceived as rejecting.

When the client entered therapy, she worked full time and paid for her sessions. At some point she lost her job and was unemployed for a few months. During this time, the therapist didn't charge her, and the client promised to pay her once she resumed work. However, this was a brief statement, with no clear agreement as to how she would repay for these sessions. At the time of the consultation, the client had been working for 3 months and still was not paying. The therapist mentioned the payment a few times and the client promised to pay the following session, but then she always "forgot." They entered into a ritual in which the therapist asked her about the payment (without stating clearly how much the client owed her), the client apologized for forgetting and promised to pay the following week, and then the client "forgot" once again.

The therapist came to supervision feeling stuck and frustrated because the debt had become quite substantial. As she spoke with a soft voice about her "frustration," it was quickly evident that she was very angry, but also feeling helpless, as though she had done everything she could to collect her debt and had reached a dead end. She wanted to continue treating the client and acknowledged that the client had made important gains, yet she felt that she could not offer therapy for free. It quickly became clear that client and therapist were re-creating a relational pattern from the client's life, in which one was rejecting (the client) and the other was feeling helpless and rejected (the therapist). Although the therapist felt she had discussed the matter many times, it seemed that she never actually negotiated the fee or revised the treatment contract at the time when the client was not working. In addition, once the client found a job (which paid a decent salary), neither of them spoke about the need for a new contract.

After some reflection in supervision, the therapist became aware that she was worried that her client might terminate therapy if she mentioned the debt and negotiated a fee. She felt that if she brought up the payment, the client would perceive it as a punishment, which would justify her decision to leave. The therapist realized that she liked this client very much and felt that she was able to do more for the client than the previous therapists, and she didn't want to "spoil things." These fears resonated very strongly with the client's relationship history and current relationships; the client felt that friends rejected her when she became needy and when she asked that her needs be fulfilled. The therapist also felt needy because she needed the money badly; however, she felt as though it was "not fair" to push the client to fulfill her own needs. These feelings also reflected her insecurity as a young therapist making her first steps as an independent practitioner. In addition, she was defending against feelings of anger, fearing disastrous consequences if she even felt angry. The client was also enacting the wish to be accepted and loved unconditionally, pushing people's limits to "prove" that they loved her.

Following the supervision and the awareness of the enactment, the therapist was able to negotiate a new fee and work out a payment plan with the client to cover the debt. She was able to address these issues as a matter of fact without feeling angry, which opened up space for inquiry about the client's behavior. The client showed no signs of wanting to leave therapy, but she did acknowledge a secret wish for "free therapy" and needed proof that she was special. However, she also became quite tense once she realized that her debt was substantial and was dreading a "backlash" from the therapist. In the end, the processing of the enactment strengthened the alliance and helped the client differentiate between regressive wishes from others (e.g., free therapy, unconditional love) and more mature relationships based on give and take.

The therapist's reluctance to collect her debt may have been responsive to the client's regressive wish but not to her current emotional and developmental needs. At this point in therapy the client needed to experience that accepting the therapy contract or conditions (payment) did not compromise their strong relationship. The client needed to feel secure in the relationship, and she realized that she could feel secure even if her regressive wishes were not fulfilled. This developmental need and the need for a secure relationship emerged clearly in experiencing and processing the enactment.

Attuning to Clients' Dissociated Self States and Defenses

Relational psychotherapists are trained to attune to self states that are dissociated (Bromberg, 1998). Therapists try to create a safe space so that clients can experience parts of themselves that seem at first to be "not me" but may later become experiences that they can own. These dissociated self states are "unformulated"; that is, they have not been consciously articulated (Stern, 1987). Thus, they are not accessible to interpretation and have to be identified and verbalized first. Therapists can identify dissociation by paying close attention to various cues such as the client's dreams, which may represent unformulated self states, and shifts in affect and body posture, as well as shifts in the therapist's own self states. The two-person model suggests that therapists and clients communicate both consciously and unconsciously, and thus shifts in the therapist's self state may signal a response to a client's unformulated relational experience.

Case Example 3: Attuning With a Client From Another Culture Who Dissociates From Her Needy Self State

In this vignette, the client was a 25-year-old woman who had immigrated to Israel from the former Soviet Union (FSU). She came to Israel as a teenager in a special program for young Jewish people who paved the way for their parents to immigrate as well. In this program, teenagers came to Israel and stayed at a special boarding school until the family arrived. In the intake, the client spoke about being "bored" while living in her home country and said that coming to Israel seemed like a new adventure. However, it seemed that her childhood and adolescence were quite lonely; her parents worked long hours, and she was encouraged to participate in numerous after-school programs in order to develop her talents and focus on academic achievement. Although she knew that her parents cared for her, she experienced very little warmth and closeness at home. Her description was quite characteristic of families from the FSU.

The client presented herself as a "hard worker" who worked weekends in order to support herself and pay for college tuition. Her parents earned low wages, and her younger brother was still living at home. She described her parents in a dry, matter-of-fact tone: "They had to work hard, so they couldn't really notice that as an adolescent I was sometimes depressed." She recalled that during one summer vacation, her parents announced that they were going away for a few days, and she had to be responsible for her 7-year-old brother. She said, "It was a real chore, but I guess I had to do it." During her high school years, she often spent time at her best friend's home, where the mother was always warm and accepting. She recalled how her friend's mother bought her a birthday gift, a shoulder bag that she had wanted for some time. The client was reluctant to accept it, explaining that it was too expensive and she could buy it herself. She explained to the friend's mother (and to the therapist in the session) that she did not want presents and it was OK not to bring her any. It seemed that this client's conscious perception of herself was as a strong and independent woman who did not need anything from anybody.

However, it gradually became clear that she had a needy self state that was characterized by longing for a safe, protective relationship in which she would be taken care of. This part of her was dissociated from her awareness. As therapy unfolded, the therapist noted that the client also "worked hard" in therapy. She was highly motivated to change and often analyzed situations very intellectually, offering different interpretations that the therapist might give her. The therapist found herself shifting between having a real appreciation for the client's efforts and sometimes tuning out and feeling guilty about it; at those times, the therapist would comfort herself with the thought that if she missed some significant content, the client would probably bring it up again. She did not admit to herself (or to the client) that she was not fully engaged in the process.

During one session, the client all of a sudden remembered a "silly dream" in which her mother was watching a video of her therapy with an expression of dismay. In the dream the client felt sorry for her mother, who was listening to her daughter talk about her painful childhood memories. The client then laughed it off, saying that of course there was no video of the therapy. She also added casually that she had not told her parents about the therapy since it was not "part of their culture." The therapist wondered aloud if she didn't feel alone sometimes since she was not supposed to "burden her parents." The client's eyes filled with tears, and she was no longer joking.

The therapist then noted a shift in her own self state, feeling more warm and engaged than she had before. She now felt that she actually wanted to connect with the client on a more personal level. She told the client that at first she was confused by her laughter about the dream, but now she felt a great deal of sadness, which touched her. She asked the client how she felt about what she had said (an intervention aimed at assessing attunement and responsiveness in the moment). The client replied that she felt closer to the therapist than she had before, and that the therapist perceived her accurately.

In the course of the next session, the client was able to acknowledge that she hated to depend on others because it made her feel weak. She couldn't trust others to contain her and was anxious about burdening them. At the same time, she also had high expectations of others and was constantly worried about being disappointed and hurt. Thus, the dream material and the therapist's attunement to shifts in the client's self states and to shifts in her own self state helped break through the dissociation. In addition, the therapist was informed by research showing that youth from the FSU living in Israel suffer from higher levels of distress compared with their Israeli peers and that the distress persists for several years (Lerner et al., 2005; Mirsky, 1997). The therapist was aware that psychotherapy in the FSU was not encouraged and was not accessible, and so it was important to attune to the client's longing for emotional support even though at first she denied such needs.

The relational approach to diversity goes beyond recognizing cultural characteristics and values and sees diversity as constantly permeating the process. It is reflected in the transference–countertransference matrix and comes to life in enactments. In this clinical example, the therapist was constantly aware that because of the client's cultural background, it was not easy for her to develop trust and to connect to her needy and lonely parts of self.

Summarizing the Key Elements of Responsiveness in the Two-Person Paradigm

Relational psychotherapy aims to help clients increase their self-awareness, connect to dissociated self states, increase their recognition of others, and develop more flexible ways of relating. In order to achieve these aims, therapists are constantly attuned to the process: to the state of the alliance, to ruptures and repair, to the transference–countertransference matrix, to enactments, and to clients' dissociated self states. Therapists are attuned to subtle shifts in clients' affect, and in their own, and to nonverbal communication in addition to overt content.

RESEARCH ON ATTUNEMENT AND RESPONSIVENESS IN THE RELATIONAL APPROACH TO PSYCHOTHERAPY

Relational theory has not produced much research; however, several areas provide support for the effectiveness of the processes described in this chapter: (a) research on dyadic processes in psychotherapy, (b) research on ruptures and rupture resolution, (c) studies on the effects of countertransference on process and outcome, and (d) studies on the impact of self-disclosure. The research in each of these areas is described briefly in the sections that follow, along with directions for future research.

Research on Dyadic Processes in Psychotherapy

In recent years, there has been a growing interest in studying dyadic processes in therapy and their relation to outcome. Most of these studies were not carried out by relational therapists; however, the idea of looking at the therapy dyad, and specifically focusing on agreement and synchrony, fits with the relational two-person paradigm. Uckelstam et al. (2020) assessed alliance from both the therapist's and the client's perspective using the Working Alliance Inventory (Horvath & Greenberg, 1989). Results showed that within-therapist variation in alliance ratings accounted for larger shares of the total variance than between-therapist variation in both therapist and client ratings. Thus, the unique relationship between therapists and their specific clients, rather than general skills or characteristics, determined the level of the alliance. The authors suggested therapist–client matching as an important subject for further investigation.

Another study, by Atzil-Slonim et al. (2015), also examined clients' and therapists' global alliance and found a "better safe than sorry" pattern: Therapists were motivated to take a vigilant approach that might lead both to underestimation of clients' alliance ratings and to increased attunement to fluctuations in the therapeutic bond. Zilcha-Mano et al. (2016) found that dyads with the highest pooled level of alliance from both partners fared best on session outcome. They concluded that these results are consistent with a two-person perspective of psychotherapy.

Research on Ruptures and Rupture Resolution

There is a growing body of research showing that unrepaired ruptures lead to poor outcomes, whereas ruptures that are resolved lead to better outcomes (Eubanks et al., 2018; Safran et al., 2011). These studies are reported at length in Chapter 4 by Eubanks et al. in this volume. In this section, I present several studies that support the relational concepts that were described above.

In their initial research on ruptures, Safran and Muran (1996) identified two broad types of ruptures corresponding to different relational needs. In *withdrawal ruptures*, clients withdraw from active collaboration in therapy by falling silent, intellectualizing, changing the subject, or becoming overly compliant. Safran and Muran found that this type of rupture masked clients' anxiety about expressing negative feelings in the relationship or difficulties communicating their wishes and needs. In *confrontation ruptures*, clients express anger or resentment toward the therapist, masking feelings of pain and a need for nurturance. In order to be responsive to clients in the course of a rupture, therapists attune to these emotions and needs to facilitate resolution.

In a series of case analyses, Safran and Muran (1996) found support for a stage process model in which resolution progressed from recognition of the rupture and exploration of its meaning to the client's expression of the need for agency or communion. Working collaboratively on ruptures and their resolution focuses on the interpersonal interaction in the room, which may not be effective for clients with different attachment styles. However, only a few studies have examined the relationship between rupture resolution and clients' attachment styles. Eames and Roth (2000) showed that the preoccupied attachment style was associated with more ruptures, whereas the dismissive attachment style was associated with fewer ruptures. Miller-Bottome and colleagues (2018) found that both securely and insecurely attached clients were involved in ruptures; however, they differed in their ability to participate in the process of rupture resolution and benefited from different resolution strategies. Secure clients disclosed their present experience openly and were particularly responsive to resolution strategies that focused on the here and now. Insecure clients minimized either their contributions to the dialogue (avoidant) or the contributions of the therapist (preoccupied). These results support the assertion that the alliance should be negotiated and interventions should fit clients' relational needs.

Coutinho et al. (2011) studied therapists' and clients' experience of ruptures and found that often a rupture event was a repetition of a previous rupture, which was a typical pattern in the therapy dyad. Ruptures occurred when clients were not prepared to respond to their therapists' interventions, which probably indicates misattunement.

Rubel and colleagues (2018) demonstrated the importance of the two-person process in resolving ruptures. Sessions in which both client and therapist perceived a rupture were especially detrimental for next-session symptom distress. However, these sessions were less damaging to next-session alliance levels than sessions in which only the client or the therapist experienced the rupture.

Studies on the Effects of Countertransference on Process and Outcome

Several studies have found associations between countertransference and therapy process and outcome. These studies have demonstrated that when therapists' unresolved conflicts or strong emotions are triggered in the therapeutic relationship, they find it difficult to be attuned and responsive to their clients. Some studies have used the Feeling Word Checklist (FWC) to examine therapists' emotions in the course of treatment and their association with outcome (e.g., Lindqvist et al., 2017; Ulberg et al., 2013). Dahl et al. (2017) used the FWC in their study on the effects of transference interpretations with clients with low or high quality of object relations. Their findings show that in the context of low therapist parental feelings, relationship work was positive for all clients. However, when parental feelings were stronger, the specific effects of such interventions were even more positive for clients with high levels of personality pathology but negative for clients with low levels of personality pathology.

In a study currently underway on the therapeutic relationship in supportive–expressive psychotherapy, I am examining the relationship between therapists' emotions before beginning the session and rupture and repair reported by both therapist and client at the end of the session. Preliminary analysis for 24 clients shows that when therapists felt "confident," there were fewer therapist and client reports of rupture and levels of rupture tension were lower. When therapists scored higher on "inadequate," they reported more ruptures and higher rupture tension levels.

In another study, Tishby and Wiseman (2014) applied the core conflictual relationship theme method (Book, 1998; Luborsky & Crits-Christoph, 1998) to study therapists' interpersonal patterns with their parents that were repeated with their clients. In that study we identified five patterns or types of countertransference based on the CCRT components that were repeated in both patterns: (a) repetition of the wish, (b) repetition of the Response of Other (RO; projecting the parent on the client), (c) repetition of the Response of Self (RS), (d) repetition of the parent RO in the RS, and lastly (e) repair, which is an RS that is the opposite of the negative parent RO. In an intensive case analysis (Tishby & Wiseman, 2014), a case with a weaker alliance and no improvement was characterized by the therapist's recurrent repetition of the wish for closeness and connection and a "repair" of the parent RO that did not fit the client's needs. In a second case with a strong alliance and significant improvement, the countertransference types that dominated the beginning of therapy became much less dominant as therapy progressed, and the therapist's perceptions of the client gradually became more flexible.

A substantial body of research has shown that managing countertransference is associated with positive outcome with a medium to large effect size, whereas countertransference that is not managed predicts poor outcome (Fatter & Hayes, 2013; Hayes et al., 2011, 2018). One of the conclusions of the Third Interdivisional American Psychological Association Task Force on Evidence-Based Relationships and Responsiveness is that managing countertransference is "probably effective," with a recommendation for further research on this construct (Norcross & Lambert, 2018).

Studies on the Impact of Self-Disclosure

Ziv-Beiman (2013) highlighted the difference between immediate and nonimmediate self-disclosure. *Immediate disclosure* consists of the articulation of self-involving feelings and the display of negative and positive attitudes toward the client and therapeutic process, as well as information regarding the therapist's education and professional approach. *Nonimmediate disclosure* pertains to the therapist's experiences outside the treatment, including biographical details, personal insights, coping strategies, and so forth Relational therapists use mostly nonimmediate disclosure addressing the therapy process. Studies show that although self-disclosure is not used frequently, clients find it very beneficial and meaningful (Curtis et al., 2004; Lane et al., 2001). Clients perceive self-disclosing therapists as warmer and more personable, particularly when the information that is disclosed is similar to their own experience (Ziv-Beiman, 2013). Hill et al. (2014) found that immediacy (which includes self-disclosure, but also other interventions) most frequently involved exploration of the client's unexpressed feelings, negotiation of tasks and goals, discussion of parallels to other relationships, and to some extent discussion of ruptures.

In contrast to these findings, several studies on the effects of therapist self-disclosure have yielded contradictory results (Henretty & Levitt, 2010) or negative results (Audet, 2004). Ziv-Beiman et al. (2017) reported that immediate therapist self-disclosure (in the course of integrative psychotherapy) reduced psychiatric symptoms among clients with elevated pretreatment symptoms (as assessed by the Brief Symptom Inventory) and bolstered a favorable perception of the therapist. Further research is needed in order to accurately define and assess self-disclosure and its effects on immediate process in terms of therapist responsiveness and its relation to outcome.

IMPLICATIONS FOR TRAINING

Training in responsiveness in relational psychoanalytic therapy focuses on increasing mutual recognition and emotional attunement, engaging in relational supervision, and identifying and managing countertransference.

Increasing Mutual Recognition and Emotional Attunement

Increased mutual recognition and emotional attunement can be achieved in different ways, such as by engaging in role play, observing therapy demonstration tapes or one's own tapes, and keeping detailed therapy notes of session process. A creative training model that one of my graduate students has used is teaching trainees theater improvisational skills. This type of training enhanced trainees' spontaneity and attunement to the other, both verbally and nonverbally. In a study conducted at the Hebrew University (Romanelli & Tishby, 2019), 35 clinical social work students participated in a semester-long course on theater improvisation skills. Measures taken at the beginning and end of the semester showed that course participants reported an increase in flexibility, therapeutic presence, and collaborative tendency. A control group from the same cohort of students did not show similar increases. Course participants reported increased mindfulness, boldness, and self-disclosure in their work following training (Romanelli et al., 2017).

Engaging in Relational Supervision

Frawley-O'Dea and Sarnat (2001) presented a model of relational supervision that consists of the core elements of relational psychotherapy; the supervisor is "an embedded participant in a mutually influencing supervisory process" (p. 41). Supervisors do not present themselves as an authority on psychodynamic psychotherapy, but rather as an expert on process. They invite the supervisee to reflect on the dyadic process with the client and on the dyadic process in supervision. In this type of supervision, differences are negotiated and the mutual influences of the client and therapist and supervisor and supervisee are recognized. Being in a relational supervision helps therapists internalize the model and hence use it in therapy. Hill and Gupta (2018) made a similar statement about the use of immediacy in supervision: "In other words, we propose that the use of immediacy in supervision is not only beneficial for the supervision relationship but is also one avenue for trainees/supervisees to learn about how to use immediacy in their provision of psychotherapy" (p. 294). They cited a qualitative study by Nelson et al. (2008) showing that supervision is a good place to learn how to manage conflict, deal with it openly, and resolve it. Supervisors in Nelson et al.'s study used techniques that are used by relational therapists: encouraging reflection, using self-disclosure, interpreting transference and countertransference, and disengaging from power struggles. Hill and Gupta noted that immediacy may not fit for supervisees or clients from cultures that refrain from (or forbid) discussing the relationship directly.

Alliance-focused training (Eubanks-Carter et al., 2015) is a training program that teaches therapists to identify alliance ruptures and apply a variety of interventions to resolve them. Therapists are trained to monitor the therapeutic relationship on an ongoing basis and to take responsibility for their own contributions to the process. Safran et al. (2014) applied alliance-focused training to cognitive behavior therapy (CBT) for Cluster C personality disorders. Following training, therapists were less likely to display controlling interpersonal process than they were during CBT training. They were also more affirming and understanding (measured using structural analysis of social behavior) than they were in CBT training. Finally, following alliance-focused training, therapists tended to self-disclose more. Clients displayed complementary shifts in interpersonal process following changes in their therapists' mode of intervention.

Identifying and Managing Countertransference

Managing countertransference entails restraining ineffective or harmful therapist behaviors and trying to derive clinically meaningful insights from internal countertransference reactions. In order to better manage countertransference, therapists need to identify it either with the help of supervision or in a process of self-reflection between sessions.

Fatter and Hayes (2013) listed five therapist factors that aid in the management of countertransference: self-insight, self-integration, empathy, anxiety management, and conceptualizing abilities. They examined different ways of developing these traits through meditation, mindfulness, and development of self-differentiation. Mindfulness was described as focusing one's attention on somatic sensations, feelings, and thoughts and was viewed as a multidimensional construct with five measurable facets: (a) observing and noticing sensations, (b) describing one's internal experience with words, (c) acting with awareness and concentration, (d) being nonreactive toward one's inner experience, and (e) being nonjudging of experience. The study was based on self-report data collected from 100 trainees and 78 supervisors who rated the facets on the Countertransference Factors Inventory Revised (CFI–R; Van Wagoner et al., 1991), a tool for assessing successful management of counter-transference. Results showed that the number of years of meditation experience was significantly correlated not only with the total score on the CFI–R ($r = .32$, $p < .01$) but also with three subscale scores: Self-Insight ($r = .36$, $p < .01$), Self-Integration ($r = .26$, $p < .01$), and Empathy ($r = .28$, $p < .01$). The authors concluded by recommending regular practice of meditation in order to foster self-awareness and insight and manage countertransference successfully.

Another method for working on countertransference in supervision is formulating the supervisee's core conflictual relationship theme (Tishby & Wiseman, 2015) and comparing it to the CCRTs of different clients in the supervisee's caseload. This is a more structured way of developing self-reflection on one's interpersonal patterns and the ways they play out with different clients. Trainees' awareness of their CCRTs can help them reflect on core issues and sensitivities that are aroused in interactions with clients.

CONCLUSION

Working in the psychoanalytic relational mode means working in a two-person model, and each therapy dyad is unique. Thus, therapists need to monitor each relationship and how it develops and fluctuates in the course of therapy. Therapists take note of ruptures and apply resolution strategies to enhance the alliance but also to explore interpersonal themes that the client is dealing with. In this type of therapy, mutual recognition is a key aspect, as is negotiation of wishes and needs. The therapist pays special attention to implicit relational processes in therapy and to transference and countertransference as reflecting the unique dance of the dyad. Therapists may use self-disclosure as a means of validating clients' experiences in therapy but also as a means of opening a meaningful dialogue as part of the therapy process. In order to be fully attuned and responsive, relational therapists must view themselves as embedded in the process as participant observers. In the course of therapy, they shift flexibly between participating in the relationship and observing it.

REFERENCES

Altman, N. (2006). Black and white thinking: A psychoanalyst reconsiders race. In R. Moodley & S. Palmer (Eds.), *Race, culture and psychotherapy: Critical perspectives in multicultural practice* (pp. 139–149). Routledge.

Aron, L. (1996). *A meeting of minds: Mutuality in psychoanalysis.* The Analytic Press.

Atzil-Slonim, D., Bar-Kalifa, E., Rafaeli, E., Lutz, W., Rubel, J., Schiefele, A.-K., & Peri, T. (2015). Therapeutic bond judgments: Congruence and incongruence. *Journal of Consulting and Clinical Psychology, 83*(4), 773–784. https://doi.org/10.1037/ccp0000015

Audet, C. T. (2004). *Client experiences of therapist self-disclosure* (UMI No. NQ96235) [Doctoral dissertation, University of Alberta]. ProQuest Dissertations and Theses Global.

Beebe, B., & Lachmann, F. M. (2002). *Infant research and adult treatment: Co-constructing interactions.* The Analytic Press.

Benjamin, J. (1999). Recognition and destruction: An outline of intersubjectivity. In S. A. Mitchell & L. Aron (Eds.), *Relational psychoanalysis: The emergence of a tradition* (pp. 181–210). The Analytic Press. (Original work published 1990)

Book, H. E. (1998). *How to practice brief psychodynamic psychotherapy: The core conflictual relationship theme method.* American Psychological Association.

Boston Change Process Study Group. (2005). The "something more" than interpretation revisited: Sloppiness and co-creativity in the psychoanalytic encounter. *Journal of the American Psychoanalytic Association, 53*(3), 693–729. https://doi.org/10.1177/00030651050530030401

Bromberg, P. M. (1998). *Standing in the spaces: Essays on clinical process, trauma, and dissociation.* The Analytic Press.

Coutinho, J., Ribeiro, E., Hill, C., & Safran, J. (2011). Therapists' and clients' experiences of alliance ruptures: A qualitative study. *Psychotherapy Research, 21*(5), 525–540. https://doi.org/10.1080/10503307.2011.587469

Curtis, R., Field, C., Knaan-Kostman, I., & Mannix, K. (2004). What 75 psychoanalysts found helpful and hurtful in their own analyses. *Psychoanalytic Psychology, 21*(2), 183–202. https://doi.org/10.1037/0736-9735.21.2.183

Curtis, R. C., & Hirsch, I. (2011). Relational psychoanalytic psychotherapy. In S. B. Messer & A. S. Gurman (Eds.), *Essential psychotherapies: Theory and practice* (3rd ed., pp. 72–106). Guilford Press.

Dahl, H. J., Høglend, P., Ulberg, R., Amlo, S., Gabbard, G. O., Perry, J. C., & Christoph, P. C. (2017). Does therapists' disengaged feelings influence the effect of transference work? A study on countertransference. *Clinical Psychology & Psychotherapy, 24*(2), 462–474. https://doi.org/10.1002/cpp.2015

Doran, J. M., Safran, J. D., Waizmann, V., Bolger, K., & Muran, J. C. (2012). The Alliance Negotiation Scale: Psychometric construction and preliminary reliability and validity analysis. *Psychotherapy Research, 22*(6), 710–719. https://doi.org/10.1080/10503307.2012.709326

Eames, V., & Roth, A. (2000). Patient attachment orientation and the early working alliance—A study of patient and therapist reports of alliance quality and ruptures. *Psychotherapy Research, 10*(4), 421–434. https://doi.org/10.1093/ptr/10.4.421

Eubanks, C. F., Muran, J. C., & Safran, J. D. (2018). Alliance rupture repair: A meta-analysis. *Psychotherapy, 55*(4), 508–519. https://doi.org/10.1037/pst0000185

Eubanks-Carter, C., Muran, J. C., & Safran, J. D. (2015). Alliance-focused training. *Psychotherapy, 52*(2), 169–173. https://doi.org/10.1037/a0037596

Fatter, D. M., & Hayes, J. A. (2013). What facilitates countertransference management? The roles of therapist meditation, mindfulness, and self-differentiation. *Psychotherapy Research, 23*(5), 502–513. https://doi.org/10.1080/10503307.2013.797124

Frawley-O'Dea, M. G., & Sarnat, J. E. (2001). *The supervisory relationship: A contemporary psychodynamic approach.* Guilford Press.

Gorkin, M. (1987). *The uses of countertransference.* Jason Aronson.

Greenberg, J. (1995). Psychoanalytic technique and the interactive matrix. *The Psychoanalytic Quarterly, 64*(1), 1–22. https://doi.org/10.1080/21674086.1995.11927441

Hayes, J. A., Gelso, C. J., Goldberg, S., & Kivlighan, D. M. (2018). Countertransference management and effective psychotherapy: Meta-analytic findings. *Psychotherapy, 55*(4), 496–507. https://doi.org/10.1037/pst0000189

Hayes, J. A., Gelso, C. J., & Hummel, A. M. (2011). Managing countertransference. *Psychotherapy, 48*(1), 88–97. https://doi.org/10.1037/a0022182

Henretty, J. R., & Levitt, H. M. (2010). The role of therapist self-disclosure in psychotherapy: A qualitative review. *Clinical Psychology Review, 30*(1), 63–77. https://doi.org/10.1016/j.cpr.2009.09.004

Hill, C. E., Gelso, C. J., Chui, H., Spangler, P. T., Hummel, A., Huang, T., Jackson, J., Jones, R. A., Palma, B., Bhatia, A., Gupta, S., Ain, S. C., Klingaman, B., Lim, R. H., Liu, J., Hui, K., Jezzi, M. M., & Miles, J. R. (2014). To be or not to be immediate with clients: The use and perceived effects of immediacy in psychodynamic/interpersonal psychotherapy. *Psychotherapy Research, 24*(3), 299–315. https://doi.org/10.1080/10503307.2013.812262

Hill, C. E., & Gupta, S. (2018). The use of immediacy in supervisory relationships. In O. Tishby & H. Wiseman (Eds.), *Developing the therapeutic relationship: Integrating case studies, research, and practice* (pp. 289–314). American Psychological Association. https://doi.org/10.1037/0000093-013

Horvath, A. O., & Greenberg, L. S. (1989). Development and validation of the Working Alliance Inventory. *Journal of Counseling Psychology, 36*(2), 223–233. https://doi.org/10.1037/0022-0167.36.2.223

Lane, J. S., Farber, B. A., & Geller, J. D. (2001, June 20–24). *What therapists do and don't disclose to their patients* [Paper presentation]. Society for Psychotherapy Research Annual Meeting, Montevideo, Uruguay.

Lerner, Y., Kertes, J., & Zilber, N. (2005). Immigrants from the former Soviet Union, 5 years post-immigration to Israel: Adaptation and risk factors for psychological distress. *Psychological Medicine, 35*(12), 1805–1814. https://doi.org/10.1017/S0033291705005726

Lindqvist, K., Falkenström, F., Sandell, R., Holmqvist, R., Ekeblad, A., & Thorén, A. (2017). Multilevel exploratory factor analysis of the Feeling Word Checklist–24. *Assessment, 24*(7), 907–918. https://doi.org/10.1177/1073191116632336

Luborsky, L. (1984). *Principles of psychoanalytic psychotherapy: A manual for supportive–expressive treatment.* Basic Books.

Luborsky, L., & Crits-Christoph, P. (1998). *Understanding transference: The core conflictual relationship theme method.* American Psychological Association. https://doi.org/10.1037/10250-000

Lyons-Ruth, K., Bruschweiler-Stern, N., Harrison, A. M., Morgan, A. C., Nahum, J. P., Sander, L., Stern, D. N., & Tronick, E. Z. (1998). Implicit relational knowing: Its role in development and psychoanalytic treatment. *Infant Mental Health Journal, 19*(3), 282–289. https://doi.org/10.1002/(SICI)1097-0355(199823)19:3<282::AID-IMHJ3>3.0.CO;2-O

Maroda, K. J. (1991). *The power of countertransference: Innovations in analytic technique.* Jason Aronson.

Maroda, K. J. (2010). *Psychodynamic techniques: Working with emotion in the therapeutic relationship*. Basic Books.

Miller-Bottome, M., Talia, A., Safran, J. D., & Muran, J. C. (2018). Resolving alliance ruptures from an attachment-informed perspective. *Psychoanalytic Psychology, 35*(2), 175–183. https://doi.org/10.1037/pap0000152

Mirsky, J. (1997). Psychological distress among immigrant adolescents: Culture-specific factors in the case of immigrants from the former Soviet Union. *International Journal of Psychology, 32*(4), 221–230. https://doi.org/10.1080/002075997400746

Mitchell, S. A. (1993). *Hope and dread in psychoanalysis*. Basic Books.

Muran, J. C. (Ed.). (2007). *Dialogues on difference: Studies of diversity in the therapeutic relationship*. American Psychological Association. https://doi.org/10.1037/11500-000

Nelson, M. L., Barnes, K. L., Evans, A. L., & Triggiano, P. J. (2008). Working with conflicts in clinical supervision: Wise supervisors' perspectives. *Journal of Counseling Psychology, 55*(2), 172–184. https://doi.org/10.1037/0022-0167.55.2.172

Norcross, J. C., & Lambert, M. J. (2018). Psychotherapy relationships that work III. *Psychotherapy, 55*(4), 303–315. https://doi.org/10.1037/pst0000193

Romanelli, A., & Tishby, O. (2019). "Just what is there now, that is what there is"—The effects of theater improvisation training on clinical social workers' perceptions and interventions. *Social Work Education, 38*(6), 797–814. https://doi.org/10.1080/02615479.2019.1566450

Romanelli, A., Tishby, O., & Moran, G. S. (2017). "Coming home to myself": A qualitative analysis of therapists' experience and interventions following training in theater improvisation skills. *The Arts in Psychotherapy, 53*, 12–22. https://doi.org/10.1016/j.aip.2017.01.005

Rubel, J. A., Zilcha-Mano, S., Feils-Klaus, V., & Lutz, W. (2018). Session-to-session effects of alliance ruptures in outpatient CBT: Within- and between-patient associations. *Journal of Consulting and Clinical Psychology, 86*(4), 354–366. https://doi.org/10.1037/ccp0000286

Safran, J. D., & Kraus, J. (2014). Alliance ruptures, impasses, and enactments: A relational perspective. *Psychotherapy, 51*(3), 381–387. https://doi.org/10.1037/a0036815

Safran, J. D., & Muran, J. C. (1996). The resolution of ruptures in the therapeutic alliance. *Journal of Consulting and Clinical Psychology, 64*(3), 447–458. https://doi.org/10.1037/0022-006X.64.3.447

Safran, J. D., & Muran, J. C. (2000). *Negotiating the therapeutic alliance: A relational treatment guide*. Guilford Press.

Safran, J., Muran, J. C., Demaria, A., Boutwell, C., Eubanks-Carter, C., & Winston, A. (2014). Investigating the impact of alliance-focused training on interpersonal process and therapists' capacity for experiential reflection. *Psychotherapy Research, 24*(3), 269–285. https://doi.org/10.1080/10503307.2013.874054

Safran, J. D., Muran, J. C., & Eubanks-Carter, C. (2011). Repairing alliance ruptures. *Psychotherapy, 48*(1), 80–87. https://doi.org/10.1037/a0022140

Stern, D. B. (1987). Unformulated experience and transference. *Contemporary Psychoanalysis, 23*(3), 484–491. https://doi.org/10.1080/00107530.1987.10746199

Tishby, O., & Wiseman, H. (2014). Types of countertransference dynamics: An exploration of their impact on the client–therapist relationship. *Psychotherapy Research, 24*(3), 360–375. https://doi.org/10.1080/10503307.2014.893068

Tishby, O., & Wiseman, H. (2015, September 24–26). *Using the CCRT in supervision: Exploring patient and therapist dynamics and enactments* [Paper presentation]. 8th European Conference on Psychotherapy Research, Klagenfurt, Austria.

Tronick, E. Z. (2003). Of course all relationships are unique: How co-creative processes generate unique mother–infant and patient–therapist relationships and change other relationships. *Psychoanalytic Inquiry, 23*(3), 473–491. https://doi.org/10.1080/07351692309349044

Uckelstam, C.-J., Holmqvist, R., Philips, B., & Falkenström, F. (2020). A relational perspective on the association between working alliance and treatment outcome. *Psychotherapy Research, 30*(1), 13–22. https://doi.org/10.1080/10503307.2018.1516306

Ulberg, R., Falkenberg, A. A., Nærdal, T. B., Johannessen, H., Olsen, J. E., Eide, T. K., Hersoug, A. G., & Dahl, H.-S. J. (2013). Countertransference feelings when treating teenagers: A psychometric evaluation of the Feeling Word Checklist–24. *American Journal of Psychotherapy, 67*(4), 347–358. https://doi.org/10.1176/appi.psychotherapy.2013.67.4.347

Van Wagoner, S. L., Gelso, C. J., Hayes, J. A., & Diemer, R. (1991). Countertransference and the reputedly excellent therapist. *Psychotherapy: Theory, Research, Practice, Training, 28*(3), 411–421. https://doi.org/10.1037/0033-3204.28.3.411

Zilcha-Mano, S., Muran, J. C., Hungr, C., Eubanks, C. F., Safran, J. D., & Winston, A. (2016). The relationship between alliance and outcome: Analysis of a two-person perspective on alliance and session outcome. *Journal of Consulting and Clinical Psychology, 84*(6), 484–496. https://doi.org/10.1037/ccp0000058

Ziv-Beiman, S. (2013). Therapist self-disclosure as an integrative intervention. *Journal of Psychotherapy Integration, 23*(1), 59–74. https://doi.org/10.1037/a0031783

Ziv-Beiman, S., Keinan, G., Livneh, E., Malone, P. S., & Shahar, G. (2017). Immediate therapist self-disclosure bolsters the effect of brief integrative psychotherapy on psychiatric symptoms and the perceptions of therapists: A randomized clinical trial. *Psychotherapy Research, 27*(5), 558–570. https://doi.org/10.1080/10503307.2016.1138334

6 RESPONSIVENESS IN CONTROL-MASTERY THEORY

GEORGE SILBERSCHATZ

Definitions of what it means to be *responsive* include concepts such as being sensitive to the needs of someone or reacting to them in the manner that is appropriate or right for that particular person. How can a psychotherapist conducting therapy with a patient know what is "right" for this particular patient? One answer can be found in the proliferation of randomized control trials in psychotherapy research that began in the 1980s and that culminated in more recent evidenced-based therapy guidelines: rely on an approach and set of techniques that have been shown to be effective for the patient's particular *DSM* (*Diagnostic and Statistical Manual of Mental Disorders*) diagnosis. If the patient suffers from posttraumatic stress disorder (PTSD), for instance, exposure therapy is "right for that particular person" according to this way of thinking about responsiveness.

Needless to say, this line of thought is not without controversy (Persons & Silberschatz, 1998). More than 2,000 years ago Hippocrates argued that it is more important to know what sort of person has a disease than to know what sort of disease a person has. Much more recently, Norcross and Wampold (2019b) pointed out that "adapting therapy to the entire person improves

https://doi.org/10.1037/0000240-007
The Responsive Psychotherapist: Attuning to Clients in the Moment, J. C. Watson and H. Wiseman (Editors)

success and decreases dropouts; the power of responsiveness exceeds that associated with Treatment Method A for Disorder Z; this represents not clinical lore but established fact" (p. 6). Relying on treatment A for disorder Z is relatively straightforward: The clinician must accurately diagnose disorder Z and competently apply treatment A. Adapting therapy responsively to the person with disorder Z is far more complex (Gazzillo, Dimaggio, & Curtis, 2019). A wide variety of approaches for responsively adapting therapy to the entire person have been proposed (for a review, see Norcross & Wampold, 2019a).

In this chapter, I describe how the San Francisco Psychotherapy Research Group (https://www.sfprg.org) uses principles from control-mastery theory to elucidate the concept of therapeutic responsiveness. I begin with a broad overview of the theory, describe the case-specific formulation method that was developed and empirically validated, and provide a brief clinical example illustrating how this approach provides a meaningful framework for understanding responsiveness and determining "what is right" for a particular patient. Next a brief overview of some research studies is presented, followed by a discussion of implications for training therapists on how to be more responsive to their patients' particular problems, goals, and needs.

OVERVIEW OF CONTROL-MASTERY THEORY

Control-mastery theory is an integrated cognitive–psychodynamic–relational theory (Sampson, 1976, 1992; Silberschatz, 2005; Weiss, 1986, 1993) of how the mind functions, how psychopathology develops, and how therapy works. The theory derives its name from two foundational premises: (a) that a person's control over their mental life is regulated by perceptions of safety and danger and (b) that patients come to therapy to master their problems and conflicts. The theory assumes that patients are highly motivated to solve their problems and pursue their goals but are in conflict about doing so. The primary sources of conflict are pathogenic beliefs or schemas that are the result of conscious and unconscious loyalty to family and loved ones, identifications, and compliance. For instance, a patient who was raised by a father who demeaned women identified (consciously or unconsciously) with his father's behavior by treating women with a dismissive, disrespectful attitude.[1] Another patient, whose parents found his incessant curiosity and inquisitiveness draining, was frequently chided for being too smart for his own good. The patient unconsciously complied with his parents' negative attitude: Despite his

---

[1] The identities of the clients in this chapter's case examples have been disguised to protect client confidentiality.

exceptional intelligence, he became a mediocre student and dropped out of college (Bugas & Silberschatz, 2005, p. 156).

A person's pathogenic beliefs stem from perceptions of danger, which are typically based on adverse or traumatic childhood experiences. Weiss (1993) described two categories of traumatic experiences: (a) discrete catastrophic childhood events that overwhelm the child's coping capacities, such as a serious accident or the death of a parent—shock trauma; and (b) persistent, inescapable traumatic experiences such as growing up in an abusive or dysfunctional family—stress trauma. Children attempt to cope with such traumatic events by constructing narratives or theories to help them understand and cope with their experiences. Due to immaturity and lack of knowledge, these theories are often filled with self-blame (R. Shilkret & Silberschatz, 2005)—for instance, "mommy got sick because I misbehaved" or "my parents ignored me because I was uninteresting." Weiss (1986, 1993) referred to such theories as "pathogenic beliefs," arguing that these beliefs play a fundamental role in the development of psychopathology.

Pathogenic beliefs are internalized cognitive–affective representations of traumatic experiences. They are extremely painful, constricting, and debilitating (Silberschatz & Sampson, 1991), and patients are highly motivated to disconfirm them:

> This fundamental motivation to solve problems and master conflicts is embedded in the concept of the "patient's plan" (Silberschatz, 2005; Weiss, 1993). Control-Mastery Theory assumes that patients come to therapy to get better, and they have a plan for doing so: the disconfirmation of their crippling pathogenic beliefs. (Silberschatz, 2008, p. 277)

Patients' plans are rarely consciously articulated; nonetheless, they organize the patients' behaviors in therapy and shape how the patients process and evaluate therapist interventions. Psychotherapy is the process by which patients work with their therapists to change their pathogenic beliefs and to pursue their adaptive goals.

Responsiveness to Client Plan Formulation

The San Francisco Psychotherapy Research Group has developed an empirically validated case formulation method, called plan formulation (Curtis et al., 1994; Curtis & Silberschatz, 2005, 2007). Plan formulations include the following elements:

- a description of the patient's adaptive goals
- pathogenic beliefs that impede goal attainment
- traumatic events that gave rise to the pathogenic beliefs

- ways in which the patient may test the therapist to disconfirm pathogenic beliefs
- insights or new experiences that may be helpful to the patient

Therapists who understand the patient's case-specific plan (i.e., the goals the patient wishes to pursue and the pathogenic beliefs impeding the patient from doing so) are more likely to react in a manner that is responsive. In other words, therapists who understand the patient's plan are likely to behave in a manner that is appropriate or "right" for the particular patient.

Consider the following example of a married woman in her late 20s who came to therapy because she frequently fought with her husband despite the fact that she loved him. She sought out a psychoanalytic therapist hoping to get help in understanding why she fought with her husband and why she couldn't enjoy their sexual relationship. She told the therapist that she grew up with an extremely narcissistic father. For instance, when her father prepared to take her and her siblings to the park, he was especially pleased if they wore outfits that he preferred, but if they chose clothing that they preferred he would become sullen and feel dejected.

She began the fifth therapy hour as follows: "I had an interesting dream last night (*pause*). I also had a fight with my husband (*silence*). Which would you like me to talk about?" The patient knew that psychoanalysts are interested in dreams, and she also made it known that she was interested in why she fought with her husband. How should the therapist respond? A rudimentary plan formulation would be a useful guide in being optimally responsive to this patient at this particular moment. The patient's goal is to understand why she fights with her husband and to get along better with him. Her pathogenic belief is that in order to preserve a loving relationship (particularly with a man), she must subjugate herself, her desires, and her preferences. Growing up with a narcissistic father was the trauma that led to her pathogenic belief, and the opening of the fifth hour represents the patient testing the therapist: "Do I need to subjugate my preferences to yours as I had to do with my father?"

Armed with this formulation, the therapist would have a clear indication of what would constitute a responsive intervention to this patient: "Whatever you'd like to talk about would be most helpful." This patient would experience such an intervention as responsive because it disconfirms her pathogenic belief that she must subjugate her interests to those of her therapist. It should be noted, however, that the identical intervention would not be considered responsive to a patient with a different set of traumas and problems. For instance, a patient whose parents were frequently overwhelmed by her questions and (appropriate) requests for help recalled them yelling at her when she was 7 years old, "We don't know what to do, why don't you just figure it out on your own." For this patient, hearing a therapist say "we should talk about whatever you want to talk about" is unlikely to be helpful or particularly responsive.

EMPIRICAL STUDIES OF THERAPIST INTERVENTIONS ON PSYCHOTHERAPY PROCESS AND OUTCOME

Control-mastery theory posits that there are three ways that patients work in therapy to disconfirm pathogenic beliefs: corrective experiences, new knowledge or insight, and directly testing the therapist (Gazzillo, Genova, et al., 2019; Silberschatz, 2008; Weiss, 1993). Patients test their pathogenic beliefs by trial actions that, according to their beliefs, are likely to affect the therapist in a particular way. They hope that the therapist will not react as the beliefs predict. For instance, a patient who was raised by an emotionally neglectful grandmother tests her therapist by offering to end a session early so that the therapist could get home; she was testing to see if the therapist would neglect her. In the example described previously, the patient tested the therapist by asking whether he'd like her to talk about a dream or about the fight with her husband; this patient was testing to see if the therapist needed her to be subservient as her narcissistic father had needed his children to be. When patients experience the therapist as disconfirming their pathogenic beliefs— that is, passing their tests—they will feel safer with the therapist, less anxious, and generally more productive in the therapy session. Similarly, any intervention that is compatible with the patient's plan can be considered optimally responsive to that patient because it helps to disconfirm the patient's pathogenic beliefs, thereby increasing feelings of safety, relaxation, and useful therapeutic work.

This hypothesis has been empirically investigated and supported by a number of process studies (for a review of these studies, see Silberschatz, 2005, 2017). In an initial study of patient tests, Horowitz et al. (1975) found that the patient consistently felt less anxious and more productive when the therapist passed a test; productivity in this study was defined as new, previously warded off contents emerging. In a subsequent study (Silberschatz, 1978, 1986), judges read through the verbatim transcripts of the first 100 hours of a tape-recorded psychoanalysis and identified all instances of the patient making an implicit or explicit demand of the analyst. Trained clinical judges read through these and identified 46 as examples of the patient testing a core pathogenic belief—that is, "key tests." Judges' ratings of the degree to which the therapist passed or failed these key tests were correlated with changes in a variety of patient process measures. The correlations showed that when the therapist passed a key test, the patient's level of involvement in the therapy session (the level of experiencing), her affect, relaxation, and productivity all increased significantly. In other words, when the therapist responded to the patient's tests by disconfirming her pathogenic beliefs, there was evidence of therapeutic progress. These results were subsequently replicated on a series of brief (16-session) psychotherapy cases (Silberschatz & Curtis, 1993).

The research described here focused on patient-initiated events in the session; the therapist responds to a testing sequence initiated by the patient. Psychotherapy sessions are filled with therapist-initiated events such as therapist interpretations. The research methods that have been employed to study patients' tests have been used to assess interventions initiated by the therapist. According to control-mastery theory, the therapist's primary task is to help patients carry out their plans to disconfirm pathogenic beliefs (Silberschatz, 2005, 2008; Weiss, 1993). Interventions are regarded as optimally responsive to the extent that they are in accord with the patient's plan; such plan-compatible interventions are hypothesized to be more effective than plan-discordant (nonresponsive) interventions. Caston (1986) and Bush and Gassner (1986) found empirical support for the hypothesis that plan-compatible interpretations (i.e., responsive interventions) were predictive of therapeutic progress.

Strong support for this hypothesis was also found by Silberschatz et al. (1986). This research was designed to compare a case-specific measure of therapeutic responsiveness—plan compatibility of interpretations—with a general technique measure—transference versus nontransference interpretation. Weiss (1993) argued that the only helpful interventions are those that are responsive to the patient's particular problems and goals. In other words, a therapist's interventions are helpful only to the extent that they disconfirm pathogenic beliefs and support the patient's plan:

> A theory of technique that prescribes roughly the same approach (or a range of related approaches) for every patient is not sufficiently flexible. It may be well suited to the treatment of some patients, but not to the treatment of others. (Weiss, 1993, p. 59)

Empirical support for this view was found in the Silberschatz et al. (1986) study: The results showed that plan compatibility, which is a measure of therapist responsiveness, was associated with in-session progress while the more general, technique measure of transference interpretation was not predictive of progress.

The psychotherapy process studies summarized above were undertaken long after the therapies were completed. The therapists were all experienced, psychodynamically trained psychologists and psychiatrists. The aim of the studies was to identify effective ingredients in the process of psychotherapy conducted by experienced therapists—not therapies conducted by control-mastery therapists. As such, the results provide a useful framework for illuminating what constitutes therapeutic responsiveness and how such interventions impact the process of therapy. However, a full and more complete account of mechanisms of change in psychotherapy requires demonstrating that changes within sessions are predictive of treatment outcome, that is, demonstrating the connection between responsive interventions and positive treatment outcomes. A recent process–outcome study (Silberschatz, 2017) examined whether patients who receive more plan compatible (responsive) interventions had better outcomes and reported more positive overall feelings about their therapy experience.

This study used data from the Mount Zion Brief Therapy Research project, which focused on time-limited (16-session) psychodynamic therapy (Silberschatz et al., 1991). The 39 patients in this study suffered predominantly from anxiety and depressive disorders. The therapists were experienced, psychodynamically trained psychologists and psychiatrists who had received specialized training in brief psychodynamic therapy. Prior to beginning therapy and following the conclusion of therapy, patients were screened by an independent clinical evaluator. The pre- and posttherapy evaluation sessions were audiorecorded and transcribed. Patients, therapists, and clinical evaluators independently completed a variety of measures pre- and post-therapy. These included symptom-based measures, individualized measures (e.g., target complaints, goal attainment scaling), and global change ratings from the patients', therapists', and evaluators' perspectives. At the conclusion of therapy, patients also completed a questionnaire that measured how they felt about their therapy experience (e.g., How freely could you talk to your therapist? How well did your therapist understand you?). This process–outcome study was initiated several years after the therapies had been completed; neither therapists who conducted the treatments nor their patients were aware of the purpose of the study or of our hypotheses.

Trained plan formulation judges read transcripts of the intake interview and prepared a plan formulation for each case. A second group of trained judges received a summary of the intake interview and the plan formulation to rate the plan compatibility of the therapist's interventions. Transcripts of all therapist utterances in the session (without any patient material) were prepared, and judges independently rated the level of plan compatibility of the therapist's interventions for the session as a whole. A 7-point Likert scale ranging from −3 (*strongly incompatible*) to +3 (*strongly compatible*) was used (this is the same scale used in the Silberschatz et al., 1986, study). Four sessions for each case were rated. These included an early session (Hour 3), early-middle (Hour 7), late-middle (Hour 11), and late session (Hour 14). An overall plan compatibility score for each of these sessions was assigned. Correlations between ratings of the plan compatibility of the interventions— that is, therapist responsiveness—and all of the outcome measures were both statistically significant and substantial in that they accounted for approximately 25% of the outcome variance on average. "The plan compatibility ratings were predictive of symptomatic improvement, ideographically assessed change measures (improvement in severity of target complaints and in goal attainment), and in overall (global) improvement ratings" (Silberschatz, 2017, p. 8). Moreover, the results showed that there were substantial correlations between how patients felt about their therapy and therapist plan compatibility: "Patients who were treated by therapists that received high plan compatibility ratings tended to view their therapies more positively, achieved greater self-understanding and self-control, and reported feeling more supported by their therapists (29% to 44% of variance explained)" (pp. 8–9). In short, patients who received more responsive (i.e., plan compatible) interventions had better outcomes and reported more positive overall feelings about their therapy experience.

Our research shows that therapist responsiveness—specifically, the degree of plan compatibility of therapist interventions—is significantly correlated with progress within sessions (process studies) as well as with treatment outcomes. These findings are noteworthy because it has been difficult for researchers to identify the effective ingredients in psychotherapy. One therapy ingredient that has received increasing attention in the research literature is the role of the therapist; there is considerable evidence showing that therapist effects predict therapy outcome (Wampold & Imel, 2015). Our findings point to one factor that likely plays a role in therapist effects: differences in responsiveness to the particular patient based on plan compatibility.

RESPONSIVENESS AND THERAPIST EFFECTS

Therapist effects are typically found in both clinical and research settings; that is, some therapists achieve consistently better results than others. Similar differences are found in many other areas: Some teachers are more effective than others, some surgeons have fewer complications for the same procedures than others, some physical therapists achieve better results than their peers, and so on. Psychotherapists who are particularly effective have been designated as "supershrinks" (Ricks, 1974) because their results are so much better than comparable peers. In one study, for instance, the outcomes of patients treated by supershrinks was nearly 10 times better than the outcomes of patients seen by less effective therapists (Okiishi et al., 2003).

This research on therapist effects leads to the intriguing question, What are the supershrinks doing that their less effective colleagues are not? To address this question, I examined the data from the process-outcome study reported by Silberschatz (2017). I grouped patient outcome scores into therapist caseloads and computed a standardized outcome score (a z-score composite of all outcome measures) for each of the 16 therapists' caseloads. These results are shown in Figure 6.1 with the 16 caseloads ranked into three groups: top, middle, and bottom outcome scores. The results are consistent with research on therapist effects (for review, see Wampold & Imel, 2015) in that the top group of therapists achieved consistently better outcomes than the middle or bottom group.

FIGURE 6.1. Therapist Caseload Ranking Grouped by Top, Middle, and Bottom Outcome Scores

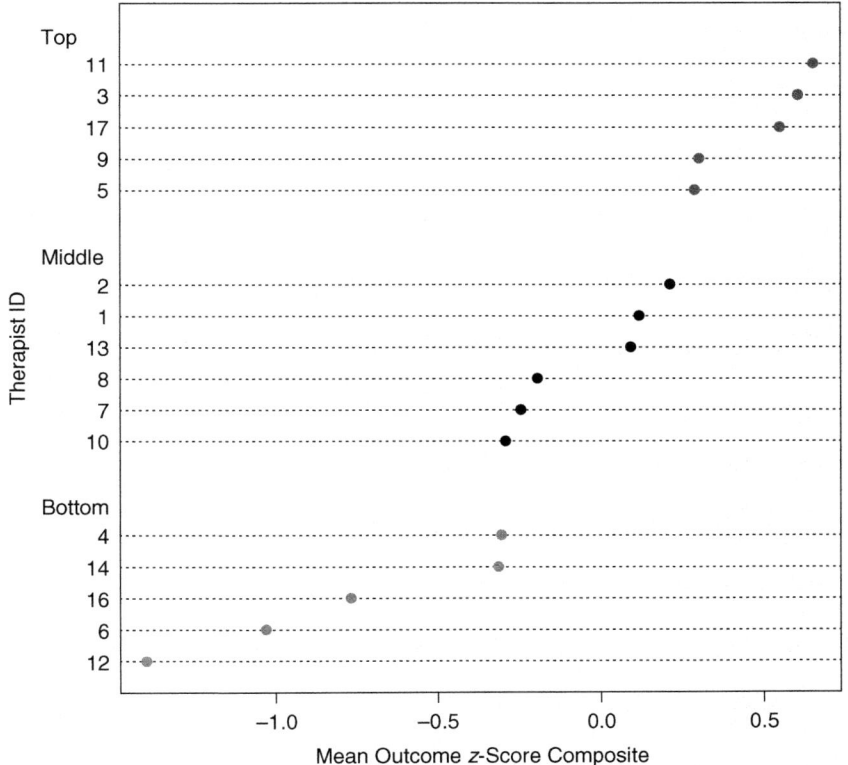

Note. Data from Silberschatz (2017).

Next, I investigated factors that could differentiate the top group from the others. Since the therapists were relatively homogenous with respect to years of clinical experience (all were experienced, with a minimum of 3 years and an average of 7 years in private practice), therapist experience levels could not account for the difference. The significant correlations we found between plan responsive interventions and outcome suggested that this variable could explain differences between more- and less-effective therapists. Therapists were divided into two groups: those who had some training in identifying pathogenic beliefs and plan formulation and those who did not.

Figure 6.2 shows the results of this grouping: Four of the five therapists in the top group had been trained in the plan formulation method; none of those who received plan formulation training had composite outcomes less than

FIGURE 6.2. Therapist Caseload Ranking Grouped by Top, Middle, and Bottom Outcome Scores

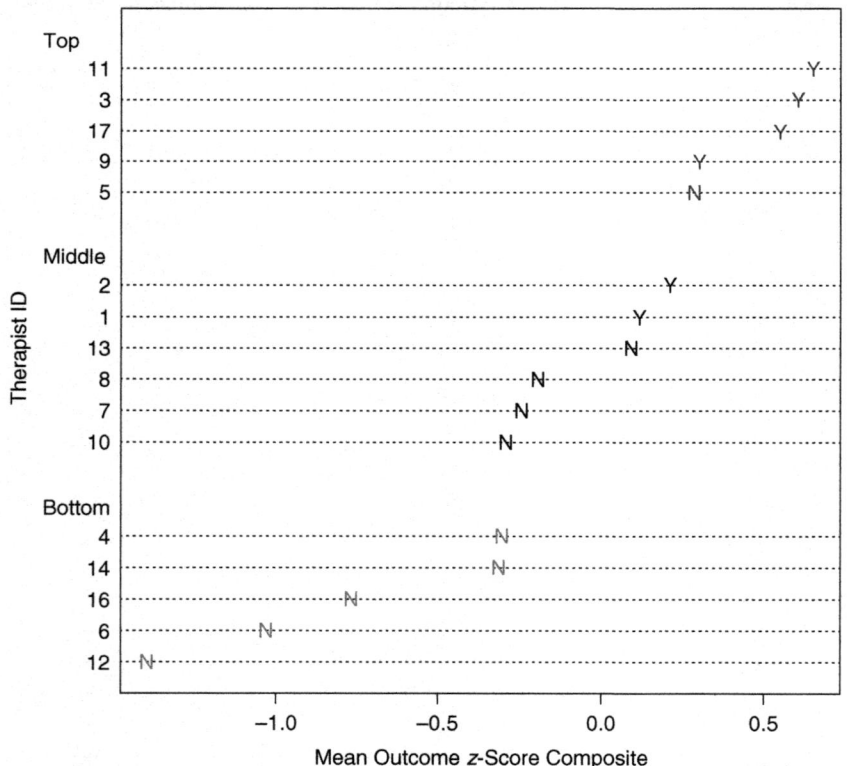

Note. Y = plan formulating training; N = no plan formulating training. Data from Silberschatz (2017).

zero. By contrast, nearly all of the therapists who had no experience using the plan formulation method had outcome scores below zero (Mann-Whitney rank sum test $p < .0005$). Did the formulation training help therapists provide more plan responsive interventions? This is clearly a critical question since our research suggests that plan compatibility is one important variable that accounts for progress in sessions and at outcome. I then examined all of the plan compatibility ratings for all of the patients in a late session (session 14) and converted the ratings to z-scores. Trained therapists all had z-scores above zero (i.e., their interventions were rated as plan-compatible) while nearly all of the untrained therapists' interventions were plan-incompatible—they had z-scores below zero (Mann-Whitney Rank Sum Test, $p < .0001$).

This is a small, preliminary study, and further research is clearly needed. These results need to be replicated on a larger sample with more consistent uniformity in therapist caseloads. Future studies will also need to consider additional variables that might be operative such as therapist relational skills or patients' and therapists' degree of emotional intelligence. Nonetheless, these results suggest that one factor differentiating supershrinks from their less effective peers is the ability to accurately respond to their patient's particular needs, problems, and goals (i.e., to their plan).

CLINICAL EXPLORATION OF THERAPIST EFFECTS

How did the treatments of the most effective therapists, the supershrinks, differ from those of their less effective counterparts? To explore this question in a more qualitative way, I reviewed therapies carried out by the most effective and least effective therapists. As noted above, four of the five supershrinks had some familiarity and training in plan formulation, and their interventions and attitudes were typically responsive to the patient's plan. Instead of following a prescribed set of techniques such as transference interpretation or resistance analysis, they tailored their approach in ways that disconfirmed pathogenic beliefs in a case-specific manner. One of these therapists was extremely active in interpreting his patient's discomfort with being more successful than her siblings and her strong resistance to acknowledging her pleasure in surpassing them; yet, this same therapist adopted a passive, listening stance with another of his patients who needed space and patience to figure things out for himself. This patient was raised by extremely intrusive parents who controlled most aspects of his life. He suffered from the pathogenic belief that others (particularly authority figures) needed to dominate him and that he needed to be submissive to sustain a relationship. The therapist's ability to allow this patient to be in control was a useful step in disconfirming the pathogenic belief. Another of these supershrinks freely gave assurance, emotional support, acceptance, advice, and affection to a patient who had been mistreated while growing up and who unconsciously complied with the mistreatment by believing that he was unworthy of respect or admiration.

In one of these highly effective treatments the therapist was unusually confrontational in her style, which the patient ultimately found reassuring and extremely helpful. The patient had been raised in a family characterized by extreme and pervasive denial. His father abused alcohol and his mother was addicted to pain medications, yet no one in the family addressed these problems. The patient would get into trouble at school and engaged in petty theft for most of high school, a pattern that also was never addressed by his parents. He developed a pathogenic belief that problems are best left ignored and hidden from others. Early in his treatment, the patient described using recreational drugs in a self-destructive way, immediately minimizing the problem and denying its severity. The therapist vigorously confronted the patient's denial—an attitude that was compatible with the patient's unconscious plan to take himself and his problems more seriously. However, this same therapist showed considerable flexibility in both her manner and her attitude with other patients. In one case of a patient who was extremely self-critical and who typically exaggerated the extent and depth of her problems, the therapist was gentle, supportive, and tried to help the patient cultivate self-compassion and kindness. The confrontational approach that this therapist adopted in the first case—which had been beneficial for that patient—would have been detrimental in this second case since the patient was so judgmental and self-critical. In reviewing these highly effective treatments it seemed that these therapists clearly understood that the same technique was simply not suitable for all patients; a technique like interpretation could be beneficial for one patient but detrimental to another (C. J. Shilkret, 2006).

In short, these supershrinks were able to tailor their attitudes and interventions to the specific problems and needs of their patients. They could be friendly, interactive, and supportive but they could also be formal, emotionally distant, or confrontational depending on the particular patient they were treating. This group of therapists seemed to understand a centuries-old aphorism (frequently attributed to Thomas Aquinas) that what is received is received in the manner of the receiver, and they were able to tailor their treatments accordingly. Their training in plan formulation provided a tool for understanding how interventions would be perceived and for optimizing responsiveness to the patient.

The therapies carried out by the less effective therapists stand in sharp contrast to those of the supershrinks. The less effective group seemed to either misconstrue their patients' plan or they frequently intervened in inconsistent ways that left patients confused. One patient, for example, sought therapy because of a troubling relationship with her older sister. She described her sister as domineering, self-absorbed, frequently emotionally abusive, and cruel. The patient wanted the therapist's help in setting appropriate boundaries to protect herself from mistreatment. Unfortunately, the therapist had a different view of the problem: the therapist was convinced that the patient's problems had more to do with anger at her deceased mother for favoring the sister over her, and when the patient disagreed with these interpretations or indicated that they did not help in solving her problems with her sister, the therapist told the patient that she was resisting a painful truth. The patient was clearly frustrated that she was not getting the help she needed and, not surprisingly, the therapy ended badly.

There were multiple cases in which therapists' interventions were inconsistent—at times, completely contradictory. These are best exemplified by the case of a woman in her early 30s who had been married for 3 years and recently had a child. Her husband had always been emotionally needy and demanded that the patient devote herself to him. She was raised by a mother who had been a caretaker to her weak father, and out of an unconscious identification with her mother she fell into a similar role with her husband. Although she bitterly resented this caretaker role, she felt too responsible for her husband's well-being and too guilty to make any changes. When she became pregnant, her husband felt emotionally abandoned and complained that time spent planning for the arrival of their child left no time to focus on him. Late in the pregnancy the husband began an affair, used recreational drugs, and recklessly spent money. When she confronted him on his reckless behavior, he moved out. The patient sought therapy because she was overwhelmed with dealing with divorce and custody arrangements, which in view of her husband's irresponsible behavior she knew would fall largely on her. The therapist focused on the feelings of loss, abandonment, and grief that the patient was likely feeling. Although she acknowledged feeling overwhelmed at finding herself in the role of a single parent, she also felt considerable relief at not needing to be a primary caretaker "for two babies," and this relief made her feel extremely guilty. The therapist interpreted her guilt as a defense against profound feelings of grief and loss that she was warding off. The patient did not find these interpretations helpful—if anything, she seemed to deteriorate. Midway through the therapy the patient told the therapist about going away for a weekend trip with her baby and how pleasant it was to get some distance from her husband. The therapist commented that perhaps she also felt guilty about having fun. She seemed to feel uplifted by this comment, but the therapist quickly returned to his view that the guilt primarily serves to protect her from more difficult feelings of loss and abandonment.

Even though all of the therapists in this study were experienced clinicians, the contrast between the most effective and least effective therapists is starkly clear. The effective therapists had an unmistakable ability to "get" their patients—they understood their goals, recognized their problems and pathogenic schemas, they were helpful in addressing them, and they did so in ways that were helpful to their patients. The ineffective therapists seemed to be more technique focused rather than patient focused. They appeared to stubbornly hold on to their views and their preferred techniques even when the patient provided evidence that it was not helpful to do so.

TRAINING AND DIVERSITY IMPLICATIONS

The empirically supported treatment movement has had a profound impact on how therapists are trained. In North America, many psychotherapy training programs offer training only in treatment protocols that have been shown to be effective in randomized controlled trials. In effect, this means that the focus is entirely on teaching particular techniques (often manualized) for particular diagnoses. It is especially ironic that this is done in the name of empirical data despite the fact that systematic research reviews show that there is no evidence that techniques contribute to treatment outcomes (Wampold & Imel, 2015). Another major problem with relying on randomized trials to decide which treatment should be offered to whom is the "homogeneity myth" (Kiesler, 1966). Therapists who assume that the therapeutic process is the same across patients from diverse cultural, socioeconomic, racial, gender, or religious backgrounds operate under the "myth of sameness" (Wilson et al., 1995, p. 101). The individualized, patient-specific approach intrinsic to control-mastery theory avoids false homogeneity assumptions; the plan formulation method in particular clearly avoids such false "sameness" risks because the emphasis is on each patient's specific goals, traumas, and pathogenic beliefs.

Sue (1998) published a paper on cultural competence in psychotherapy that has become a classic in the field, and many of the points he made pertain to broader issues of addressing diversity in psychotherapy. An effective therapist, according to Sue, is one who takes issues of diversity into account and strenuously avoids the pitfalls of sameness assumptions. He raised the question of what constitutes competence in dealing with diverse cultures. The first characteristic he identified is "scientific mindedness," which refers to "therapists who form hypotheses rather than make premature conclusions about the status of culturally different clients, who develop creative ways to test hypotheses, and who act on the basis of acquired data" (p. 445). This kind of scientific attitude is intrinsic to the plan formulation method and results in therapies that are tailored to the patient's specific needs, problems, and goals. With the diversity of patients seeking psychotherapy rapidly increasing, therapists need to be trained in how to individualize treatment. The plan formulation method offers one useful framework for doing so.

Control-mastery theory provides an evidence-based approach for conceptualizing responsiveness; research on the theory strongly supports the proposition that plan formulation training enhances therapists' responsiveness, which has been shown to play an important role in the process and outcome of psychotherapy. Therapists who understand the patient's plan and who intervene in ways that are responsive (i.e., disconfirm pathogenic beliefs) are effective therapists; their patients achieve better outcomes and they report more positive experiences of their therapies. One important implication of these findings is that therapists should receive more training in case formulation—in particular, plan formulation—rather than in using prescribed techniques for various disorders. In other words, training programs should focus more on what kind of person has a "disease" than what kind of disease the person has and what techniques should be used to treat the disease. Therapists can be trained to understand and formulate a patient's plan, and such training allows them to be more responsive to the patient. The supershrinks described previously had such training, and their interventions and treatment outcomes reflected it. Since the data for the study were collected, the plan formulation method has been refined and training procedures have been further standardized (Curtis & Silberschatz, in press).

SUMMARY

I have described how principles from control-mastery theory elucidate the concept of therapeutic responsiveness. The plan formulation method—which addresses the patient's conscious and unconscious goals, the pathogenic schemas that are obstructions, the traumas that give rise to these schemas, and how the patient will work in therapy to overcome them—provides a meaningful framework for determining "what is right" for a particular patient and for assessing therapist responsiveness. Research studies show that therapist interventions that are compatible with the patient's plan (disconfirm pathogenic beliefs) are associated with treatment effectiveness. Moreover, a comparison of therapists' caseloads suggests that the most effective therapists (those whose patients have the best outcomes) have training in plan formulation and consistently deliver more plan compatible interventions.

Instead of training therapists to adopt a specified technique for patients who share a diagnosis, therapists need to receive more training on how to be more responsive to their patients' particular problems, goals, and needs.

REFERENCES

Bugas, J., & Silberschatz, G. (2005). How patients coach their therapists in psychotherapy. In G. Silberschatz (Ed.), *Transformative relationships: The control-mastery theory of psychotherapy* (pp. 153–167). Routledge.

Bush, M., & Gassner, S. (1986). The immediate effect of the analyst's termination interventions on the patient's resistance to termination. In J. Weiss, H. Sampson, & The Mount Zion Psychotherapy Research Group (Eds.), *The psychoanalytic process: Theory, clinical observations, and empirical research* (pp. 299–322). Guilford Press.

Caston, J. (1986). The reliability of the diagnosis of the patient's unconscious plan. In J. Weiss, H. Sampson, & The Mount Zion Psychotherapy Research Group (Eds.), *The psychoanalytic process: Theory, clinical observations, and empirical research* (pp. 241–255). Guilford Press.

Curtis, J. T., & Silberschatz, G. (2005). The assessment of pathogenic beliefs. In G. Silberschatz (Ed.), *Transformative relationships: The control-mastery theory of psychotherapy* (pp. 69–91). Routledge.

Curtis, J. T., & Silberschatz, G. (2007). Plan formulation method. In T. D. Eells (Ed.), *Handbook of psychotherapy case formulation* (2nd ed., pp. 198–220). Guilford Press.

Curtis, J. T., & Silberschatz, G. (in press). Plan formulation method. In T. D. Eells (Ed.), *Handbook of psychotherapy case formulation* (3rd ed.). Guilford Press.

Curtis, J., Silberschatz, G., Sampson, H., & Weiss, J. (1994). The plan formulation method. *Psychotherapy Research, 4*(3–4), 197–207. https://doi.org/10.1080/10503309412331334032

Gazzillo, F., Dimaggio, G., & Curtis, J. T. (2019). Case formulation and treatment planning: How to take care of relationship and symptoms together. *Journal of Psychotherapy Integration.* Advance online publication. https://doi.org/10.1037/int0000185

Gazzillo, F., Genova, F., Fedeli, F., Curtis, J. T., Silberschatz, G., Bush, M., & Dazzi, N. (2019). Patients' unconscious testing activity in psychotherapy: A theoretical and empirical overview. *Psychoanalytic Psychology, 36*(2), 173–183. https://doi.org/10.1037/pap0000227

Horowitz, L. M., Sampson, H., Siegelman, E. Y., Wolfson, A., & Weiss, J. (1975). On the identification of warded-off mental contents: An empirical and methodological contribution. *Journal of Abnormal Psychology, 84*(5), 545–558. https://doi.org/10.1037/h0077139

Kiesler, D. J. (1966). Some myths of psychotherapy research and the search for a paradigm. *Psychological Bulletin, 65*(2), 110–136. https://doi.org/10.1037/h0022911

Norcross, J. C., & Wampold, B. E. (Eds.). (2019a). *Psychotherapy relationships that work: Vol. 2. Evidence-based responsiveness* (3rd ed.). Oxford University Press.

Norcross, J. C., & Wampold, B. E. (2019b, September). Relationships and responsiveness in the psychological treatment of trauma: The tragedy of the APA Clinical

Practice Guideline. *Psychotherapy, 56*(3), 391–399. https://doi.org/10.1037/pst0000228

Okiishi, J., Lambert, M. J., Nielsen, S. L., & Ogles, B. M. (2003). Waiting for supershrink: An empirical analysis of therapist effects. *Clinical Psychology & Psychotherapy, 10*(6), 361–373. https://doi.org/10.1002/cpp.383

Persons, J. B., & Silberschatz, G. (1998). Are results of randomized controlled trials useful to psychotherapists? *Journal of Consulting and Clinical Psychology, 66*(1), 126–135. https://doi.org/10.1037/0022-006X.66.1.126

Ricks, D. F. (1974). Supershrink: Methods of a therapist judged successful on the basis of adult outcomes of adolescent patients. In D. F. Ricks, M. Roff, & A. Thomas (Eds.), *Life history research in psychopathology*. University of Minnesota Press.

Sampson, H. (1976). A critique of certain traditional concepts in the psychoanalytic theory of therapy. *Bulletin of the Menninger Clinic, 40*(3), 255–262.

Sampson, H. (1992). The role of "real" experience in psychopathology and treatment. *Psychoanalytic Dialogues, 2*(4), 509–528. https://doi.org/10.1080/10481889209538948

Shilkret, C. J. (2006). Endangered by interpretations: Treatment by attitude of the narcissistically vulnerable patient. *Psychoanalytic Psychology, 23*(1), 30–42. https://doi.org/10.1037/0736-9735.23.1.30

Shilkret, R., & Silberschatz, S. A. (2005). A developmental basis for control-mastery theory. In G. Silberschatz (Ed.), *Transformative relationships: The control-mastery theory of psychotherapy* (pp. 171–187). Routledge.

Silberschatz, G. (1978). Effects of the analyst's neutrality on the patient's feelings and behavior in the psychoanalytic situation. *Dissertation Abstracts International, 39*(6-B), 3007.

Silberschatz, G. (1986). Testing pathogenic beliefs. In J. Weiss, H. Sampson, & The Mount Zion Psychotherapy Research Group (Eds.), *The psychoanalytic process: Theory, clinical observations, and empirical research* (pp. 256–266). Guilford Press.

Silberschatz, G. (2005). *Transformative relationships: The control-mastery theory of psychotherapy*. Routledge.

Silberschatz, G. (2008). How patients work on their plans and test their therapists in psychotherapy. *Smith College Studies in Social Work, 78*(2–3), 275–286. https://doi.org/10.1080/00377310802114528

Silberschatz, G. (2017). Improving the yield of psychotherapy research. *Psychotherapy Research, 27*(1), 1–13. https://doi.org/10.1080/10503307.2015.1076202

Silberschatz, G., & Curtis, J. T. (1993). Measuring the therapist's impact on the patient's therapeutic progress. *Journal of Consulting and Clinical Psychology, 61*(3), 403–411. https://doi.org/10.1037/0022-006X.61.3.403

Silberschatz, G., Curtis, J. T., Sampson, H., & Weiss, J. (1991). Research on the process of change in psychotherapy: the approach of the Mount Zion psychotherapy research group. In L. Beutler & M. Crago (Eds.), *Psychotherapy research: An international review of programmatic studies* (pp. 56–64). American Psychological Association. https://doi.org/10.1037/10092-006

Silberschatz, G., Fretter, P. B., & Curtis, J. T. (1986). How do interpretations influence the process of psychotherapy? *Journal of Consulting and Clinical Psychology, 54*(5), 646–652. https://doi.org/10.1037/0022-006X.54.5.646

Silberschatz, G., & Sampson, H. (1991). Affects in psychopathology and psychotherapy. In J. Safran & L. Greenberg (Eds.), *Emotion, psychotherapy, and change* (pp. 113–129). Guilford Press.

Sue, S. (1998). In search of cultural competence in psychotherapy and counseling. *American Psychologist, 53*(4), 440–448. https://doi.org/10.1037/0003-066X.53.4.440

Wampold, B. E., & Imel, Z. E. (2015). *The great psychotherapy debate: The evidence for what makes psychotherapy work* (2nd ed.). Routledge/Taylor & Francis Group. https://doi.org/10.4324/9780203582015

Weiss, J. (1986). I. Theory and clinical observations. In J. Weiss, H. Sampson, & The Mount Zion Psychotherapy Research Group (Eds.), *The psychoanalytic process: Theory, clinical observation, and empirical research* (pp. 3–138). Guilford Press.

Weiss, J. (1993). *How psychotherapy works.* Guilford Press.

Wilson, M. N., Phillip, D., Kohn, L. P., & Curry-El, J. A. (1995). Cultural relativistic approach toward ethnic minorities in family therapy. In J. E. Aponte, R. Y. Rivers, & J. Wohl (Eds.), *Psychological interventions and cultural diversity* (pp. 92–108). Allyn & Bacon.

7

CONTEXT-RESPONSIVE PSYCHOTHERAPY INTEGRATION APPLIED TO COGNITIVE BEHAVIORAL THERAPY

MICHAEL J. CONSTANTINO, BRIEN J. GOODWIN,
HEATHER J. MUIR, ALICE E. COYNE, AND JAMES F. BOSWELL

If *required* to state a clinical identity, we would all define ourselves as psychotherapy integrationists dedicated to clinical flexibility. In one way or another, at some stage of our training and/or career, we each became disillusioned with the sometimes-peddled notion that evidence-based practice (EBP) primarily reflects the faithful delivery of standardized treatments (and their supposed theory-consistent active ingredients) to classes of patients. Our own clinical experiences, and our consumption of and contributions to the psychotherapy research base, fed our challenges to this assumption. To us, therapist flexibility and the ongoing, responsive personalization of treatment to patient and context represent more nuanced EBP and are consistent with contemporary American Psychological Association (2006) guidelines. In this chapter, we present our evolving *context-responsive psychotherapy integration* (CRPI; Constantino et al., 2013) framework, both in its general, pantheoretical format and as applied more specifically to contexts somewhat specific to cognitive behavioral therapy (CBT). As we elaborate herein, CRPI privileges therapist flexibility in making informed and collaborative decisions about the shape of treatment, adherence to a treatment for as long as it seems well-suited to the patient, and a fundamental willingness to shift course (away from the

https://doi.org/10.1037/0000240-008
The Responsive Psychotherapist: Attuning to Clients in the Moment, J. C. Watson and H. Wiseman (Editors)

current plan, such as a CBT agenda) when the treatment, or the relationship in which it is grounded, are not working (i.e., *if* this contextual process marker occurs, *then* try this clinical departure strategy).

More specifically, we first review general research that establishes the need for therapist responsivity and the necessarily evolving attunement to the moment and patient. Next, we present the conceptual CRPI framework in more detail. To do so, we discuss responsivity across the "lifespan" of a treatment course, including first-step responsiveness as *getting off on the right foot*, during-session responsiveness as *doing more of the same*, and during-session responsiveness as marker-driven *departure*. We reference common clinical processes that can conceptually guide therapist and dyad action in ways that heed the research base and eschew the rigid implementation of treatment plans/agendas. Following this presentation of the general, pantheoretical CRPI framework, we provide examples of such responsivity in the specific context of CBT. That is, we discuss scenarios where CBT therapists may need to depart from model-specific foci in order to address evidence-based markers that would confer risk if unattended. We also discuss the intersection of responsiveness and patients' cultural identities. Next, we provide research findings (nonexhaustive) that support our notions of contextual responsivity, again across the treatment lifespan, and we also propose pertinent future research directions. Finally, we offer training strategies for maximizing clinicians' responsiveness in a manner that applies to CBT but that can also be applied pantheoretically.

RESEARCH ESTABLISHING THE NEED FOR RESPONSIVITY AND ATTUNEMENT IN PSYCHOTHERAPY

From varied angles, the literature supports the importance of a provider's contextual responsivity and attunement to the patient, the relationship, and/or the moment. For example, patient factors (e.g., treatment-related beliefs), therapist factors (e.g., emotional expression), and relationship qualities (e.g., the working alliance) that cut across treatment orientations explain significant variance in patients' outcomes, sometimes more so than putative theory-unique variables (Wampold & Imel, 2015). Additionally, meta-analyses indicate that neither a therapist's global adherence to specific, manual-prescribed techniques nor competence in delivering them (the two components of treatment *integrity*; Cox et al., 2019) relates significantly to patients' outcomes (Webb et al., 2010). Supporting responsivity, this lack of effect makes sense when considering that some patients within a latent class, such as diagnosis, will need more, less, or an average amount of a given technique or process to benefit comparably, thus negating a linear integrity-outcome correlation (Stiles, 2013).

Underscoring these notions, several studies have shown that when a therapist demonstrated more flexibility in technique use *within the context of a single case*, that dyad showed better therapy process (Goldman et al., 2013), and that patient demonstrated more improvement (Katz et al., 2019). Notably, such flexibility involved using techniques that might typically be considered proscribed if the provider's goal was to remain theoretically faithful. Research has also explicitly revealed the risk of therapist rigidity. For example, therapist *perseverative* adherence in the face of alliance tensions has been shown to relate to worse outcomes (e.g., Castonguay et al., 1996). Conversely, when therapists move away from strict adherence to treatment agendas in such moments, and instead are more emotionally supportive and autonomy granting, it facilitates improvement (e.g., Elkin et al., 2014). In fact, experimental tests of such "departure modules" precipitated by a specific marker (e.g., a dyad's alliance rupture) have indicated a superior effect over standard treatments that lack specific guidance on how to depart from an a priori treatment plan to negotiate disruptive process (e.g., Constantino et al., 2008). Because these additive designs can demonstrate cause and effect, they establish the departure module (the singular manipulation) as a mechanism of patient change.

Research is also emerging that measures relational *attunement* more precisely and captures its beneficial effect. For example, studies have demonstrated that when patients and therapists become more similar over time in their respective rating of their relationship (viz. alliance convergence), including in the context of CBT, the patient shows greater subsequent improvement (e.g., Coyne et al., 2018). Addressing a long-standing shortcoming of measuring a relationship construct from individual perspectives only (e.g., *I* myself believe that *we* the dyad agree on something), these findings spotlight the importance of true agreement (e.g., when *we each* rate *our* relationship on a parallel scale, *we each* agree, or disagree, that *we* the dyad agree, or disagree, on something). Coyne (2016) noted that

> Unique information may be gained by taking both the patient and therapist perspectives into account to create a true dyad-level alliance variable, and that future research should continue to develop methods to capture the relationship, rather than two individual experiences. (p. 10)

In sum, there is a growing research base that establishes the importance of operationalizing and scientifically evaluating therapist flexibility, contextual responsivity, and dyadic attunement.

CONTEXT-RESPONSIVE PSYCHOTHERAPY INTEGRATION BROADLY DEFINED

The need for a therapist's responsivity and attunement can have notable salience *before* treatment begins (e.g., administering one treatment over others when taking into account a patient's interpersonal style), *during* a treatment moment (e.g., uttering a sensitive response to a patient's affective reaction), and/or *across* time (e.g., using multiple sessions to address a persistent alliance rupture). Inherent in these examples is the notion of being responsive *to* something (for which there is some clue, or marker), as well as being responsive *with* something, such as a particular decision, intervention, or stance. Combined, these actions represent a given therapist doing so-called *right* or *right enough* things at *right* times with a given patient in the context of a given treatment (Stiles & Horvath, 2017). Of course, this notion is necessarily complex given that treatment is often nonlinear and self-correcting; that said, progress is being made, both conceptually and empirically, on how to apply certain right/right-enough things at certain right times. In this section, we focus on *conceptual* advances of responsivity across the lifespan of a treatment course, providing just a few representative examples.

As exemplified across this volume, responsivity can take different shapes, all of which have an undercurrent of adapting treatments in appreciation of idiographic information about the person of the patient, the person of the therapist, and the nature of their relationship and treatment "contract." As noted previously, we term our framework CRPI (Constantino et al., 2013), which privileges therapist flexibility via (a) making informed and collaborative decisions about what nature a treatment should take, how best to start it, and who should deliver it; (b) staying a treatment course when it seems indicated (ideally determined not just by clinical judgment but also by case-specific or generalizable evidence); and (c) possessing a fundamental willingness to shift course when the treatment, or the relationship in which it is grounded, are not working (ideally determined not just by judgment, but also by patients' disclosures and/or a routine outcome or process measure).

Responsiveness as Getting Off on the Right Foot

CRPI considers responsiveness as a crucial element of a therapy dyad getting off on the right foot. This is where a clinician's knowledge of and facility with different theoretical orientations may be most useful, as it is important to present patients with an illness conceptualization and a proposed (and well-aligned) therapy rationale that is compelling enough to instill a belief that the provider and their approach can help (King & Boswell, 2019). Without this, the therapist's attunement to patients' needs and belief systems is immediately misaligned, which creates a risk of low perceived credibility and low outcome expectation (OE)—both beliefs that can undermine initial engagement and efficacy (Coyne, Constantino, & Muir, 2019).

Even when collaboratively selecting a treatment that aligns well with a patient's treatment-related beliefs, there can be other markers calling for first-step responsivity. For example, patients' motivational language can be an important indicator of their readiness to engage effectively in a treatment (again, even when said treatment is conceptually a good fit). When patients are using more change-talk (CT), or language that favors adaptive behavior revision ("It's just a spiral of worry that's so unnecessary"), they may be prepared to engage fully in a treatment contract that implies removal of maladaptive patterns/behaviors. However, when patients are articulating more counter change-talk (CCT), or language that favors maintaining the problem feature ("I mean, worrying can be a good thing to a point"), they may require a different first step than the explicitly change-oriented treatment. The key is that change readiness is an individual difference variable. When such change readiness is low (perhaps signaled by high CCT), patients may benefit from a motivational focus (e.g., a motivational interviewing [MI] *pretreatment*) that supports and validates their questions or ambivalence about relinquishing familiar, albeit maladaptive, patterns (Miller & Rollnick, 2013).

First-step responsiveness could also have more to do with the therapist and their match to the patient. Not only can therapists differ from one another in their general and/or problem domain-specific effectiveness, they can also possess relative strengths and weaknesses within their *own* caseloads depending on their patients' presenting problems (Kraus et al., 2016). For example, Therapist A's average depressed patient may show more improvement than Therapist A's average anxious patient. If this inherent strength becomes stable over numerous cases, such information can be made actionable in the form of certain stakeholders using provider performance indices to match patients to clinicians with a known track record of efficacy in treating the primary problem(s) with which the patients present. This represents a type of responsiveness that would go overlooked if only considering adaptation *after* a treatment begins.

Responsiveness as Doing More of the Same

Presuming that therapy is off and running on a reasonably good foot, CRPI next centers on in-session processes. Specifically, it reframes common factors as frequently occurring clinical situations that therapists need to assess and to which they will need to respond sensitively. Notably, the responsive "read" here could be to continue as planned. For example, with cues such as a good-enough treatment rationale that the patient seems to trust, patient language that appears to reflect a readiness to change in the way a treatment model outlines, and a seemingly good enough working relationship with a therapist who is practicing within her efficaciousness "wheelhouse," responsivity may rather straightforwardly require acting in a way that supports the trusted treatment contract and frame.

Doing more of the same is consistent with *plan compatibility*, or therapist behavior that aligns with an ideographic case formulation (Silberschatz, 2017). To ensure such compatibility, therapists and patients would need to arrive at a case formulation that a patient understands and that can be revisited as treatment unfolds, and therapists would need to be open to their behavior being evaluated (perhaps through patient feedback and/or independent observation) in relation to the plan. To be responsive, the dyad would also need to appreciate that the plan/formulation can shift, and that in-session compatibility would necessarily be redefined throughout treatment. Thus, open discussion of such shifts would need to remain on the "front burner" over time.

Another "stay-the-course" indicator relates to overall relational health. Drawing on social psychological research that healthy dyads tend to perceive and experience things more similarly over time (Anderson & Keltner, 2004), it may be useful for clinicians and patients to regularly monitor how aligned they are on perceptions of their own working relationship (e.g., the degree to which each agrees on feeling bonded) and treatment processes (e.g., the degree to which each agrees that progress is being made). As noted, clinicians could use parallel measures to obtain this attunement snapshot; if aligned, the dyad is likely on a good track on which it should remain.

Of course, the efficacy of these staying-the-course responsivity examples needs to be evaluated in relation to target outcomes. To this end, clinicians might turn to a routine outcome tool as an ongoing check for success versus relying on judgment or biased self-assessment. To us, this would be a version of *doing the same* because of practice-based evidence that it works, as opposed to being motivated simply to perform in a standardized way to heighten a sense that one is mastering a therapeutic approach.

Responsiveness as Clinical Departure

Common in-session situations can also call for the responsive read of doing something different. In these scenarios, CRPI proposes an *if-then* guidance system; *if* this cue presents itself, *then* try this departure response to address it. We believe immense benefit can come from therapists using evidence-backed, replicable, and modular behaviors that have a facilitative impact in precise moments (Constantino et al., 2013). For example, *if* a patient reports that his beliefs in the treatment rationale and/or expected outcome are waning (despite having once been cultivated to the point of getting off on a good foot), *then* the therapist can respond by limiting the given treatment (such as CBT) to those elements that the patient continues to find credible (e.g., the B more than the C; see Boswell & Schwartzman, 2018), or by shifting the treatment more fully (e.g., adopting a more integrative or interpersonal approach; Coyne, Constantino, & Muir, 2019).

Or, *if* a patient uses motivational language signaling ambivalence (e.g., language high in CT *and* CCT), *then* the therapist may need to adjust treatment to match this likely stage of "unreadiness." For example, a CBT clinician may need to shift from being change-oriented ("As we discussed, let's continue with exposure exercises until your panic extinguishes") to becoming more validating ("I appreciate that sometimes giving up something familiar, even if problematic, can be complicated") and discovery-oriented ("I wonder if your panic ever promotes or detracts from important goals that you have"; Goodwin et al., 2019).

As another example, *if* a patient's diminished OE and/or growing ambivalence about change manifests behaviorally as resistance to the therapist or therapy, *then* the therapist might shift to a person-centered response. For example, the CBT clinician could address this misattunement by momentarily stepping away from her valued direction (the change agenda) and instead validating the patient's lived experience, supporting his autonomy, and eliciting his own motivation for pursuing personally valued directions when ready. Such sensitive responsiveness might even have special interpersonal relevance for some patients, such as those with generalized anxiety disorder (GAD; Gomez Penedo et al., 2017) who may excessively defer in relationships in a way that pulls for others (including a therapist) to take charge and perpetuate a maladaptive pattern. In this scenario, a patient may muster the rare courage to assert their own direction (via resistance), and a validating, supportive, and deferent therapist (using MI responsively) could be catalyzing a relationally corrective experience.

As just a few other responsive departure examples, *if* an alliance rupture emerges, *then* a therapist might depart from her current agenda and apply rupture-repair strategies to address it (Eubanks et al., 2018). Or, *if* a routine outcome measure signals that a patient is not on track for response, *then* a clinician can use this feedback to explore the patient's experience and employ clinical support tools as course changers (e.g., assessing and attempting to heighten external social supports; Slade et al., 2008). Drawing on these examples, the overarching theme is that dissemination and implementation of therapy methods becomes less about packaged treatment integrity and more about the timely delivery of process-attuned, modular interventions (that can span from temporary shifts to more permanent revisions) vis-à-vis specific markers/moments (Hatcher, 2015).

CONTEXT-RESPONSIVE PSYCHOTHERAPY INTEGRATION AS APPLIED TO CBT

Although CRPI is inherently pantheoretical in its focus on common occurrences that can happen in any foundational treatment, it can take unique shapes depending on that treatment's orientation. Thus, CRPI can be tailored to, or distinctively reflective of, CBT. Like any approach, CBT requires starting on the right foot in a way that can be facilitated by first-step responsiveness. Moreover, like any treatment, responsiveness as doing more of the same can be guided by the previously discussed indicators. However, where CBT may be most unique in relation to responsiveness is with regard to therapist departure in the face of disruptive process.

More specifically, with its transparent agenda-driven nature (explicitly anchored to reducing problematic cognitions and/or behaviors), markers for when CBT is not working may have more immediate salience than treatments that are more patient centered or for which session foci are typically more fluid. In CBT, these moments may be especially potent for some patients for whom a therapist's willingness to be less change oriented could represent a corrective experience (such as the aforementioned therapist allowing a patient who may be maladaptively deferent to others to take the treatment reigns). These moments may also be particularly challenging for CBT therapists in that they need to be willing to "change their stripes," by either temporarily or more permanently moving away from their home orientation for which agenda compliance may have typically been their marker that treatment is moving efficiently and going well. In the face of disruptive process, efficiency may take a different shape than moving through preplanned steps, whereas the notion of going well may be more tied to flexibility than "textbook" delivery.

CLINICAL ILLUSTRATIONS OF CBT THERAPISTS' RESPONSIVE ATTUNEMENT

Here we provide hypothetical case material demonstrating the *if* marker of patient resistance that calls for *then* responsiveness of shifting out of CBT and into timely MI.[1] For these examples, we draw on our clinical experiences

---

[1]All clinical case material represents an amalgam of different patient interactions with all potentially identifying information disguised to protect client confidentiality.

of treating patients with GAD. The first example follows a 22-year-old patient named Chris who demonstrated resistance because of his diminishing belief in the logic and/or efficacy of CBT, despite being highly motivated to reduce worry and related symptoms. Then, astutely observing this verbal marker, the therapist shifted away from CBT (remaining open to this shift being temporary or more permanent) and instead prized Chris's doubt, collaboratively got alongside the resistance to explore rather than oppose it, and honored Chris's own illness conceptualization and beliefs about what would be helpful for reducing worry and distress.

PATIENT: I know I initially agreed to this approach, but I'm really doubting that constantly monitoring my thoughts and doing thought records make a whole lot of sense for me.

THERAPIST: Oh, okay. I'm really glad you brought this up, as your outlook on therapy is so central to it working. I can appreciate that the thought records are not for everyone and seem off the mark for you. Am I capturing that accurately?

PATIENT: Yeah, definitely not feeling those. Generally speaking, I don't think that I "distort" any more than anyone else, so to me this thought process is not the cause of my worry.

THERAPIST: Right. So, to you, the idea that you think in extremes or distort reality doesn't really fit your experience. Thus, again, my trying to help you work on changing those thoughts would seem to be off base for you.

PATIENT: Exactly.

THERAPIST: Okay. Can you help me understand directions we could take that you might be more optimistic about, whether it's something that we have discussed so far, or some new focus altogether?

PATIENT: Sure. Actually, the idea of improving my ability to relax, especially during times that I worry a lot, made good sense to me. To me, the worry escalates not because of how I think, but because I'm unable to relax or destress effectively. Maybe we could skip right to that step! (*laughing*)

THERAPIST: Yes, that makes sense, and it actually fits nicely within the larger realm of CBT. Let's try it; however, I also invite you to keep expressing any additional concerns that might emerge openly and freely. Finding the things that work best for you and your life can be an ongoing process and one that I value greatly in my work.

A second example follows a 35-year-old patient, Renee, who demonstrated resistance because of underlying ambivalence about actually relinquishing her worry (as evidenced by CCT), despite wanting to eliminate the distress that followed its excessive and uncontrollable nature (as evidenced by CT). By attending to patient language and recognizing ambivalence as the cause of Renee's resistance, the CBT therapist departed to MI to validate this internal conflict, evoke Renee's emotional reaction to it, empathize with such emotion, and foster Renee's own autonomy and valued treatment direction (as a means to increasing her *internal* vs. *external* motivation to improve).

PATIENT: Let me start by acknowledging that I have missed a few sessions. I'm sorry, but to be honest, I'm not sure this is working. This treatment [CBT] focuses on essentially eliminating my worry, but I kind of depend on it . . . at least somewhat. I mean, as a nursing student, I need to stay on top of many, many things, and worrying kind of holds me accountable. I mean, it sucks to worry all the time, but I rarely let anyone down. So, in that sense, it's helpful too. I know you're right that worry is a problem for me, so I've been avoiding talking to you about this . . . quite literally by skipping our sessions!

THERAPIST: First, I really appreciate your openness; I imagine it wasn't easy to share with me.

PATIENT: No, I lost a little sleep over it. (*laughing*)

THERAPIST: Second, it must be so difficult to hold two strong, but competing, feelings at the same time. On the one hand, a lot of worrying does suck; but, on the other, it can also come in handy . . . especially for someone who has so many professional and personal responsibilities like you do. I wonder if you could say more about how this bind feels?

PATIENT: Well, it's tough. It can feel heavy and hopeless . . . like I have to accept that I will never feel truly calm if I am going to be successful in my career. Like it's one or the other—a peaceful but underachieving life or a worrisome yet successful one. (*becoming tearful*)

THERAPIST: (*after a pause*) When you put it like that, I can really sense that hopelessness. That's indeed a heavy burden to carry, and I can hear in your voice how hard this is for you.

PATIENT: It is, which is why I feel bad for missing sessions. I need to be in therapy. I need to get this worry at least somewhat under control, as it has kept me from having good relationships and from enjoying things that I know I inherently like.

THERAPIST: I completely understand; however, therapy, and me, also need to meet your needs and see both sides of the coin. I can see how it was not terribly useful for me to convince you only of the merits of reducing your worry when this symptom has actually served you well in some ways! I missed the mark on that, and you telling me this today is such an important step in our relationship.

PATIENT: Well, thanks for that. I feel better for having said it, but it was not easy.

THE INTERSECTION OF RESPONSIVENESS AND CULTURAL DIVERSITY

CRPI also accommodates cultural diversity (Goodwin et al., 2018). Notably, it is important to consider that not every resistance moment links straight-forwardly to perceptions of a treatment's credibility or ambivalence about change. Instead, resistance might indicate cultural misattunement. For example, a treatment, even when viewed as credible and relevant, might also be viewed as culturally limited or misaligned (e.g., in failing to incorporate family or spirituality), which might prompt a patient to dig in their heels. Or, it is possible that a therapist inadvertently says something insensitive regarding a patient's cultural identities, which could trigger an overt disagreement or subtle rupture.

In any of these scenarios, the nature of the resistance creates the need for a therapist's unique and culturally specific form of responsivity. For example, *if* resistance results from a disparity between a patient's cultural worldview (e.g., change only makes sense through the lens of family and/or faith) and a key feature of traditional CBT (i.e., individually focused revisions to intrapsychic thought processes), *then* a therapist may need to depart from tradition and gravitate toward personalization. And, in this case, simply using the aforementioned MI approach that targets a presumed ambivalence about change, lack of motivation, and/or a deferent interpersonal style (in an ostensibly responsive manner) would actually represent inappropriate and ineffectual responsiveness. Even when engaging the patient's resistance with a generally validating and supportive stance, unless the clinician made the connection to the cultural mismatch, the resistance will likely go unresolved. Instead, therapists could use a multicultural orientation to guide their responsiveness; namely, they can draw on the evidence-informed pillars of cultural humility (e.g., relinquishing one's sense of superiority by being open and curious toward the patient's identities), cultural opportunity (e.g., by attending to the contextual resistance as an opportunity to connect organically and demonstrate a willingness to learn from the patient), and cultural comfort (e.g., by exhibiting a sense of ease working with diverse others and their diversity-salient dynamics; Davis et al., 2016).

RESEARCH SUPPORTING CRPI ACROSS THE LIFESPAN

Here we focus on a few representative examples of *empirical* advances of responsivity across the lifespan of a treatment, including research specific to CBT.

Responsiveness as Getting Off on the Right Foot

Two meta-analyses have supported the need to assess and address patients' treatment beliefs as first-step responsivity. One statistical aggregation established an association between patients' greater early-therapy perception of treatment credibility and better posttreatment outcome (Constantino, Coyne, et al., 2018). The other established an association between patients' more positive presenting or early treatment OE and their posttreatment improvement, which was even stronger when therapists practiced according to a manual, a hallmark of CBT (Constantino, Vîslă, et al., 2018). Related to treatment selection, responsivity could be informed by research on treatment x patient aptitude interactions, including those which reveal an advantage of CBT over other options, or vice versa. For example, when taking into account patients' baseline interpersonal problems, standard and directive CBT may be less effective for patients who have pronounced problems of nonassertiveness; for these patients, it may be more helpful to use an integrative form of CBT for which the therapist is less directive and fosters more collaboration (Gomez Penedo et al., 2017).

Research has also supported the need to attend to patients' early motivational language. For instance, in one study for GAD, CBT patients with higher versus lower CT had a faster rate of worry reduction (Goodwin et al., 2019). Also, whether receiving CBT or CBT integrated with MI, CT was associated with a greater likelihood of clinically significant response, whereas more CCT was associated with a lower likelihood of response. This predictive validity of observer-coded language replicated previous studies that pointed to such language as a better clinical cue for existing motivation than patients' own self-report (e.g., Poulin et al., 2019). Finally, as previously discussed, initial responsiveness may need to heed the research that therapists possess relative strengths and weaknesses in treating different types of presenting problems, with past performance stably predicting future performance (e.g., Kraus et al., 2016). Such findings can be made actionable by stakeholders using provider performance indices to refer patients to clinicians with a known track record of stable efficacy in treating the primary problem(s) with which they present.

Responsiveness as Doing More of the Same

Some research also supports the notion that responsivity could involve doing more of the same once therapy is underway. For example, when an initial case formulation resonates with a patient, the more a therapist behaves in a way that is compatible with that formulation the better their outcome (Silberschatz, 2017). In addition, as we discussed, social psychological research on healthy, close relationships can translate to the clinical situation. For example, researchers have demonstrated an association between patients and their therapists perceiving their alliance quality more similarly over time and subsequent patient improvement, including in CBT (e.g., Coyne et al., 2018; Laws et al., 2017). Thus, with appropriate dyadic assessments, therapists can stay abreast of relational health and use it as a marker for staying the course when high.

Responsiveness as Clinical Departure

Although much more work is needed to understand how best to respond to waning treatment beliefs, some research has indicated that delivering (or revisiting) a clear treatment rationale that has persuasion elements, like emphasizing its broad impact on affect, cognition, and behavior, can help patients to see a treatment as more credible and to have a higher prognostic expectation for its personal helpfulness (Ametrano et al., 2017). However, where research has perhaps advanced the most with regard to informing departure relates to relational markers that manifest during the course of treatments like CBT. For example, our team showed that CBT integrated with MI (specifically to address moments of patient resistance) outperformed standard CBT over a 12-month follow-up (Westra et al., 2016). Moreover, over 75% of this effect was transmitted through MI-CBT promoting, as hypothesized, less observer-reported patient resistance (Constantino et al., 2019). Further underscoring this, when focusing on the CBT-only group, we found that even a small increase in naturally varying MI "spirit" during precise moments of patient–therapist disagreement had 10 times the influence on worry reduction than similar spirit displayed at randomly selected times (Aviram et al., 2016).

To us, this is what makes this *if-then* approach different from previous interpretations of common factors research. For example, one might suggest that based on a theoretical common factor like empathy (a key component of MI spirit) correlating with outcome, therapists need to be more empathic *in general*. But actually, work like Aviram and colleagues (2016) suggests that it is most important be empathic *when a patient disagrees with you* (i.e., an evidence-informed microadjustment to an observable dyadic process; again, right thing/right time). This notion squares with research on adjustments in CBT that are specifically used to address alliance ruptures. In another randomized trial that points to specific departure mechanisms, our team found that temporarily putting CBT strategies on the shelf and instead using interpersonal and humanistic repair strategies when a rupture marker was revealed was more effective in both process (patient ratings of alliance and therapist empathy) and outcome (depression reduction) than using traditional CBT measures straight through such process (Constantino et al., 2008).

Future Research Directions

Although research on responsiveness across the three lifespan elements exists to some level of maturity, it is fair to say that evidence-informed responsivity remains in its infancy. Thus, replication and extension are essential for continuing to clarify the precise *if/whens* and *then/hows* of responsiveness as getting off on the right foot, doing more of the same, or departing from the initial plan. Though future relevant research can take many guises, we spotlight two.

First, researchers can try to identify mechanisms of effective treatments that do or do not assimilate marker-driven departures. Although such departures can causally augment standard CBT's efficacy, we have also shown that there are mechanisms that explain why *standard* CBT can work well as is in some circumstances. For example, we found that, on average, standard CBT for GAD promoted more patient friendly compliance than MI-CBT, which in turn promoted better outcomes—a type of *competing indirect effect* to MI-CBT promoting less resistance that in turn fostered better outcomes (Coyne, Constantino, Westra, & Antony, 2019). Thus, people can derive therapy benefit in different ways (see Boswell & Bugatti, 2016). As stated throughout this chapter, sometimes it can help when a therapist embodies responsivity as continuing with a direction that the patient trusts, whereas sometimes it can help when a therapist embodies responsivity as going off-protocol

Second, it will be important to learn more about whether responsivity largely resides in the eye of the patient. If so, we need to know what patient characteristics predict it, so that clinicians can attempt to foster such factors with each of their patients to increase being experienced as responsive. Alternatively, responsivity might largely reside at the between-therapist level. In this case, we need to (a) discover therapist-level factors that determine responsiveness, (b) harness those factors, and (c) teach therapists to consistently draw on, or employ, them consistently across their patients. Most likely, though, we will learn that responsivity exists at the patient *and* therapist levels; consequently, we will need to appreciate that determinants of both between-patient and between-therapist effects may often coexist.

TRAINING IMPLICATIONS FOR MAXIMIZING THERAPIST RESPONSIVITY AND ATTUNEMENT

We believe that a major shift in training methods is needed. Rather than the historical focus on teaching trainees to *deliver* a finite number of named therapies that trainers evaluate on dimensions of integrity or skill, we see the need to teach trainees to *engage* in psychotherapy in all of its complex and contextualized glory. To this end, we still value teaching theory (e.g., the cognitive and behavioral underpinnings of CBT), and perhaps especially pathways to theoretical integration (e.g., ways in which interpersonal notions, like objective transference, can relate to cognitive and behavioral practice). However, we see this not in the service of establishing a preferred identity and orientation solely for oneself, such as experiencing a sense of mastery or feeding the self-conception that "I am a staunch cognitive behaviorist." Rather, we see learning such theories as being in the service of articulating a palette of treatment rationales to patients in a way that allows them to select which align best with their conceptualizations of their problems, human change, cultural identities, etc. Once selected, clinicians can then administer principle-based interventions that best align with those rationales, including with an off-on-the-right-foot and staying-the-course assist from existing manuals.

Most uniquely, though, training that aligns with CRPI would incorporate evidence-based teachings on how to attune (to markers) and adjust (via stances and behaviors) to patients' contextualized pathology and nondiagnostic characteristics, as well as to during-therapy experiences or relational interactions. In terms of how to execute such complementary teachings, we envision brief, focused workshops/in-services on marker recognition and therapist response sequences. Not only does this if-then learning paradigm promote cognitive uptake (Parks-Stamm & Gollwitzer, 2009), but it also allows for efficient lifelong learning (e.g., busy professionals tuning into 30-min trainings vs., say, weeklong workshops) of continually evolving content that mirrors the evolution of research on therapists' local adaptations to individual patients and their contexts (Constantino et al., 2017). Reshaping training toward these *bottom-up*, microresponsivity modules holds promise for improving our long-standing methods, as there is currently no evidence that therapist effectiveness improves with experience or following traditional *top-down* theoretical trainings (Tracey et al., 2014).

CONCLUSION

Although articulations of therapist competence have grown to include elements of adaptability, they typically suggest the idea of being pliable within the same overarching model (e.g., using more exposures in CBT vs. relying as heavily on Socratic questioning). In this chapter, we discussed a more encompassing form of responsivity, including departures from the overarching model (e.g., abandoning, at least temporarily, exposures and Socratic questioning to use MI spirit and strategy in the face of resistance or metacommunicating in the face of a cultural opportunity). With this broader focus on evidence-informed responsiveness, dissemination and implementation efforts would shift away from questions about how best to employ treatment packages in more naturalistic settings toward how best to track responsivity across the lifespan of a given case and to respond in ways that the evidence most supports at a given time. Of course, the evidence will evolve, thereby necessitating that dissemination and implementation efforts will constantly need to be reshaped. In this vein, as we revisit our identities, perhaps we are better classified not as psychotherapy integrationists, but as psychotherapy "contextualists" dedicated to the exploration, testing, and use of evidence-informed responsiveness and fluid treatment personalization.

REFERENCES

American Psychological Association. (2006). Evidence-based practice in psychology: APA Presidential Task Force on Evidence-Based Practice. *American Psychologist, 61*(4), 271–285. https://doi.org/10.1037/0003-066X.61.4.271

Ametrano, R. M., Constantino, M. J., & Nalven, T. (2017). The influence of expectancy persuasion techniques on socially anxious analogue patients' treatment beliefs and therapeutic actions. *International Journal of Cognitive Therapy*, *10*(3), 187–205. https://doi.org/10.1521/ijct.2017.10.3.187

Anderson, C., & Keltner, D. (2004). The emotional convergence hypothesis: Implications for individuals, relationships, and cultures. In L. Z. Tiedens & C. W. Leach (Eds.), *Studies in emotion and social interaction. The social life of emotions* (pp. 144–163). Cambridge University Press. https://doi.org/10.1017/CBO9780511819568.009

Aviram, A., Westra, H. A., Constantino, M. J., & Antony, M. M. (2016). Responsive management of early resistance in cognitive-behavioral therapy for generalized anxiety disorder. *Journal of Consulting and Clinical Psychology*, *84*(9), 783–794. https://doi.org/10.1037/ccp0000100

Boswell, J. F., & Bugatti, M. (2016). An exploratory analysis of the impact of specific interventions: Some clients reveal more than others. *Journal of Counseling Psychology*, *63*(6), 710–720. https://doi.org/10.1037/cou0000174

Boswell, J. F., & Schwartzman, C. M. (2018, August). An exploration of intervention augmentation in a single case. *Behavior Modification*. https://doi.org/10.1177/0145445518796202

Castonguay, L. G., Goldfried, M. R., Wiser, S., Raue, P. J., & Hayes, A. M. (1996). Predicting the effect of cognitive therapy for depression: A study of unique and common factors. *Journal of Consulting and Clinical Psychology*, *64*(3), 497–504. https://doi.org/10.1037/0022-006X.64.3.497

Constantino, M. J., Boswell, J. F., Bernecker, S. L., & Castonguay, L. G. (2013). Context-responsive integration as a framework for unified clinical science: Conceptual and empirical considerations. *Journal of Unified Psychotherapy and Clinical Science*, *2*(1), 1–20.

Constantino, M. J., Coyne, A. E., Boswell, J. F., Iles, B. R., & Vîslă, A. (2018). A meta-analysis of the association between patients' early perception of treatment credibility and their posttreatment outcomes. *Psychotherapy*, *55*(4), 486–495. https://doi.org/10.1037/pst0000168

Constantino, M. J., Coyne, A. E., & Gomez Penedo, J. M. (2017). Contextualized integration as a common playing field for clinicians and researchers: Comment on McWilliams. *Journal of Psychotherapy Integration*, *27*(3), 296–303. https://doi.org/10.1037/int0000067

Constantino, M. J., Marnell, M. E., Haile, A. J., Kanther-Sista, S. N., Wolman, K., Zappert, L., & Arnow, B. A. (2008). Integrative cognitive therapy for depression: A randomized pilot comparison. *Psychotherapy*, *45*(2), 122–134. https://doi.org/10.1037/0033-3204.45.2.122

Constantino, M. J., Vîslă, A., Coyne, A. E., & Boswell, J. F. (2018). A meta-analysis of the association between patients' early treatment outcome expectation and their posttreatment outcomes. *Psychotherapy*, *55*(4), 473–485. https://doi.org/10.1037/pst0000169

Constantino, M. J., Westra, H. A., Antony, M. M., & Coyne, A. E. (2019). Specific and common processes as mediators of the long-term effects of cognitive-behavioral therapy integrated with motivational interviewing for generalized anxiety disorder. *Psychotherapy Research*, *29*(2), 213–225. https://doi.org/10.1080/10503307.2017.1332794

Cox, J. R., Martinez, R. G., & Southam-Gerow, M. A. (2019). Treatment integrity in psychotherapy research and implications for the delivery of quality mental health services. *Journal of Consulting and Clinical Psychology, 87*(3), 221–233. https://doi.org/10.1037/ccp0000370

Coyne, A. E. (2016). The alliance: Recovering the dyad and deconstructing its parts. *The Integrative Therapist, 2*(4), 10–12. https://cdn.ymaws.com/www.sepiweb.org/resource/resmgr/Integrative_Therapist/Integrative_Therapist-v2-4.pdf

Coyne, A. E., Constantino, M. J., Laws, H. B., Westra, H. A., & Antony, M. M. (2018). Patient–therapist convergence in alliance ratings as a predictor of outcome in psychotherapy for generalized anxiety disorder. *Psychotherapy Research, 28*(6), 969–984. https://doi.org/10.1080/10503307.2017.1303209

Coyne, A. E., Constantino, M. J., & Muir, H. J. (2019). Therapist responsivity to patients' early treatment beliefs and psychotherapy process. *Psychotherapy, 56*(1), 11–15. https://doi.org/10.1037/pst0000200

Coyne, A. E., Constantino, M. J., Westra, H. A., & Antony, M. M. (2019). Competing indirect effects in a comparative psychotherapy trial for generalized anxiety disorder. *Psychotherapy, 56*(4), 549–554. https://doi.org/10.1037/pst0000163

Davis, D. E., DeBlaere, C., Brubaker, K., Owen, J., Jordan, T. A., II, Hook, J. N., & Van Tongeren, D. R. (2016). Microaggressions and perceptions of cultural humility in counseling. *Journal of Counseling & Development, 94*(4), 483–493. https://doi.org/10.1002/jcad.12107

Elkin, I., Falconnier, L., Smith, Y., Canada, K. E., Henderson, E., Brown, E. R., & McKay, B. M. (2014). Therapist responsiveness and patient engagement in therapy. *Psychotherapy Research, 24*(1), 52–66. https://doi.org/10.1080/10503307.2013.820855

Eubanks, C. F., Muran, J. C., & Safran, J. D. (2018). Alliance rupture repair: A meta-analysis. *Psychotherapy, 55*(4), 508–519. https://doi.org/10.1037/pst0000185

Goldman, R. E., Hilsenroth, M. J., Owen, J. J., & Gold, J. R. (2013). Psychotherapy integration and alliance: Use of cognitive-behavioral techniques within a short-term psychodynamic treatment model. *Journal of Psychotherapy Integration, 23*(4), 373–385. https://doi.org/10.1037/a0034363

Gomez Penedo, J. M., Constantino, M. J., Coyne, A. E., Westra, H. A., & Antony, M. M. (2017). Markers for context-responsiveness: Client baseline interpersonal problems moderate the efficacy of two psychotherapies for generalized anxiety disorder. *Journal of Consulting and Clinical Psychology, 85*(10), 1000–1011. https://doi.org/10.1037/ccp0000233

Goodwin, B. J., Constantino, M. J., Westra, H. A., Button, M. L., & Antony, M. M. (2019). Patient motivational language in the prediction of symptom change, clinically significant response, and time to response in psychotherapy for generalized anxiety disorder. *Psychotherapy, 56*(4), 537–548. https://doi.org/10.1037/pst0000269

Goodwin, B. J., Coyne, A. E., & Constantino, M. J. (2018). Extending the context-responsive psychotherapy integration framework to cultural processes in psychotherapy. *Psychotherapy, 55*(1), 3–8. https://doi.org/10.1037/pst0000143

Hatcher, R. L. (2015). Interpersonal competencies: Responsiveness, technique, and training in psychotherapy. *American Psychologist, 70*(8), 747–757. https://doi.org/10.1037/a0039803

Katz, M., Hilsenroth, M. J., Gold, J. R., Moore, M., Pitman, S. R., Levy, S. R., & Owen, J. (2019). Adherence, flexibility, and outcome in psychodynamic treatment of depression. *Journal of Counseling Psychology, 66*(1), 94–103. https://doi.org/10.1037/cou0000299

King, B. R., & Boswell, J. F. (2019). Therapeutic strategies and techniques in early cognitive-behavioral therapy. *Psychotherapy*, *56*(1), 35–40. https://doi.org/10.1037/pst0000202

Kraus, D. R., Bentley, J. H., Alexander, P. C., Boswell, J. F., Constantino, M. J., Baxter, E. E., & Castonguay, L. G. (2016). Predicting therapist effectiveness from their own practice-based evidence. *Journal of Consulting and Clinical Psychology*, *84*(6), 473–483. https://doi.org/10.1037/ccp0000083

Laws, H. B., Constantino, M. J., Sayer, A. G., Klein, D. N., Kocsis, J. H., Manber, R., Markowitz, J. C., Rothbaum, B. O., Steidtmann, D., Thase, M. E., & Arnow, B. A. (2017). Convergence in patient–therapist therapeutic alliance ratings and its relation to outcome in chronic depression treatment. *Psychotherapy Research*, *27*(4), 410–424. https://doi.org/10.1080/10503307.2015.1114687

Miller, W. R., & Rollnick, S. (2013). *Motivational interviewing: Helping people change* (3rd ed.). Guilford Press.

Parks-Stamm, E. J., & Gollwitzer, P. M. (2009). Goal implementation: The benefits and costs of if–then planning. In G. B. Moskowitz & H. Grant (Eds.), *The psychology of goals* (pp. 362–391). Guilford Press.

Poulin, L. E., Button, M. L., Westra, H. A., Constantino, M. J., & Antony, M. M. (2019). The predictive capacity of self-reported motivation vs. early observed motivational language in cognitive behavioural therapy for generalized anxiety disorder. *Cognitive Behaviour Therapy*, *48*(5), 369–384. https://doi.org/10.1080/16506073.2018.1517390

Silberschatz, G. (2017). Improving the yield of psychotherapy research. *Psychotherapy Research*, *27*(1), 1–13. https://doi.org/10.1080/10503307.2015.1076202

Slade, K., Lambert, M. J., Harmon, S. C., Smart, D. W., & Bailey, R. (2008). Improving psychotherapy outcome: The use of immediate electronic feedback and revised clinical support tools. *Clinical Psychology & Psychotherapy*, *15*(5), 287–303. https://doi.org/10.1002/cpp.594

Stiles, W. B. (2013). The variables problem and progress in psychotherapy research. *Psychotherapy*, *50*(1), 33–41. https://doi.org/10.1037/a0030569

Stiles, W. B., & Horvath, A. O. (2017). Appropriate responsiveness as a contribution to therapist effects. In L. G. Castonguay & C. E. Hill (Eds.), *How and why are some therapists better than others? Understanding therapist effects* (pp. 71–84). American Psychological Association. https://doi.org/10.1037/0000034-005

Tracey, T. J. G., Wampold, B. E., Lichtenberg, J. W., & Goodyear, R. K. (2014). Expertise in psychotherapy: An elusive goal? *American Psychologist*, *69*(3), 218–229. https://doi.org/10.1037/a0035099

Wampold, B. E., & Imel, Z. E. (2015). *The great psychotherapy debate: The evidence for what makes psychotherapy work* (2nd ed.). Routledge. https://doi.org/10.4324/9780203582015

Webb, C. A., Derubeis, R. J., & Barber, J. P. (2010). Therapist adherence/competence and treatment outcome: A meta-analytic review. *Journal of Consulting and Clinical Psychology*, *78*(2), 200–211. https://doi.org/10.1037/a0018912

Westra, H. A., Constantino, M. J., & Antony, M. M. (2016). Integrating motivational interviewing with cognitive-behavioral therapy for severe generalized anxiety disorder: An allegiance-controlled randomized clinical trial. *Journal of Consulting and Clinical Psychology*, *84*(9), 768–782. https://doi.org/10.1037/ccp0000098

8 RESPONSIVENESS IN EMOTION-FOCUSED THERAPY

JEANNE C. WATSON

Responding to the tugs and pulls of different currents is essential in any treatment, but it is particularly so in emotion-focused therapy (EFT), with therapists navigating between providing the therapeutic relationship conditions and working with more active techniques. In this chapter, the concept of responsiveness in EFT will be explored, and a developmental model of the self, highlighting zones of proximal development, is presented to guide therapists' responsiveness (Watson & Greenberg, 2017). Additional micromarkers and the qualities that inform responsiveness when working with clients from diverse backgrounds and multiple intersecting identities are discussed. The chapter concludes with some thoughts about the implications of responsiveness for research and training.

Stiles and Horvath (2017) suggested that responsiveness requires an active ongoing assessment of what the client needs in the moment and overall, as therapists attempt to find the right response. This requires therapists to be flexible and open to changing direction. As they attune and attend with sensitivity in the moment, experiential therapists work to effectively tailor their treatments to their clients' cognitive and affective states (Kramer &

https://doi.org/10.1037/0000240-009
The Responsive Psychotherapist: Attuning to Clients in the Moment, J. C. Watson and H. Wiseman (Editors)

Stiles, 2015). This calls for high levels of mastery and expertise as therapists synthesize knowledge from a number of different sources and across different timelines (see Chapters 1 and 2 of this volume). Responsive therapists are fully alive and present with their clients, letting go of their own concerns and conflicts, to mobilize all their resources to focus on what the client is bringing to the session. It is this quality of presence that Rogers (1980), in his later writings, characterized as the essence of an empathic, accepting, prizing, and genuine therapeutic relationship and is an essential aspect of EFT (Geller & Greenberg, 2012).

DEFINITION AND CONCEPTUALIZATION OF RESPONSIVENESS IN EFT

Like the other therapeutic conditions identified by Rogers (1957), responsiveness can be conceptualized as an attitude or a way of being with another that is characterized as a willingness or capacity to be flexible and fluid. Like responsive caretakers (Wade et al., 2018), responsive therapists are constantly assessing and adjusting to their clients' needs and states of readiness. They are carefully attuned to what is happening with their clients in the moment, while attending to their experience within the session and over time. Responsiveness in EFT is characterized by thoughtful, caring responses drawing on a deep empathic understanding of the client. However, it is more than empathy, because as therapists constantly attune to understand and track their clients' experiences, they are adjusting and modulating their responses as they attend to feedback from their clients and assess how best to respond.

To better understand the process of being responsive, five expert experiential therapists were interviewed about their experience at moments of optimal responsiveness in the session. They reported that they were aware of actively *tracking* and *following* their clients and carefully *attuning* and *assessing* how to respond most appropriately at these moments. They drew on their knowledge of the client and their treatment methods as well as their own theoretical and personal knowledge to find the "right response." They were aware of balancing the needs and goals of the client with their treatment methods, their moment-by-moment observations, their place in the treatment trajectory, their assessment of the quality or state of the therapeutic alliance, and the interpersonal pulls they experienced in the session. This delicate balancing act is informed by different markers that provide clues about clients' emotional processing capacity, the quality of their self-organizations, the completeness and coherence of their narratives and their attachment histories, as well as their sense of autonomy and mastery. All of this information and possibly more that is beyond conscious awareness (Schore, 2003) informs EFT therapists' responsiveness.

Tracking and Following

The emphasis on tracking and following the client's direction in EFT is rooted in the writings of Rogers (1980) and other experiential psychotherapists, in which they emphasize the therapeutic attitudes of empathy, acceptance, warmth, and genuineness. Experiential therapists try to convey these attitudes as they empathically follow what their clients are sharing and continuously test their understandings with them using empathic reflections. EFT therapists try to support clients' autonomy, seeing them as active self-healers. They trust and believe that clients' inner organismic tendency will enable them to self-right given the right conditions (Bohart & Tallman, 1996; Tallman & Bohart, 1999).

Empathically tracking and following clients requires therapists to maintain high levels of concentration and perceptive attention to listen to their clients' narratives, distill the essence of their experience, and continuously check their understanding with their clients. The process of distilling and checking understanding maintains contact with the client and guides the therapist to make minute corrections to maintain connection and guard against veering off course. These small corrections to keep aligned with the client moment to moment in the session characterize one facet of responsiveness in EFT.

Therapists' empathic following and reflecting what their clients are saying not only demonstrates that they are listening and trying to remain connected, but it also provides both participants with the opportunity to reflect on what the client has said and to evaluate and adjust if necessary. For example,[1] one therapist recalled that the small window of time that was provided as she reflected back her understanding to the client allowed her to assess and adjust her response. Her client had described all the people who had abandoned her while she was growing up, including her sisters, her mother, and a grandfather, the one person on whom she had been able to rely for support and comfort, who passed away suddenly. Since his death, she had been unable to grieve and express her sadness. Within an EFT model, the losses she identified are markers of unfinished business that might prompt a therapist to suggest an empty chair dialogue to allow the expression and resolution of some negative feelings about being abandoned. Usually after suggesting an empty chair

---

[1]The identities of the clients in this chapter's case examples have been disguised to protect client confidentiality.

task, therapists ask their clients to choose with whom they would like to dialogue in the empty chair. However, in this case as the therapist began to formulate her response, she recalled how the client had teared up at mention of her grandfather. Acutely aware that this was a single session, the therapist thought it might be easier for the client to work with a significant other who had provided love and support, did not intentionally abandon her, and whose memory had evoked tears. Thus, midsentence, the therapist changed course and specifically asked the client if she would like to work with her grandfather. After expressing some hesitation about talking about her feelings, but reiterating her goal to be more expressive and open, the client agreed.

This example shows the therapist deciding, in the moment, to modify her usual way of working to accommodate her emerging understanding of the client, including the clients' nonverbal behavior, the nature and timing of the session, as well as her understanding of the specific technique that was being suggested. What stood out for the therapist was that by taking the time to reflect back to the client what she had heard, she had a split second to reflect on and modify her response. The space and the opportunity to slow down reactions that is afforded by active listening dialogues has long been recognized as useful in couples therapy, enabling people to modulate their emotions and facilitate greater understanding (Hendrix, 2007). In the preceding example, it provided a useful way for the therapist to recalibrate during a session to be more attuned and responsive to the client.

Actively Attuning and Assessing

Attuning in the moment is an active process as therapists watch their clients attentively, try to sense what they are feeling, and listen for poignancy as thresholds to pain (Elliott et al., 2004). In the process of attuning, experiential therapists' sense into their client's experiences and are aware of their own reactions as they resonate with what their clients are sharing. They attend to indicators of pain and distress as revealed by clients' verbal and nonverbal behaviors including body language, voice, and language use, their own bodily felt sense, and how they are resonating with their client's experiences as well as their personal reactions in the moment (Watson, 2007).

As they attune and become aware of different pulls, experiential therapists actively assess what the best response might be for their clients in the moment, especially at times when their clients are distressed, hesitant, reluctant, or at odds with them about specific techniques. The therapists who were interviewed noted that when they sensed distress or hesitation and reluctance in their clients, they would slow down and actively question what their clients needed in that moment. They would question where they should focus their attention as they searched for a fitting response. They consciously tried to balance their assessment of the therapeutic alliance with their clients' attachment histories and the interpersonal pulls that they were experiencing, along with their techniques. This balancing act can be supported by experiential therapists working within clients' zones of proximal development (TZPD), including emotional processing capacity, self-organizations, and level of differentiation. These skills or capacities can be fostered in psychotherapy and are necessary to engage productively in the process to enhance functioning.

Leiman and Stiles (2001) suggested that to be optimally responsive, therapists should try to work within clients' therapeutic zone of proximal development (TZPD). Applying the concept of specific ZPDs in EFT, Watson and Greenberg (2017) recently proposed a developmental model of the self that includes four capacities that form and develop across the lifespan as individuals grow toward maturity and that, if stalled or are underdeveloped as a result of adverse circumstances, may be fostered in psychotherapy. These capacities include clients' ability to *process and regulate their emotions*, the quality of their *self-organizations*, their *understanding* of their lived experience as reflected in the completeness and coherence of their narratives, and their interpersonal process, including their capacity to be optimally *differentiated* from others, *agentic*, and *self-governing*. These theorists posit that to thrive, people need to be able to process and regulate their organismic and affective experience, develop positive self-organizations, make sense of their experience, and establish relationships with others that balance their needs for connection, autonomy, and agency. Some of the primary tasks in EFT are focused on fostering these capacities, including focusing, chair dialogues, empathic reflections, and systematic evocative unfolding, as discussed below.

TASK MARKERS TO ENHANCE RESPONSIVENESS IN EFT

An important way that EFT therapists align with their clients' goals and demonstrate responsiveness in the moment is with the identification of specific tasks based on different problem statements shared by clients (Rice & Greenberg, 1984). Markers and the pathway to resolve different problem states have been described and modelled using task analysis. These models provide maps to therapists to alert them to moments when clients may be ready to work on specific issues and illuminate the experiential questions their clients are posing to guide exploration. Markers of problem states include, among others, negative self-statements reflective of negative self-organizations or statements of unfinished business indicating compromised differentiation of self and other. A primary focus of the different tasks is to heighten clients' emotions in the session, to facilitate their access to and awareness of their subjective experiencing, so that it can be symbolized and relevant needs identified in order to change behavior and resolve problematic issues, for example, increasing emotional processing capacity to facilitate understanding and modulation of emotion, or increasing self-compassion and self-acceptance as antidotes to negative and critical voices.

While these tasks help to facilitate therapists' responsiveness, if used in a rote and mechanical manner, they can be experienced by clients as overly controlling and directive. In addition, when markers emerge and clients are hesitant or resistant to engage in chair work or focus inwardly on their feelings, therapists may feel frustrated, self-critical, and hopeless as their efforts seem blocked. These negative feelings can serve as an indication to therapists that they are out of alignment with their clients. To try to ensure collaboration and maintain alignment, EFT therapists frame the problems and propose tasks tentatively while attending closely to how their clients respond. For example, a therapist might ask, "Feelings of resentment seem to emerge whenever we speak of your brother, is that so?" or "It seems to me that you are very self-critical, does that fit for you?" If clients agree with the proffered formulation, therapists can suggest a specific task to address it more explicitly. However, if clients do not agree, responsive therapists attend to the feedback, step back, and continue to try to work toward a shared view of the problem.

When clients are reluctant or hesitant, therapists' primary aim should be to better understand their client's perspective. Questions therapists might ask themselves at these times include, "How come the frame does not fit?" "Does the client feel self-conscious?" "Is the client scared that they will lose voice by following my suggestions?" Each client concern will call for a different response from the therapist and provide opportunities for open discussion about how clients see their problems and hopefully establish a shared view and better fit in terms of what the therapist can offer. Some clients, after discussing their concerns, may be willing to continue as their therapists suggest, while others may need their therapists to update their paradigm and gather more information to understand their clients' focus and align better with their goals. Stepping back and relinquishing control can assist therapists to get back on course and reconnect with their clients and allow the necessary time to reassess the timing and appropriateness of suggested tasks.

WORKING WITHIN CLIENTS' TZPD IN EFT

Even with task maps that illuminate when and how to intervene at specific times, EFT therapists can feel challenged if their clients do not move through the different stages of each task smoothly and easily. Moments when clients are unable to proceed through a specific stage of a task can indicate to therapists that they are working outside their clients' TZPD, including their clients' emotional processing capacity, their self-organizations, their understanding of their lived experience, and the level of differentiation between self and other. To be optimally responsive, EFT therapists adjust and scaffold their interventions to their clients' level of functioning or TZPD. Each of these capacities is elaborated further below with examples that indicate when therapists and clients are outside the latter's TZPD, and alternative ways of responding are suggested.

Emotional Processing and Regulation

EFT theorists emphasize the importance of emotional processing in therapy. An important objective in experiential therapy is to enhance clients' emotional processing capacity and modulation so that they can better meet their needs, feel more confident overall, and deal more effectively with their environments. Effective emotional processing and regulation may be broken down into a number of steps (Gratz & Roemer, 2004; Greenberg, 2007; Watson et al., 2011): first, the capacity to attend inwardly to the body and become aware of emotions as distinct from other physiological states such as hunger or tiredness; second, the capacity to symbolize and express these feelings using labels, images, and metaphors; third, the capacity to modulate levels of inner arousal and the expression of emotions; and fourth, the capacity to reflect on feelings to solve problems in living in order to survive and thrive. These capacities or skills are developed both implicitly and explicitly in interpersonal environments, particularly with caretakers (Schore, 2003). This type of learning also occurs in therapy, sometimes explicitly and often implicitly. In EFT, therapists empathically reflect their clients' experience and attune to their affect, as clients turn their attention inward, become aware of and try to symbolize their affective experience and bodily felt sense, and develop ways of regulating it more effectively (Elliott et al., 2004; Rogers, 1957; Schore, 2003). As they explore their experiences, the emotion schemes that inform clients' behaviors become apparent as does their role in creating problems in the present. Clients acquire an understanding of the origin of those schemes and process their experiences, which includes developing an understanding of their life histories to make sense of experience, symbolizing and expressing the emotional impact of events, identifying their needs and goals, and modifying them to support their aims and goals in relationship with a supportive, empathic other.

When clients' emotional processing capacity is underdeveloped, experiential therapists try to foster it using empathic responding as well as specific techniques such as focusing (Gendlin, 1982). This technique actively teaches clients to focus on their organismic experience, to increase their awareness of their bodies and facilitate the symbolization of their bodily felt sense. The capacity to attend to the body and represent feelings and express them is foundational to other experiential techniques, including chair dialogues, systematic evocative unfolding, and relational dialogues (Elliott et al., 2004; Greenberg et al., 1993). If clients have difficulty accessing and expressing what they feel in any of these other tasks or techniques, therapists may need to step back and work to develop clients' awareness of their organismic experience, tolerance of their emotions, as well as their capacity to symbolize and label their organismic experience. In this process, as therapists respond empathically, clients acquire the skills to modulate their levels of arousal and expression and make sense of their experience in the context of a positive therapeutic relationship characterized by empathy, acceptance, prizing, and genuineness.

Developing Positive Self-Organizations

In his personality theory, Rogers (1959) observed that people develop self-concepts partly based on introjected conditions of worth from interactions with significant others and their environments. These shape a person's sense of self-esteem and confidence. In addition, attachment theorists and interpersonal theorists (Benjamin, 1974; Sullivan, 1947) suggest that how others, particularly caretakers, respond to us affects how we process our affective experience and relate to ourselves and others. Thus, whether we relate positively with acceptance, warmth, and concern or negatively with control and indifference to our feelings and emotions is rooted in our attachment experiences. One way that EFT addresses problems with negative self-organizations and the negative ways that clients relate to themselves and their experience is with two-chair dialogues (Greenberg et al., 1993; Watson & Greenberg, 2017).

However, clients and therapists can be challenged at different stages in the resolution of two-chair dialogues. For example, when working in two chairs to address negative treatment of self (e.g., self-criticism or self-silencing), clients are asked to express negative statements to an imagined self to activate an emotional response in the "experiencing chair." The process of activating emotions in the experiencing chair requires clients to be aware of, tolerate, and label their experience. However, if this emotional processing capacity is underdeveloped, clients may collapse and be unable to respond effectively to the critic. This is a clear marker that therapists are working outside clients' TZPD in terms of their emotional processing capacity. Recognizing this, therapists may need to change direction and focus on working with their clients to increase their emotional processing capacity, including awareness and tolerance of their emotions and the capacity to symbolize them and express them in words, using a mix of empathic responding, focusing tasks, and narrative reconstruction.

Another stage in two-chair work when clients' capacities may be challenged is when the critical or negative side fails to soften or respond to the pain and needs that have been expressed in the experiencing chair. Softening requires reserves of self-compassion and self-acceptance. However, if clients have strong negative self-organizations with underdeveloped positive introjects and ways of treating the self, then they may be unable to soften into compassion and self-acceptance. This can be a cue to therapists to refocus their efforts to provide the relationship conditions and encourage and support their clients to internalize the therapeutic attitudes of empathy, acceptance, and positive regard (Watson & Greenberg, 2017; Watson et al., 2007). One way to facilitate this is by continuing to explore clients' experiences, working with them to develop their understanding of how they were impacted along with supporting clients to develop enhanced emotional processing capacity in the context of an empathic, accepting, and warm relationship. In addition, experiential therapists try to scaffold the development of self-compassion using self-soothing dialogues, "clearing a space," and psychoeducation. Building more positive self-organizations is essential if clients are to successfully resolve two-chair dialogues and transform negative ways of treating the self. Once this foundational work has taken root, then they can once again work with two-chair dialogues to foster more compassionate, protective, and nurturing ways of being with the self.

Making Sense of Experience: The Role of Clients' Narratives

Stories make sense of experience. People describe experiences to know and understand them better and to see what is salient and meaningful for them. Naming and describing experience enables them to apprehend their environments and together with their affective experience respond effectively to meet the demands of their environment and their personal needs. Stories are informed by our memories and life histories. However, memories and the consolidation of life experiences are highly sensitive to stress, and some life experiences and early environments may not support their formation and consolidation, resulting in confusion, misunderstanding, and anxiety (Sapolsky, 2004; Schore, 2019).

One way that experiential therapists assess their clients' narratives is in terms of their completeness and coherence (Angus & Greenberg, 2011). One marker of incompleteness that is salient for experiential therapists is when clients spend hours describing and detailing the events and interactions in their lives without fully accounting for feelings or transforming their experience. Having clients circle "the same old story" can be experienced as repetitive and frustrating. Therapists may become impatient and critical as they listen to clients revisit painful and challenging life experiences and express reluctance to engage in other tasks, such as chair dialogues, to resolve painful feelings. However, clients' circling of the same material may be a useful signal for therapists to be more responsive and reassess their clients' TZPD in terms of their understanding or representation of what has happened to them.

Some clients may be searching to symbolize their experience more fully. They may feel that aspects of their experience have not been adequately represented, or an aspect of experience and its impact have not been symbolized. Some clients may need to revisit old ground and continue to share their stories, to build the neural connections that will enable them to consolidate memories and experiences to understand themselves and their world in a different way. At times when clients seem stuck, it can be helpful for therapists to remember that the creation of neural connections may require several firings to reach necessary thresholds (Sapolsky, 2004). Alternatively, clients' circling the same material may reflect a lack of trust in their perceptions and/or experience, and it is only with continual validation and attention to it that they will be able to trust themselves, their feelings, and their perceptions. When they are feeling frustrated, therapists may need to slow down, to fall in line with their clients' pace, until the latter feel more confident and trusting of their perceptions and reactions and able to stride forth more quickly and confidently. Once clients feel more trusting of themselves, the process will flow as they actively change how they present and respond to painful experiences.

New understandings can emerge as clients elaborate their narratives. The revised understandings and new information they acquire often make it easier to see the triggers of their pain and the maladaptive emotion schemes that are driving some of their experiences in the present (Greenberg et al., 1993; Rogers, 1959). Armed with this information and engaging in the necessary emotional processing, they can learn ways to effectively modulate and soothe their emotions. This, in turn, will enable them to build trust and confidence in themselves and their therapists as they develop a greater sense of agency and self-regulation while becoming more hypothetical in their interpretation of events.

Differentiating Self and Other and Becoming Self-Regulating

Developing the capacity to self-regulate and become autonomous and differentiated from others while maintaining connection is an essential aspect of a mature organism. This capacity is supported and fostered in EFT. As clients change their negative self-organizations, they begin to relate differently to others. They are able to be more self-accepting and self-protective. A better balance between the needs of self and the needs of others is achieved, as clients become more compassionate toward themselves and assertive with others. In the process of differentiation they become more responsible for self and more effectively self-governing such that they attend to their needs and try to meet them and are able to attend better to the needs of others.

Times when clients are unable to fully resolve empty chair dialogues or are unable to fully integrate the needs of the experiencing chair and the negative side in two-chair dialogues may be an indication that they need to develop more confidence in themselves, their feelings, and their perceptions as well as develop confidence in their ability to take care of themselves and meet their needs. The capacity to be self-governing and fully responsible for self and other is another TZPD to which experiential therapists are sensitive. Patience is required as they work with their clients to build this capacity so that the latter can fully resolve empty chair dialogues, differentiate from significant others, and engage autonomously and independently in the world with the strength and confidence to meet their needs in interaction with others. To be optimally responsive, experiential therapists recognize and respond appropriately to clients' varying TZPD to facilitate their goals and objectives for therapy and enable them to thrive. This requires understanding and patience so that clients do not feel pushed or coerced to respond in specific ways and therapists do not feel defeated and hopeless when their clients do not respond as the task maps indicate they should at different stages of the process toward resolution. Being aware of and sensitive to clients' TZPD can help experiential therapists remain on track and stay attuned to their clients as they recognize these developmental markers.

MICROMARKERS FOR THERAPISTS' RESPONSIVENESS

In addition to attending to specific task markers as well as clients' TZPD, experiential therapists attend to other micromarkers to guide them moment to moment. These include clients' emotions; their expressions of pain and distress; their nonverbal behaviors and feedback; as well as therapists' reactions in the moment, their sense of felt flow, and their assessment of the therapeutic relationship and the interpersonal pulls they experience with clients.

Emotions

EFT emphasizes that emotions serve as a compass to alert therapists to clients' pain and draw attention to what is salient to clients' moment-to-moment in the session as well as highlight the experiences that need to be processed.

Rice (1974) observed that the poignancy of clients' language serves as a portal to their emotional experience in the session. To attune to poignancy, EFT therapists attend to the images and metaphors clients use as well as their idiosyncratic use of language (Elliott et al., 2004; Watson, 2015). EFT therapists may heighten clients' emotions to assist clients to process them in the session. Alternatively, they may work with empathic responding or self-soothing tasks if clients feel too overwhelmed.

Clients' Expressions of Pain and Distress

Responding to expressions of pain and distress is common to the human experience more generally, especially in relationships characterized by care and protection (e.g., parents and children, doctors and patients), and it is central to being optimally responsive in EFT. Experiential therapists attend to the painful memories that clients recall as well as clients' facial expressions of pain, including sadness, shame, fear, rejection, and injury. They acknowledge their clients' distress and acknowledge these moments of intense vulnerability with empathic validation and prizing (Greenberg et al., 1993). Experiential therapists' responsiveness to pain not only provides clients with the opportunity to process painful experiences but also provides soothing in the moment, as it reduces clients' levels of arousal and allows for new interpersonal learnings and corrective experiences to occur to transform the pain and forge new ways of relating to self and other.

Clients' Nonverbal Behavior

Other micromarkers that alert experiential therapists to be responsive include clients' voice, posture, and facial expressions. Experiential therapists listen to changes in clients' vocal quality to alert them to moments that require attention. For example, they listen for breaks in speech, hesitation, hoarseness, or soft raggedness that might convey emotion or the emergence of a new felt sense (Elliott et al., 2004; Rice, 1965). In addition to vocal characteristics, EFT therapists attend to their clients' facial expressions, for example, when eyes crinkle or tear up, or expressions of surprise, pain, or despair. They also watch their clients' body movements—their slumping or upright postures, shallow breathing, or the position of their hands and feet—to alert them to moments of pain and vulnerability. They attend to whether the different nonverbal cues are consistent with clients' narratives and what they are sharing in the moment or are incongruent to assess clients' readiness to engage in treatment as well as their emotional processing capacity in the moment.

At these moments, EFT therapists tentatively mirror and reflect their clients' nonverbal behavior, for example, by asking, "Is that tears I see?" or "Your face looks sad, is that what you are feeling?" Responding in this manner can validate feelings that may not be in awareness or fully expressed. Being responsively attuned to clients' affective communications is an important way of remaining connected with them in the session, demonstrating presence and responsiveness in the moment, and encouraging clients to deepen their emotional processing. However, there may be times when clients are not open to exploring these aspects of experience. They may feel too vulnerable or be unwilling to confront painful experiences at that time. At these moments, experiential therapists change course and pull back following their clients' lead, trusting that clients will return, if and when they are ready to explore those aspects of experience that are outside awareness. The choice is theirs and is respected.

Attending to Client Feedback

Experiential therapists continually watch how clients respond to their suggestions, reflections, reframes, questions, etc. Client feedback may be either verbal or nonverbal. Verbal feedback can be clear, for example, the client who responds that there are not two parts of the self, only one part that expects them to excel, after the therapist has proposed that there is a conflict between one side that needs rest and another that wants to achieve. Another example is when a client insists that the therapist use the former's words exactly when they are reflecting back their understanding of what the client said. Therapists may experience this request as controlling. However, if the therapist can step back and try to understand the client's aims and needs, it may be easier to adjust. By shifting perspective, the therapist might recognize that the client has great difficulty maintaining a sense of self and experiences the use of different words as intrusive, deflecting them from their own experience. Sensitive to their clients' needs and attachment histories, experiential therapists try to work within their clients' TZPD and what they can tolerate moment to moment, while remaining attentive and alert to those moments when their clients may be ready to move to the next level and be open and receptive to a more differentiated therapist response.

Clients' feedback can be negative or positive. Examples of positive feedback include smiling and looking relieved, lighter, and less worried. They continue to elaborate their experiences while nodding their heads in recognition and agreement, or they readily engage with their therapists' suggestions. These behaviors are in sharp contrast to negative feedback, times when clients shake their heads, go quiet, pull back, look shut down or defeated, or seem impatient, irritated, or hostile. Positive responses provide therapists with feedback that their clients are experiencing them as responsive and helpful and confirm that they are on the right track, while negative responses require therapists to become more self-reflective, to reassess and attend to what is happening. At times, therapists may defer to clients' requests to stop engaging in chair work, or, alternatively, therapists might inquire about what is transpiring in the moment and talk about the relationship and what they are doing more explicitly to see if they can come to a better understanding and agreement about the work of therapy (see Chapter 4 by Eubanks et al. in this volume; see also Safran et al., 2011; Watson & Greenberg, 1995).

Being responsive may not always mean accommodating to the client in the moment. Sometimes, therapists may decide to challenge clients' feedback and objections to address an agreed-on goal of therapy or to encourage them to view their situation differently. For example, one therapist spoke about challenging a client to consider that a major life-threatening illness provided him with the opportunity to do "a reckoning of his life." The client had engaged in self-defeating patterns for many years, and his therapist was trying to encourage him to let go of these behaviors and to find more satisfying ways of being in the world as he faced the threat of a terminal illness. The client framed the goal of therapy as an opportunity to review his life, which his therapist challenged, saying, "No, it is a reckoning, providing you with the opportunity to change your behavior and heal," at which point the client paused and then agreed. It is important to note that this confrontation followed a prior session in which the client had said how much he appreciated his therapist challenging him and encouraging him to take risks and requested that he continue to do this as they progressed in treatment.

Therapists' Reactions

At moments of optimal responsiveness, experiential therapists said they attended to their own feelings to alert them to clients' needs and to guide them in the moment. Therapists attend to two different types of responses: first, how they resonate with their clients' experiences, and second, their own more personal reactions, both positive and negative. Experiential therapists try to resonate with their clients' experience as they actively imagine their clients' stories. Their personal responses and reactions can illuminate aspects of the story not fully elaborated and provide clues to what their clients might be feeling. Therapists attend to their own bodily reactions, aware that they can sense their clients' feelings, for example, hostility or sadness, sometimes before they are named, enabling them to be more responsive in the moment (Watson, 2007).

Therapists also attend to their negative and positive reactions in the session. They recognize that negative feelings can be a sign that they need to be more responsive and attuned to their clients' experience. Negative feelings of boredom, irritation, and helplessness can be important indicators that they are off track and need to realign with their clients. Therapists also attend to their positive feelings to navigate their relationships with their clients and remain responsive in the moment. One therapist shared that he would attend to his own feelings of acceptance or rejection to gauge whether he was being received by clients. He observed that when he felt feelings of acceptance he would continue on track, while feelings of rejection would inform him that he should let go, change course, and check in with his client. While trusting in one's perceptions and senses is important, these should nonetheless be held and offered tentatively so as not to override clients' feedback and view of what is happening.

Felt Flow

Experiential therapists attend to the felt flow of the relationship. They assess whether the flow feels smooth or rough. This includes assessing whether their clients are open and engaged or hesitant and reluctant to share their experiences and focus on certain issues. Clients' feedback and reactions as described previously contribute to the felt flow. As therapists begin to establish a treatment framework, the flow can be choppy with the stop-and-go quality of rush-hour traffic. When things are smooth, clients respond positively, actively nodding and saying yes when therapists get it right and when therapists' responses fit their experience. There is little hesitation except for moments of productive silence or deep reflection. For therapists there is a sense of being in the "zone." However, when things are rough, clients are hesitant, express reluctance to engage in tasks, refuse to disclose information, and seem resistant or stuck. There is a sense that they are shut down and withdrawn from the interaction and the process. Some of these responses have been identified as alliance ruptures indicating a need for active repair (see Chapter 4 by Eubanks et al. in this volume; see also Watson & Greenberg, 1995), but they also alert therapists to the need to adjust and reassess the overall quality of the therapeutic relationship and how they are working with their clients, as well as clients' TZPD, and their working relational capacity to find a way to carry the work forward.

When clients demur and challenge therapists' suggestions, it can be useful for therapists to step back and try to realign with their clients, while taking time to reflect and reassess what is happening. For example, if the client disagrees with the therapist's suggestion that she is too self-critical and demanding of herself, this may indicate that they do not have a shared framework, or that the client is not attending to their organismic experience, or that they lack self-compassion, or all of the above. If this is the case, then the focus of work is to build a shared framework of the clients' problems, develop clients' capacities to be aware of and accept their organismic experience to process their emotions, or develop self-compassion and self-acceptance before moving on to engaging in more active techniques such as two-chair work.

Assessing the Relationship

Responsive therapists are constantly gauging the strength of the therapeutic relationship to determine when and how to intervene in therapy. Early in therapy, a therapist may be less inclined to address a clients' emotional processing style, waiting instead until the therapeutic relationship is formed before observing that a client silences or interrupts their emotions. For example, one therapist, seeing a client for the first time, was conscious of proceeding slowly. The client had come to therapy to mourn the death of his wife, which was amplified by the prior death of their daughter. After his wife's death, the client had immersed himself in his work to remain available for his patients. However, on retiring, he wanted to process his grief. As he shared his story, his therapist was aware of a "wall of silence" and that the client was practiced in putting up a brave front. However, she did not focus on his difficulty expressing his sadness and pain in the session, deciding instead to focus on building a strong therapeutic relationship before tackling the way he coped and processed his emotions. Later in therapy, when therapists are more confident about the relationship, they may be more active and introduce tasks more quickly.

Interpersonal Pulls

Experiential therapists are aware of clients' interpersonal pulls based on what is happening in the moment and assess these in terms of clients' attachment histories and relational capacity. Therapists attend to their own reactions in the moment, for example, feeling controlled or feeling vulnerable and at risk, and question what these feelings are about. In one case, a therapist recalled having the sense of wanting to protect herself and curl up into a ball in a session as she listened to her client describe her experience. This prompted her to ask the client to assume a position that would best fit her feelings in the moment. The client assumed the position of a fetus and curled up in the chair and began to cry. As she did this, the client became aware of feeling intensely vulnerable, experiencing the world as dangerous and overwhelming. Once the client acknowledged and expressed her feelings, her therapist was able to work with her to modulate and soothe them.

In another example, a client said she felt like she was drowning and experiencing a deep sense of hopelessness along with suicidal thoughts toward the end of the session. At that moment, the therapist felt a strong feeling to be protective along with an image of teaching her young children to swim in a lake. Aware that the client had a history of sexual abuse and was extremely sensitive to boundaries and being intruded upon, the therapist shared an image of her swimming nearby and said that she was there to support her if she needed it. She asked the client if she could see her in the water nearby. The client nodded and in the next session told her therapist how helpful and comforting the image had been. In this example we see the therapist actively synthesizing her understanding of her client across different domains as she found the optimal response to support her client in the moment and between sessions.

RESPONSIVENESS TO DIVERSITY IN EFT

Clients come to therapy with multiple identities and different life experiences that intersect and constitute each person's uniqueness. The complexity and uniqueness of each individual needs to be respected and valued in therapy. Fuertes et al. (2006) suggested that an in-depth understanding of clients' specific location within society includes sensitivity to issues of race, oppression, socioeconomic status, gender, sex, religion, as well as other sociopolitical forces. To acquire this understanding, therapists need to interrogate their assumptions and be aware of the multiple lived experiences of each client, including their joys and sorrows, their struggles and triumphs. Interrogating one's beliefs, attitudes, knowledge, and skills requires therapists to be sensitive, humble, open, and curious to all of their clients' experiences and to be sensitive to behaviors that might injure or silence others.

These attitudes are foundational to experiential practice; however, as human beings we are all subject to blind spots and to being limited by various frameworks, paradigms, and ways of viewing the world. To work effectively with diverse peoples, it is necessary to subject ourselves and our experiences to reflection and to be open and aware of the myriad ways that people can be injured and impacted by the various individuals and systems with which they come into contact, including families, friends, strangers, and cultural, political, and social institutions including schools, police, hospitals, the media, and the world at large. The lived experience of our clients might mean that our techniques are challenged and our ways of working experienced as foreign and unhelpful. At these times, it is important for experiential therapists, if they are to be responsive, to put their assumptions, tools, and ways of thinking aside and work toward a better understanding of their clients to explore their lived experience to collaborate effectively to realize their clients' goals in therapy.

KEY RESEARCH FINDINGS IN EXPERIENTIAL THERAPY

Schore (2019) proposed that the study of responsiveness requires a two-person research paradigm to identify how clients and therapists impact each other moment to moment in the session and over the course of psychotherapy. A growing number of studies have investigated the interaction between therapist and client using third-party ratings of in-session process. Sachse and colleagues showed that therapist processing proposals had an impact on the depth of clients' exploration (Sachse, 1990). Similarly, Adams and Greenberg (1996) found that clients were more likely to move to deeper levels of experiencing if their therapists directed attention to clients' inner experience at moments when they were externally focused. Toukmanian and colleagues found that therapists' empathy, attunement, and exploration were each associated with higher levels of client experiencing and client perceptual processing in the session (Gordon & Toukmanian, 2002). Taken together, these microanalytic studies suggest that the manner in which therapists respond to their clients exerts a significant influence in the session and can provide active assistance to support clients' processing efforts (Watson, 2018).

More recently, researchers have examined shifts in clients' narrative process in psychotherapy. Mendes et al. (2016), using the Assimilation of Problematic Experiences Scale (APES; Stiles, 2001), found that in a good outcome case the therapist used a "balanced strategy" such that either participant could change focus or direction in the session. Similarly, Ribeiro et al. (2016), studying a client who achieved a higher level on APES, found that the therapist used a balance of supportive and challenging interventions. In another study, Gonçalves et al. (2011) found that therapists' use of action skills was more often associated with clients' innovative moments or shifts in their narratives across all phases of therapy and especially in the final phase for good outcome clients. Studying moments of optimal responsiveness, when therapists respond to markers alerting them to alter course or attend differently, illuminates optimal interactional cycles in therapy from which we can derive principles of practice.

Other researchers have identified productive episodes of psychotherapy interaction and subjected them to study using task analysis. Rice and Greenberg (1984) used task analysis to analyze productive episodes in process-experiential psychotherapy to describe the actions of both client and therapist on a moment by moment basis to develop maps or models of change, including two-chair dialogues (Greenberg, 1984), systematic evocative unfolding (Rice & Saperia, 1984; Watson, 1996), and empty chair dialogues (Greenberg & Foerster, 1996). Subsequently, Safran and Muran (1996) used this method to study alliance ruptures and repair strategies (see Chapter 4 by Eubanks et al. in this volume). Moving forward, task analysis could be used to investigate optimal moments of responsiveness based on the markers that have been described in this and other chapters, with the objective of describing and developing models of client-therapist process that would provide procedural maps of positive interaction to inform theory and practice. In addition, it will be important to demonstrate the links between proximal and distal changes using sequential designs.

IMPLICATIONS FOR TRAINING

Responsiveness requires therapists to be flexible, fluid, and hypothetical in their formulations, to constantly assess and readjust what they are doing to fit clients' states of readiness. While this capacity to read and attune to others is rooted in empathy, being responsive is more than empathy as it requires careful tracking, attuning, and assessment to find the best response. Several therapist qualities that can be cultivated during training to enhance responsiveness include openness, humility, and the capacity to regulate negative affect. In addition, therapists can become more aware of their own nonverbal behavior including their postures, facial expressions, and vocal quality as well as their assumptions about the world and their place in it.

Openness

To be optimally responsive, therapists need to be open to their own and their clients' experiences. Therapists must be confident and curious enough to let go of their own worldviews and apprehend their clients' worlds. They must have a high tolerance for ambiguity and uncertainty so they can trust their clients' process even as they remain attentive to negative feedback and continue to navigate the process. A quality that has been identified as central to empathy is verbal fluency or the capacity not only to have quick access to varied ways of representing experiences but also the capacity to "break set" swiftly. This means being able to form new gestalts and understandings quickly and easily, and just as quickly to let them go and allow others to emerge and form. This quicksilver, malleable way of interacting, while remaining grounded and centered, may be the essence of being responsive in psychotherapy.

Humility

The capacity to be open and to break set and revise preconceptions requires a certain humility, a willingness to decenter from one's concerns and world-view and to be fully present with the client. At times this requires us to detach from our theories and ways of working as we try to be optimally responsive and work with clients in their singular and unique problem spaces. Sometimes, this may mean revisiting episodes of interpersonal interactions numerous times as clients try to find their way out of the forest, hacking their way through to clarity and understanding. At other times, it may mean saying sorry or acknowledging that we were wrong, off track, or too attached to a specific outcome. All of these are vulnerable and challenging experiences for therapists in the session with little support or opportunity to reflect in the moment. Some strategies therapists can use to attend to themselves to preserve their openness and presence in the moment include cultivating mindfulness as a practice, accessing peer support, acquiring strategies for self-care, and developing the ability to regulate negative affect (Geller & Greenberg, 2012).

Regulating Negative Affect

To be optimally responsive requires therapists to modulate their negative affect. As therapists we know that one of the quickest ways to silence another is to show distress or anxiety in the face of their pain. How many clients report feeling isolated, lonely, and shut down when a parent was unable to bear witness to their distress and offer support without becoming overly activated, taking charge, or disintegrating? Other negative feelings include lack of confidence in ourselves and our work. Feeling stuck and helpless can make us self-critical and impatient with clients. We may begin to question our effectiveness and view clients as difficult or resistant. Acquiring the skills to intercept these feelings and modulate them is vital to maintaining a positive therapeutic relationship and to remaining responsively attuned in the session. To modulate negative feelings, trainee therapists require the support of peers and mentors.

Therapists' Nonverbal Behavior

While much attention has been paid to identifying markers to guide therapists' responsiveness in the session, training needs to focus on how responsiveness is communicated. Communicating responsiveness includes facial expressions, whether of concern or indifference, expressiveness, or impassivity. Impassive expressions may leave clients feeling confused and uncertain that their pain is understood. Similarly, words are not always enough to convey concern. Words are supported by vocal tone. Using voices expressively, including variations in pitch, tempo, timbre, rhythm, tone, and color, can augment our techniques and ways of working so that they are experienced as responsive and caring. Training can be helpful to make trainees more aware of how they use their voices and teach them to vary the pitch, modulation, and rhythm of their voices while still remaining congruent and authentic in the moment. Trainee therapists need support and encouragement to cultivate these qualities so they can lay aside their need to be correct and helpful. Client-centered methods of responding are central to training responsive clinicians in EFT and provide a necessary foundation for all effective therapeutic work.

CONCLUSION

In this chapter, several ways of enhancing therapists' responsiveness in EFT were identified and discussed. The awareness and understanding of expert therapists, including their thoughts, feelings, and perceptions at moments when they were trying to be optimally responsive in the session, was described and illustrated. The activities of tracking, following, attending, and assessing were highlighted, as well as therapists' capacities to remain flexible and open in order to revise hypotheses and goals in line with clients' feedback and responses to specific treatment suggestions and techniques. EFT task markers to guide therapists' responses were described, and a model to assess clients' TZPD was provided as a framework to track clients' process overall in therapy and in the session in the context of specific task markers. The model of clients' TZPD alerts therapists to moments when they may need to scaffold their interventions and refocus their work to fit within their clients' therapeutic zones before they can move forward to resolve problematic issues. Attention to clients' TZPD can safeguard against feelings of frustration and helplessness when clients' process seems stalled. Additional micromarkers to guide moment-to-moment practice were identified, and ways to enhance responsiveness in training programs, taking account of clients' diversity along with directions for future research, were discussed. Given its essential role in all relationships, it is important that we continue to study responsiveness and highlight its role in psychotherapy to improve treatment outcomes.

REFERENCES

Adams, K. E., & Greenberg, L. S. (1996, June). Therapists' influence on depressed clients' therapeutic experiencing and outcome. Paper presented at the 43rd annual convention of the Society for Psychotherapeutic Research, St. Amelia, FL.

Angus, L. E., & Greenberg, L. S. (2011). *Working with narrative in emotion-focused psychotherapy: Changing stories, healing lives.* American Psychological Association.

Benjamin, L. S. (1974). Structural analysis of social behavior. *Psychological Review, 81*(5), 392–425. https://doi.org/10.1037/h0037024

Bohart, A. C., & Tallman, K. (1996). The active client: Therapy as self-help. *Journal of Humanistic Psychology, 36*(3), 7–30. https://doi.org/10.1177/00221678960363002

Elliott, R., Watson, J. C., Goldman, R. N., & Greenberg, L. S. (2004). *Learning emotion-focused therapy: The process-experiential approach to change.* American Psychological Association. https://doi.org/10.1037/10725-000

Fuertes, J. N., Stracuzzi, T. I., Bennett, J., Scheinholtz, J., Mislowack, A., Hersh, M., & Cheng, D. (2006). Therapist multicultural competency: A study of therapy dyads. *Psychotherapy: Theory, Research, & Practice, 43*(4), 480–490. https://doi.org/10.1037/0033-3204.43.4.480

Geller, S. M., & Greenberg, L. S. (2012). *Therapeutic presence: A mindful approach to effective therapy.* American Psychological Association. https://doi.org/10.1037/13485-000

Gendlin, E. T. (1982). *Focusing.* Bantam.

Gonçalves, M. M., Ribeiro, A. P., Mendes, I., Matos, M., & Santos, A. (2011). Tracking novelties in psychotherapy process research: The innovative moments coding system. *Psychotherapy Research, 21*(5), 497–509. https://doi.org/10.1080/10503307.2011.560207

Gordon, K., & Toukmanian, S. (2002). Is *how* it is said important? The association between quality of therapist interventions and client processing. *Counselling and Psychotherapy Research, 2*(2), 88–98. https://doi.org/10.1080/14733140212331384867

Gratz, K. L., & Roemer, K. (2004). Multidimensional assessment of emotion regulation and dysregulation: Development, factor structure, and initial validation of the Difficulties in Emotion Regulation Scale. *Journal of Psychopathology and Behavioral Assessment, 26*(1), 41–54. https://doi.org/10.1023/B:JOBA.0000007455.08539.94

Greenberg, L. S. (1984). A task analysis of intrapersonal conflict resolution. In L. N. Rice & L. S. Greenberg (Eds.), *Patterns of change: Intensive analysis of psychotherapy process* (pp. 67–123). Guilford Press.

Greenberg, L. S. (2007). Emotion coming of age. *Clinical Psychology: Science and Practice, 14*(4), 414–421. https://doi.org/10.1111/j.1468-2850.2007.00101.x

Greenberg, L. S., & Foerster, F. S. (1996). Task analysis exemplified: The process of resolving unfinished business. *Journal of Consulting and Clinical Psychology, 64*(3), 439–446. https://doi.org/10.1037/0022-006X.64.3.439

Greenberg, L. S., Rice, L., & Elliott, R. (1993). *Process-experiential therapy: Facilitating emotional change.* Guilford Press.

Hendrix, H. (2007). *Getting the love you want: A guide for couples.* St. Martin's Griffin.

Kramer, U., & Stiles, W. B. (2015). The responsiveness problem in psychotherapy: A review of proposed solutions. *Clinical Psychology: Science and Practice, 22*(3), 277–295. https://doi.org/10.1111/cpsp.12107

Leiman, M., & Stiles, W. B. (2001). Dialogical sequence analysis and the zone of proximal development as conceptual enhancements to the assimilation model: The case of Jan revisited. *Psychotherapy Research, 11*(3), 311–330. https://doi.org/10.1080/713663986

Mendes, I., Rosa, C., Stiles, W. B., Caro Gabalda, I., Gomes, P., Basto, I., & Salgado, J. (2016). Setbacks in the process of assimilation of problematic experiences in two cases of emotion-focused therapy for depression. *Psychotherapy Research, 26*(6), 638–652. https://doi.org/10.1080/10503307.2015.1136443

Ribeiro, E., Cunha, C., Teixeira, A. S., Stiles, W. B., Pires, N., Santos, B., Basto, I., & Salgado, J. (2016). Therapeutic collaboration and the assimilation of problematic experiences in emotion-focused therapy for depression: Comparison of two cases. *Psychotherapy Research, 26*(6), 665–680. https://doi.org/10.1080/10503307.2016.1208853

Rice, L. N. (1965). Therapist's style of participation and case outcome. *Journal of Consulting Psychology, 29*(2), 155–160. https://doi.org/10.1037/h0021926

Rice, L. N. (1974). The evocative function of the therapist. *Innovations in Client-Centered Therapy, 570,* 289–311.

Rice, L. N., & Greenberg, L. S. (Eds.). (1984). *Patterns of change: Intensive analysis of psychotherapy process.* Guilford Press.

Rice, L. N., & Saperia, E. P. (1984). Task analysis of the resolution of problematic reactions. In L. N. Rice & L. S. Greenberg (Eds.), *Patterns of change: Intensive analysis of psychotherapy process* (pp. 29–66). Guilford Press.

Rogers, C. R. (1957). The necessary and sufficient conditions of therapeutic personality change. *Journal of Consulting Psychology, 21*(2), 95–103. https://doi.org/10.1037/h0045357

Rogers, C. R. (1959). A theory of therapy, personality, and interpersonal relationships as developed in the client-centered framework. In S. Koch (Ed.), *Psychology: A study of science: Vol 3. Formulations of the person and the social context* (pp. 184–256). McGraw-Hill.

Rogers, C. R. (1980). The foundations of a person-centered approach. In *A way of being* (pp. 113–136). Houghton Mifflin.

Sachse, R. (1990). The influence of therapist processing proposals on the explication process of the client. *Person-Centered Review, 5*(3), 321–344.

Safran, J. D., & Muran, J. C. (1996). The resolution of ruptures in the therapeutic alliance. *Journal of Consulting and Clinical Psychology, 64*(3), 447–458. https://doi.org/10.1037/0022-006X.64.3.447

Safran, J. D., Muran, J. C., & Eubanks-Carter, C. (2011). Repairing alliance ruptures. *Psychotherapy: Theory, Research, & Practice, 48*(1), 80–87. https://doi.org/10.1037/a0022140

Sapolsky, R. M. (2004). *Why zebras don't get ulcers: The acclaimed guide to stress, stress-related diseases, and coping—now revised and updated.* Holt.

Schore, A. N. (2003). *Affect regulation and the repair of the self* (Vol. 2). W. W. Norton.

Schore, A. N. (2019). *The development of the unconscious mind.* W. W. Norton.

Stiles, W. B. (2001). Assimilation of problematic experiences. *Psychotherapy: Theory, Research, Practice, Training, 38*(4), 462–465. https://doi.org/10.1037/0033-3204.38.4.462

Stiles, W. B., & Horvath, A. O. (2017). Appropriate responsiveness as a contribution to therapist effects. In L. G. Castonguay & C. E. Hill (Eds.), *How and why are some therapists better than others? Understanding therapist effects* (pp. 71–84). American Psychological Association. https://doi.org/10.1037/0000034-005

Sullivan, H. S. (1947). *Conceptions of modern psychiatry.* William Alanson White Psychiatric F.

Tallman, K., & Bohart, A. C. (1999). The client as a common factor: Clients as self-healers. In M. A. Hubble, B. L. Duncan, & S. D. Miller (Eds.), *The heart and soul of change: What works in therapy* (pp. 91–131). American Psychological Association. https://doi.org/10.1037/11132-003

Wade, M., Jenkins, J. M., Venkadasalam, V. P., Binnoon-Erez, N., & Ganea, P. A. (2018). The role of maternal responsiveness and linguistic input in pre-academic skill development: A longitudinal analysis of pathways. *Cognitive Development, 45*, 125–140. https://doi.org/10.1016/j.cogdev.2018.01.005

Watson, J. C. (1996). An examination of clients' cognitive-affective processes during the exploration of problematic reactions. *Journal of Consulting and Clinical Psychology, 63*, 459–464.

Watson, J. C. (2007). Facilitating empathy. *European Psychotherapy, 7*(1), 59–65.

Watson, J. C. (2015). Empathy. In D. Cain, K. Keenan, & S. Rubin (Eds.), *Humanistic psychotherapies: Handbook of research and practice* (2nd ed.). American Psychological Association.

Watson, J. C. (2018). Mapping patterns of change in EFT: Implications for theory, research, practice and training. *Psychotherapy Research: Psychopathology, Process and Outcome, 28*(3), 389–405. https://doi.org/10.1080/10503307.2018.1435920

Watson, J. C., Goldman, R. N., & Greenberg, L. S. (2007). *Case-studies in the experiential treatment of depression: A comparison of good and bad outcome.* American Psychological Association.

Watson, J. C., & Greenberg, L. (1995). Alliance ruptures and repairs in experiential therapy. *In Session: Psychotherapy in Practice, 1*(1), 19–32.

Watson, J. C., & Greenberg, L. S. (2017). *Emotion focused psychotherapy for generalized anxiety disorder.* American Psychological Association.

Watson, J. C., McMullen, E. J., Prosser, M. C., & Bedard, D. L. (2011). An examination of the relationships among clients' affect regulation, in-session emotional processing, the working alliance, and outcome. *Psychotherapy Research, 21*(1), 86–96. https://doi.org/10.1080/10503307.2010.518637

9 RESPONSIVENESS AND THERAPEUTIC COLLABORATION IN NARRATIVE THERAPY

EUGÉNIA RIBEIRO, MIGUEL M. GONÇALVES, AND DULCE PINTO

First it's strange, then it gets into you!

—Fernando Pessoa

The concept of *therapeutic responsiveness* has been defined as the therapist's attentive behavior being influenced by the evolving context, including client's characteristics and emergent behavior (e.g., Elkin et al., 2014; Kramer & Stiles, 2015; Stiles et al., 1998; Stiles & Horvath, 2017). In this chapter, we approach the concept of therapeutic responsiveness at an immediate interactive context (Kramer & Stiles, 2015) based on the therapeutic collaboration model (TCM; E. Ribeiro et al., 2013). We engage with the responsiveness phenomenon from a microlevel perspective, by focusing on the therapeutic dyad in-session and moment-to-moment interaction, and we provide an illustration of therapeutic responsiveness in a narrative therapy session with Stephen Madigan (2010). Our conception of responsiveness is supported by the empirical studies that we have been doing with the TCM.

https://doi.org/10.1037/0000240-010
The Responsive Psychotherapist: Attuning to Clients in the Moment, J. C. Watson and H. Wiseman (Editors)

THERAPEUTIC COLLABORATION: CLIENTS' THERAPEUTIC ZONE OF PROXIMAL DEVELOPMENT AND RESPONSIVENESS

The TCM (E. Ribeiro et al., 2013) integrates the concept of zone of proximal development proposed by Vygotsky (1978) and adapted for psychotherapy by Leiman and Stiles (2001) in the context of the assimilation model (Stiles, 2001), along with the conceptualization of narrative change according to the innovative moments model (Gonçalves et al., 2009). The assimilation model suggests that the self is a community of voices. Psychological functionality is featured by an easy communication between different voices that enter into dialogue and arrive at shared meanings. However, there are instances in which voices are not easily assimilated into the community, as they menace the self's main meanings. When this occurs, these nondominant voices become problematic, and emotional suffering and symptoms emerge. According to this model, change in psychotherapy occurs by the progressive assimilation of the problematic voices into a cohesive self—by their smooth integration into the community of voices (Stiles, 2001; Stiles et al., 1998). The innovative moments model is based on the assumption that people organize the important meanings of their lives into self-narratives (that they may or may not share with others). There is a bidirectional influence between experiences and narratives constructed, in the sense that narratives organize the experience and experience influences what is narrated (Habermas & Bluck, 2000; McAdams, 2001, 2015; McLean et al., 2007). According to this model, emotional suffering occurs when peoples' experiences are shaped by rigid self-narratives that reduce the diversity of experiences and meanings. The complexity of the self is reduced to very repetitive and detrimental meanings (e.g., "I as incapable person"), in which alternative meanings are ignored or rejected (see White, 2007; White & Epston, 1990). Change in psychotherapy occurs as innovative moments that disrupt the hegemony of these rigid self-narratives are perceived, narrated, and integrated into the self, leading the way to more flexible forms of meaning making (Gonçalves et al., 2009, 2017). Thus, the innovative moments model assumes two points in a development continuum, from the problematic self-narratives that organize clients' experiences at the beginning therapy (and may be operationalized by a problem list in a case formulation) to what clients may achieve during effective treatment (e.g., alternative forms of meaning making). The first stage is what in the TCM is regarded as the actual development and the latter is the potential development level. From the perspective of the assimilation model, the first stage is the absence of assimilation of the problematic voices and the latter is the assimilation of the problematic voices into the self. Although the TCM is framed in developmental and narrative principles of therapeutic relationship and change, it has been theoretically assumed and empirically supported as a transtheoretical model (e.g., Cardoso et al., 2020; A. P. Ribeiro et al., 2014, 2016; E. Ribeiro et al., 2013, 2014, 2016; E. Ribeiro, Silveira, et al., 2019; Pinto et al., 2018; Stiles et al., 2016).

Moreover, the TCM proposes a therapeutic collaboration concept that is in line with definitions presented by other authors (e.g., Hatcher, 1999; Kazantzis & Kellis, 2012; Tryon et al., 2019; Tryon & Winograd, 2002, 2011), which emphasize the mutual contribution of the therapist and client to an active process of change and involvement in a helping relationship. The main specificity of the TCM refers to the operationalization of the therapeutic collaboration based on the developmental concept of therapeutic zone of proximal development (TZPD). From this perspective, therapeutic collaboration is conceived of as a joint effort by therapists and clients to maintain the therapeutic focus within the limits of clients' TZPD (Leiman & Stiles, 2001; E. Ribeiro et al., 2013). Clients' TZPD ranges from their problematic perspectives—their actual developmental level—to alternative and innovative perspectives—their potential developmental level. Usually, this upper limit of a client's TZPD matches the treatment goals, which are negotiated by the therapeutic dyad in early sessions and are being pursued, specified, and actualized throughout the therapy process.

At the beginning of therapy, a client's actual level is limited by their demoralization, hopelessness, and reduced self-efficacy (Frank & Frank, 1991), but with therapist's help, the client can progressively reach higher levels of flexibility, complexity, and integration of experiences, as well as independent understanding and performance of new experiences (E. Ribeiro et al., 2013, 2016; Stiles et al., 2016). Theoretically, through collaborative dyadic interaction, what at a given time represents a client's potential level (e.g., to have insight into their problematic perspective) gradually becomes their actual level, and what was previously nonfamiliar and inaccessible becomes possible and familiar. At the same time, the potential level rises too, allowing the client to have new experiences emerging in the horizon of the therapy work and the client's daily life. For example, based on clients' new insights into their problematic perspective, therapists may help clients to develop new actions with implications into their work, family, and/or personal life. Therefore, the concept of TZPD is intrinsically dynamic and interactive, because it necessarily makes reference to clients' and therapists' mutual engagement toward the change of the clients (Leiman & Stiles, 2001; Muntigl, 2004; E. Ribeiro et al., 2013; Wilson & Weinstein, 1996).

According to the TCM, therapists help clients change throughout their TZPD by supporting or challenging clients' perspectives (problematic or alternative). On one hand, when appropriately supporting clients' perspectives, therapists' interventions are expected to facilitate clients' experiences of feeling safety (closer to the TZPD client's actual level). On the other hand, when appropriately challenging clients' perspectives, therapists' interventions are expected to facilitate experiences of tolerable risk (closer to the TZPD client's potential level). In either case, it is expected that the clients will accept (validate in TCM terms) therapists' interventions and that the therapeutic communication will occur within clients' TZPD. However, therapeutic communication can occur outside of clients' TZPD, if clients invalidate or express ambivalence (oscillation between validation and invalidation) regarding therapists' interventions.

Taking the TCM as theoretical background, when we think of therapeutic responsiveness, we aim to respond to a body of questions, ranging from those focused on how therapists do their job to help clients to go further within their TZPD, to those focused on how therapists adjust and correct their interventions after a previous intervention was found to be outside clients' TZPD. As we have said elsewhere (e.g., A. P. Ribeiro et al., 2014; E. Ribeiro et al., 2013, 2016) therapists do not have a priori knowledge about clients' TZPD limits, but following an implicit principle of "push where it moves," they can adjust their interventions to help clients progress along their TZPD. The general question is how can therapists do "the right thing at the right time" (Kramer & Stiles, 2015, p. 278) in the context of the therapeutic collaboration.

From our perspective, therapeutic responsiveness involves the therapist's sensitivity to understanding the client's signals of their actual and potential developmental levels (e.g., are clients persisting with their current problematic perspectives or are they willing to go further toward alternative perspectives?). In addition, therapists' responsiveness involves their ability to maintain or retreat from previous interventions by continually adjusting them based on clients' previous responses (E. Ribeiro et al., 2013; Stiles et al., 2016). In our view, the concepts of therapeutic collaboration and of therapeutic responsiveness are intrinsically related. We suggest that "appropriate responsiveness" (Kramer & Stiles, 2015, p. 278) is the inherent property of therapeutic collaboration, which in turn is bounded by clients' TZPD limits (Leiman & Stiles, 2001; E. Ribeiro et al., 2013). In a broad context, clients' TZPD is influenced by characteristics, beyond the diagnosis or specific problems, that clients bring to therapy. Clients' perspectives on their experiences are developed in culturally, socially, and spiritually diverse contexts that shape their needs and preferences. Responsive therapists must be sensitive to broader limits of their clients' TZPD by appropriately tailoring their interventions to specific clients' diversities. The TCM helps to operationalize how therapists' interventions, contextualized in the immediate circumstance of the ongoing dyadic interaction, are responsive to the emergent clients' requirements and needs, and clients' responses (e.g., validation, invalidation, ambivalence) are the privileged indicators of therapists' appropriate responsiveness (Kramer & Stiles, 2015). Before introducing a case illustration, we briefly characterize narrative therapy.

RESPONSIVENESS IN NARRATIVE THERAPY

Narrative therapy (NT) assumes a collaborative stance in which therapists and clients not only cooperate, as in other forms of therapy (e.g., cognitive therapy, emotion-focused therapy), but are seen as partners in constructing conversational realities (White, 2007). Actually, from a constructionist point of view, social and psychological realities are always the output of a coconstruction process, from proximal contributions (e.g., significant others) to distal ones (e.g., culture). Therapy is just a specific context for exercising this joint construction of meaning, in which clients and therapists make an effort to transform the life narratives of the clients, in dialogue with absent partners, from the more concrete ones (e.g., my deceased father) to the more abstract and cultural immanent beliefs (e.g., competition is a natural process; see Konopka et al., 2019).

This constructionist position has two implications: first, a specific conception of the therapeutic relationship (congruent in several aspects with the TCM); and second, an alternative perspective of change itself when compared to the more traditional models of therapy. In terms of the therapeutic relationship, NT is suspicious when expert knowledge is applied to people's experience and sees in this knowledge a potential for alienation; NT prefers a more horizontal power relationship between a therapist and their clients. This is consistent with NT political positioning, summarized in White's (1994) assertion that therapists should exercise a special form of curiosity toward their clients' narratives:

> This is not just curiosity. It is curiosity about how things might be otherwise, a curiosity about that which falls outside of the totalizing stories that persons have about their lives, and outside of those dominant practices of self and of relationship. (p. 146)

Thus, this collaborative stance of NT is guided by a position of political activism, mostly organized from its Foucauldian background (Madigan, 1998) that lead McLeod (2004) to refer to this model as a postpsychological therapy. NT involves a way of doing therapy that tends to refuse the *psy* language (see Danziger, 1990), as this expert knowledge could be part of the dominant practices of self and relationships referred to earlier. For instance, according to White (2007), all the notions that position people as devoid of intentionality, with their actions "explained" by their internal psychological constructs, has the potential to contribute to further alienation. Thus, narrative therapists favor conceptions that put people in charge of their lives, as actors and authors of their own life narratives (Sarbin, 1986).

The second implication is centered on change itself. Language has a pivotal role in its multiple forms in the meaning-making processes. However, from this perspective, language is not seen as a reflection of the reality out there or the reality inside clients' minds (to which therapists have a privileged access), but as a social tool that constitutes realities (Rorty, 1979). This makes therapists (hopefully) experts on language use, facilitating the emergence of new meanings, by the questions that are formulated, the tasks that are proposed, or the suggestions that are tentatively offered. NT emphasizes the use of questions as a main strategy of doing therapy, as questions facilitate a more horizontal power relationship. However, in accordance with the TCM, the therapist may formulate these questions with the intention of supporting or challenging (in NT language, "deconstructing," as discussed later) the client's perspectives.

The Three-Stage Change Process in NT

NT suggests (see White, 2007; White & Epston, 1990) that changes in psychotherapy follow a three-stage process, starting with deconstructing the problematic self-narratives, moving to reconstruction in which alternative meanings are rehearsed, and then to consolidation in which the alternative meanings lead to the construction of alternative self-narratives.

Stage 1: Deconstructing Problematic Self-Narratives

According to NT, a problem may be considered as a "system of meanings that interferes with preferable direction of someone" (Zimmerman & Dickerson, 1996, p. 30). This system of meanings, organized around problematic self-narratives, should first be the target of therapist deconstructing efforts—the therapist must try to make it clear that the taken–for-granted truths support the problematic meanings. For instance, often problematic self-narratives naturalize meanings such as success, competition, or being the best instead of meanings that value community and cooperation. The well-known narrative therapeutic strategy used for deconstructing problematic meanings is externalizing conversations, although there are many other strategies a narrative therapist may use. When therapists use externalization, they try to facilitate, through activities (e.g., interviewing the problem) and questions (e.g., "what is the effect of *depression* in the way you see yourself?"), the separation between clients' identities and their problems. This form of conversation may lead, for example, to a client responding to questions about the main objectives of depression for his life, that "depression wants to rob my entire life" (i.e., instead of saying that "I want to kill myself"). Externalization is usually achieved with clients by the way the questions are asked, with the narrative therapist avoiding an internalizing framework in which the client is perceived as someone with psychological deficits responsible for the problem. It is very important to understand that externalizing the conversation is not a simple therapeutic "trick," but rather is a framework of seeing and understanding the client, in which the main aim is to understand how the problematic system of meanings was constructed and is currently maintained. The entire logic of externalization is maintained by the therapist, even if the specific strategy of externalization is not used and another therapeutic strategy is preferred as a tool for deconstruction in that specific case. It is not possible for us to analyze other therapeutic strategies that are used to produce deconstruction, but it is probably sufficient to say that the aim of the deconstruction is to separate metaphorically the client from the problem, allowing the client to reimagine their life without the influence of the problem.

In sum, when externalization is successful, therapists and clients witness the problematic self-narrative losing its strength, as its meaning system is challenged by clients and a new reality is experienced. Importantly, the idea that our reality is language-based cannot be confused with the idea that externalization is purely a cognitive activity, in which language magically changes and therapeutic transformation follows. The change that occurs with externalizing activities, or for that matter with other deconstruction activities, involves an enactment from the client. Similar to chair work (Greenberg & Goldman, 2019), the client really imagines part of their self, or significant other, in the other chair and proceeds *as if* this is the reality. From this stance, we claim that the power of any therapeutic technique to prompt changes in clients is dependable from this "as if" quality that allows clients to change their current experience, even if just temporarily. We often use a metaphor when starting externalizing interviews, telling clients that this interview would be like taking the car to a mechanic (you walk away and leave the car): "Imagine that you leave your problem here and go away for a walk. Today, I would like to speak with your problem and not with you." Of course, other forms of starting an externalizing conversation or activity are possible (e.g., creating a sculpture of the problem, drawing the problem) in addition to our preferable one.

Stage 2: Reconstructing Self-Narratives and Rehearsing New Meanings
During the reconstruction phase, the client already has created some distance from the problematic self-narrative and no longer experiences it as

themself. The problem becomes an influence on the client, it is not *the* client. Previously, as the problem was internalized, there was confusion between the problem and the client's identity ("I am a depressive person"); at this stage, the therapist aims at a separation of both ("I am a person in relation to depression"). Often, this change in the experience of the problem creates a distinction between two possibilities: (a) events in which the client may support the problem, perpetuating it in their life; and (b) events in which the client decides what is preferable for him or her. We have here a kind of bifurcation point, in which exceptions start to emerge—what White and Epston (1990) termed "unique outcomes"—exceptions that emerge and create a disruption in the problematic pattern (we have been studying these occurrences empirically with the concept of innovative moments; see, e.g., Gonçalves et al., 2009, 2017). This opens the door for the reconstruction of life narratives. Now the client has the possibility to reflect on the values and the preferences that should guide the client's life. There are clear similarities between this and the concept of values clarification in acceptance and commitment therapy (Hayes et al., 2009).

Before deconstructing the problem, there was apparently no decision to be made, just complying with the implicit rules of the problem. Now that the rules of the problem are no longer implicit and dominating the life of the client, new options emerge. Freedman and Combs (1996), Parry and Doan (1994), and White (2007), among many others, have offered clear guidelines on how to proceed during this phase of therapy. Identifying unique outcomes with the client, amplifying unique outcomes (increasing the client's awareness of them), asking questions about if these events may be related with other relevant events of the past, trying to connect these current occurrences with future ones, and asking what new avenues may open unique outcomes in the client's life are just a few examples of how the therapist may proceed.

Stage 3: Consolidating New Self-Narratives

The final stage is consolidation, and it represents another clear distinctive position of this therapy when compared with other models. This stage helps clients to validate the new knowledge that was acquired during therapy, circulating it on their social network, and making public not their deficits but their new competencies. A client may decide to implement a final ceremony to celebrate change, write letters to their future self about change, inform significant others about their new ways of functioning, be involved in political action against social systems that favor the problem (e.g., an antianorexia league), or even write letters to other clients with similar problems (we always ask clients to do to it anonymously). The framework for implementing good consolidation practices involves anchoring the new story, creating audiences that validate change, and facilitating a flexible position toward the new self-narrative, thus making it easier for future changes to occur (see Parry & Doan, 1994).

NT and Therapeutic Collaboration

We assert that there are connections between NT and TCM. Clearly, deconstructing the problem is akin to challenging clients' problematic self-narrative. Of course, we suggest that all therapies use strategies to promote challenging, be it Socratic questioning in cognitive therapy, interpretation in psychodynamic therapy, or chair work in emotion-focused therapy. From the NT perspective, these are tools to promote the deconstruction of problems. The TCM assumes that supporting the problem may be a necessary step in exploring the problematic perspective, which is also congruent with NT practices. Reconstruction is akin to supporting alternative meanings, in which the new meanings are expanded and moves the client along the TZPD.

AN ILLUSTRATION OF THE CHANGE PROCESS IN NARRATIVE THERAPY: THE CASE OF DAVID

Drawing on six sessions of psychotherapy delivered by Stephen Madigan as a demonstrative video of NT (Madigan, 2010), in this section we illustrate the therapist's responsiveness as a dynamic property of the therapeutic collaboration. This illustration is based only on the first of these six sessions. The session was fully transcribed, according to the video captions, and then coded while observing the video employing the Therapeutic Collaboration Coding System (TCCS) procedures—the procedures of the observational coding system directly derived from the TCM (E. Ribeiro et al., 2013; E. Ribeiro, Pinto, et al., 2019).

David (a pseudonym) was a man in his early 50s who was struggling with what he named anxiety, fear, nervousness, lack of worth, and negative imagination.[1] The story David told about his problems (i.e., the problematic self-narrative that he presented at the beginning of the therapy, which corresponded to his actual developmental level on the TZPD) has kept him inside his home for 2 full years, has prohibited him from holding a job for 10 years (he did some on-and-off driving and janitorial work), and has prevented

---

[1] Details regarding client identity were omitted or changed to protect client confidentiality.

him from meeting other people and developing close relationships (with both friends and romantic attachments).

Exhibit 9.1 presents a dialogue from the beginning of the session and demonstrates how, at that point, David told the story of his problems. In addition, it indicates Madigan's orientation toward a very close-up interview, in order to get David's own definition of his problems. Mostly it is based on questions (e.g., Lines 1–2, 4, and 15–17) and repetitions of David's own words (e.g., Lines 10, 11, and 13), thus reflecting the curious and coconstructing stance that usually characterizes NT (White, 2007). The TCCS codes are in brackets beside each of Madigan's interventions and David's responses (for all of the TCCS codes, see E. Ribeiro et al., 2013; E. Ribeiro, Pinto, et al., 2019).

From the TCM perspective, in every therapeutic interaction represented in this illustration (i.e., each pair of therapist–client adjacent speaking turns), Madigan's interventions were aimed at supporting David's problematic perspective as they explored and captured a good understanding of the way David himself conceptualized his problems. David's validating responses, confirming Madigan's reflections and offering relevant information in relation to the questions Madigan raised, seem indeed to support Madigan's appropriate responsiveness to David's momentary TZPD. This is because Madigan's interventions were attuned with David's actual developmental level (and closer to his problematic perspective) and contributed to the interaction unfolding within David's TZPD limits.

In line with Exhibit 9.1 and with David's problematic perspective, Exhibit 9.2 shows that not talking, not acting, and isolating himself were strategies David adopted in childhood (at approximately age 5, when his parents got divorced), primarily because of fear that he would be abandoned or verbally abused Again, mostly through questioning (e.g., Lines 1, 2, 6–9, 11–13), as it is characteristic of NT (e.g., White, 2007), Madigan tried to facilitate the development of a richer meaning-making process of the story David was telling about his problems and coping strategies. Indeed, what we might observe is that, as a child, what David did in order to prevent and/or survive verbal abuse and possible abandonment was actually a reasonable and adaptive strategy. However, until the point in his life when he entered therapy, David only conceptualized it as a failure, instead of as once being a means of survival, that nevertheless has persisted over the years and was not that helpful anymore. In terms of the TCM (E. Ribeiro et al., 2013), Madigan was pushing David toward the upper limit of his TZPD (i.e., toward his potential developmental level), which was then defined by the potential change point he could achieve within the therapeutic interaction. This would be achieved through the emergence of a new, alternative, and more adaptive meaning, thus fostering the deconstruction of his usual and problematic perspective (self-narrative).

EXHIBIT 9.1. Responsive Therapist's Supporting Problem Intervention

1 2	T	The anxiety . . . I'm not exactly sure what anxiety is. Is that your word or someone else's word? [Supporting the problematic perspective–questioning]
3	C	Well, I make it up but . . . [Validating the intervention–giving information]
4	T	You make it up? [Supporting the problematic perspective–reflecting]
5 6	C	I noticed I have a lot of nervousness. [Validating the intervention–giving information]
7	T	Okay. [Supporting the problematic perspective–minimal encouragement]
8 9	C	Sometimes to the point of feeling scared or frightened. [Validating the intervention–giving information]
10 11	T	Nervousness and sometimes you feel scared. [Supporting the problematic perspective–reflecting]
12	C	Yes. [Validating the intervention–confirming]
13	T	And frightened. [Supporting the problematic perspective–reflecting]
14	C	Yes. [Validating the intervention–confirming]
15 16 17	T	And is there anything else you can tell me about what you are calling this experience of nervousness? [Supporting the problematic perspective–questioning]
18 19	C	Just uncomfortable. It's mostly around people. [Validating the intervention–giving information]
20	T	It's mostly around people? [Supporting the problematic perspective–reflecting]
21 22	C	Yeah, mostly in social situations or performing in front of people. [Validating the intervention–giving information]
23 24	T	How do you mean performing? [Supporting the problematic perspective–questioning]
25 26	C	Well, one would be work, working somewhere. [Validating the intervention–giving information]
27 28	T	And would work be one of these social situations? [Supporting the problematic perspective–questioning]
29 30 31 32	C	It wouldn't be only because. . . . Yeah, it would be social situation but it's not only because it's social. It's just performing, doing things in front of people with my hands, stuff like that, whatever . . . [Validating the intervention–giving information]
33 34	T	Okay. What do you do for your work? [Supporting the problematic perspective–questioning]
35	C	I used to drive. [Validating the intervention–giving information]

Note. T = Therapist (Madigan); C = Client (David). Transcribed and adapted from *Narrative Therapy Over Time*, by S. Madigan, 2010, American Psychological Association. Copyright 2010 by the American Psychological Association.

EXHIBIT 9.2. Responsive Therapist's Challenging Intervention

1	T	So, it was safer not to talk than to talk? [Supporting the problematic
2		perspective–reflecting]
3	C	Not only talk. Not to do anything. You know, move. . . . You know, drink a glass
4		of milk. . . . Whatever. [Validating the intervention–giving information]
5		(. . .)
6	T	Do you think that it was wise of you as a young person to adopt the strategy to
7		survive and remain safe by not talking and by not acting? [Challenging the
8		problematic perspective–inviting to explore hypothetical scenarios, as
9		Madigan is offering an alternative meaning for David's behaviors]
10	C	I think, yeah, it was wise. [Validating the intervention–confirming]
11	T	Yeah. Why do you think it was wise? [Challenging the problematic
12		perspective–changing the level of analysis as Madigan is going deeper
13		on the meaning exploration]
14	C	Because I think if I would have done something that he would have
15		disapproved of, and if it would have been harsh, I would hurt and I would
16		have emotional pain. [Validating the intervention–giving information]
17	T	Okay. So, adopting this strategy to be safer and not to talk and not to act, it
18		allowed you to remain safe, remain in the home? Am I right in thinking that?
19		[Challenging the problematic perspective–interpreting]
20	C	Uh-hmm. Right. [Validating the intervention–confirming]
21	T	Yeah. So . . . [Challenging the problematic perspective–minimal encouragement]
22	C	I think any more disapproval from him would have hurt like I said, emotionally.
23		But I think there was a fear for maybe abandoning me a hundred percent,
24		not coming home at all. Because I think throughout the years, there's a part
25		of me hoping he would come back of me, hoping he would come back
26		and my ma' would get back together. [Validating the intervention–giving
		information]
27		(. . .)
28	T	And is this a strategy that you held on to through the course of your life?
29		[Challenging the problematic perspective–changing the level of analysis
30		from David's behavior as a child to David's behavior through life]
31	C	I think so. I think it might be still going on now. [Validating–giving information]
32	T	Yeah. Yeah. In what ways do you see it continuing to go on now? [Challenging
33		the problematic perspective–changing the level of analysis, as Madigan asks
34		for current specifics of the same strategy]

EXHIBIT 9.2. Responsive Therapist's Challenging Intervention (*Continued*)

35	C	The way I isolate, the way I could be in a meeting and frightened to talk, and
36		sometimes I won't talk, depending on the level of my anxiety. [Validating the
37		intervention–giving information]
38	T	Right. [Challenging the problematic perspective–minimal encouragement]
39	C	Because of the fear of rejection . . . [Validating the intervention–giving
40		information]
41	T	Yeah . . . [Challenging the problematic perspective–minimal encouragement]
42	C	And ridicule and stuff like that. [Validating the intervention–giving information]
43	T	Right. [Challenging the problematic perspective–minimal encouragement]
44	C	That pretty much controls me. [Validating the intervention–giving information]

Note. T = Therapist (Madigan); C = Client (David). Transcribed and adapted from *Narrative Therapy Over Time,* by S. Madigan, 2010, American Psychological Association. Copyright 2010 by the American Psychological Association.

In fact, across all interactions in Exhibit 9.2, Madigan's interventions were intended to challenge David's problematic perspective. The interventions were designed to promote insight into the way David conceived his coping strategies until that moment, as well as to propose an alternative meaning to them (i.e., not talking, not acting, and isolating himself as means of survival during his childhood instead of seeing it as failures in his adulthood). Again, David's validating responses, accepting Madigan's invitations to explore such alternative meanings (i.e., inviting to explore hypothetical scenarios TCCS marker; e.g., Lines 6–9), and providing relevant information to the questions he raised to bring to the surface David's meaning attributions (i.e., changing the level of analysis TCCS marker; e.g., Lines 11–13, 28–30, 32–34), seem indeed to support Madigan's appropriate responsiveness, as his interventions contributed for the interaction unfolding within David's TZPD limits, in attunement with his potential developmental level (closer to a potential alternative self-narrative). According to NT, this interaction is an effort of deconstructing the problematic self-narrative, in which the client starts seeing some value in the way he used to act (protecting himself, given the fear of rejection), although externalizing conversation is not used in here. What was from the perspective of the problematic perspective a deficit or an inability is now being reconstructed as a tool of survival. Notice also how the first meaning was an "explanation," whereas the second is an intentional explanation and, as such, repositions David as an actor in his narrative (not yet as an author, to use the distinction from Sarbin, 1986).

Exhibit 9.3 shows an interaction that occurred right after the one represented in Exhibit 9.2.

If in the second interaction we could observe Madigan working to promote David's construction of meaning regarding the usefulness of his strategy not to talk, not to act, and isolating himself back in his childhood—which he validated as it was responsive to his TZDP limits at the time—in this third interaction, Madigan proceeds with the attempt to deconstruct the usefulness of that same strategy in David's adult life. He also starts using externalizing reformulation of the problem as in "it continues to tell you that it's safe." However, regarding the first interaction (i.e., the first pair of Madigan and David's adjacent turns; Lines 1–7), from the TCM perspective, David was unable to move forward into his TZPD, as he invalidated Madigan's invitation to explore such alternative perspective by adding that such strategy was not only useful in his younger years but was still useful, probably more than anything in his life at that moment. Indeed, David's response signaled that Madigan's intervention was not responsive to the upper limit of his TZPD, and

EXHIBIT 9.3. Nonresponsive Therapist's Challenging Intervention and Its Repair

1 2 3 4	T	So even though this was a very . . . what you consider to be a safe strategy when you were young, as you grow older . . . are you saying that it may not serve your needs as well as it once did when you were younger? [Challenging the problematic perspective–interpretation]
5 6 7	C	I would say it's more helpful to me than anything now. [Invalidating the intervention–disagreeing with therapist's proposal/defending the problematic perspective by intolerable risk]
8 9	T	So, a strategy that was quite helpful has, through the years, turned harmful. [Challenging the problematic perspective–interpretation]
10 11	C	Right, even though there still feels like there's a safety in it, you know. [Showing ambivalence towards the intervention]
12 13	T	Yeah. So, something that was once safe has become harmful . . . [Supporting the problematic perspective–reflecting]
14	C	Right. [Validating the intervention–confirming]
15 16	T	But, somehow, it continues to tell you that it's safe. [Supporting the problematic perspective–reflecting]
17	C	Right. I'll be safer, yeah. [Validating the intervention–giving information]
18	T	You'll be safer. [Supporting the problematic perspective–reflecting]
19	C	Right. [Validating the intervention–confirming]

Note. T = Therapist (Madigan); C = Client (David). Transcribed and adapted from *Narrative Therapy Over Time*, by S. Madigan, 2010, American Psychological Association. Copyright 2010 by the American Psychological Association.

instead entailed a threatening experience for him (i.e., of intolerable risk, in TCCS terms). Theoretically, such an exchange between Madigan and David corresponded to a therapeutic collaboration break (see, e.g., Cardoso et al., 2020), which might be seen as a clinical error as it exceeded David's TZPD (Stiles et al., 2016) and may lead to nonproductive work if the therapist does not recognize and repair it. However, if not persistent and the collaboration is responsively reestablished, it might also be seen as a strategy to test the flexibility of clients' TZPD limits, promoting contact with unfamiliar and alternative experiences and meanings.

Framed in our conceptualization of responsiveness as a process that occurs in the immediacy, at a moment-to-moment level, it is curious to notice that, despite David's response, Madigan persisted in his agenda of challenging the usefulness of David's current strategy to not talk, to not act, and to isolate himself (Lines 8, 9). In fact, adopting a more purposive stance, Madigan affirmed, in form of a conclusion ("So . . ."), that David's strategy, which although once was quite useful, has become harmful through the years. Although David softened his position by starting to give the impression that he was about to validate Madigan's intervention, his perspective still persisted ("Right, even though . . .")—for him, his strategy still entailed a meaningful sense of safety (Lines 10, 11). Following the TCCS procedures, once David's response presupposed a movement from validating to invalidating it, we considered it as indicating ambivalence in relation to Madigan's intervention. That said, in this illustration, Madigan's second intervention (Lines 8, 9) continued to exceed David's TZPD. The intervention was nonresponsive to its limits at that moment, as well as to David's previous intolerable risk experience, contributing to the continuing noncollaborative stance between them. However, it is likely that Madigan was testing the limits of the David's TZPD by persisting with his challenging intervention.

In the following interactions (Lines 12, 13, 15, 16), however, it is clear that Madigan adjusted his intervention to David's perspective, as he retreated from his agenda and reflected the main content of David's previous response (namely, his ambivalence; see Lines 10–11). By doing that, and having David validated such interventions (Lines 14, 17), the therapeutic interaction was relocated inside David's TZPD, respecting its limits and reestablishing the climate of safety and collaboration shown in the following interaction (Lines 18, 19), as well as in the previous two interactions (Exhibits 9.1 and 9.2) and, in general, in the remaining interactions of the session.

That said, from Exhibit 9.1 to Exhibit 9.2 (that sequentially occurred in the session), an alternative self-narrative to the way David used to tell his story started to emerge, entailing a new meaning of his behavior as a child (i.e., to not talk, to not act, and to isolate himself), which then started to be conceptualized as helpful, instead of useless and problematic. In retrospect, this review of meanings about experiences established the ground for the emergence of a new comprehension focused on how David currently lived his life (shown in Exhibit 9.3, later in the session). After all, what had, in fact, been very adaptive and helpful in his childhood has persisted over the years and was now constraining his movements. According to the TCM (E. Ribeiro et al., 2013), we argue that at that point in therapy, David's assimilation of the helpfulness of his behavior as a child that, however, has now become a useless and harmful strategy, established the upper limit of his TZPD—closer to his potential developmental level.

RESEARCH ON TCM AND RESPONSIVENESS IN NT

We recognize the extensive empirical literature on the topic of therapeutic collaboration and its relation to therapy outcomes (see Tryon et al., 2019, for an updated review), as well as its contribution to the recognition of the collaboration as an effective element of the therapeutic relationship (Norcross, 2002; Norcross & Lambert, 2019). However, for the sake of coherence with the theoretical framework and the purpose of this chapter, here we restrict the focus on the research based on the TCM. The interested reader may check other sources, namely, to see the results from meta-analytic evidence on the relation between collaboration and therapeutic outcomes.

A number of studies using the TCM (E. Ribeiro et al., 2013) have supported the conceptualization of therapeutic responsiveness based on clients' TZPD. These studies were based on the theory-building research strategy (Stiles, 2007, 2009, 2010) and aimed to describe the therapeutic interaction with reference to clients' TZPD (i.e., therapeutic collaboration) throughout the therapy process, describing patterns of therapeutic exchanges that differentiate good and poor outcome cases with different types of termination (completers versus dropouts) and of a diversity of therapy approaches, including narrative therapy (Cardoso et al., 2020; Ferreira et al., 2015; A. P. Ribeiro et al., 2014, 2016; E. Ribeiro et al., 2013, 2014, 2016; E. Ribeiro, Silveira, et al., 2019).

Based on detailed and idiographic clinical observations, these case studies have helped us to highlight how therapists appropriately adjusted (or not) their interventions to clients' responses on a moment-to moment basis throughout the therapy processes. A general contribution of a comparative case study in narrative therapy (Ferreira et al., 2015) supporting the TCM is that, compared with a poor outcome, the therapist of a good outcome case (both completer cases) seems to have been appropriately responsive to clients by adjusting the therapist's interventions to the client's previous immediate responses and being able to maintain or quickly return to work within the client's TZPD. In contrast, in narrative poor outcome dropouts, we have found a pattern of therapist's insistence on interventions that exceeded clients' TZPD, and this behavior increased in predropout sessions (e.g., A. P. Ribeiro et al., 2016; Pinto et al., 2018). In addition, the same narrative case studies support the notion that, in different phases of therapy, responsive therapists may consider the use of different strategies (e.g., supporting or challenging clients' perspective) based on specific clients' experiences and progress. Consistent with case studies of other therapy approaches (E. Ribeiro et al., 2016; E. Ribeiro, Silveira, et al., 2019) using TCM, narrative comparative case studies have shown that, in the middle and final phases of therapy and in contrast with poor outcome cases, the therapist of good outcome cases were more able to balance the supporting and challenging interventions with a progressive increase in the latter, which suggests that they were sensitive to the client's growing tolerance for innovation.

In another study focused on breaks in therapeutic collaboration throughout the therapy of a narrative recovered case, Cardoso and coauthors (2020) studied the therapist's actions after therapeutic collaboration breaks in sequences in which therapeutic collaboration was or was not re-established. The authors were interested in studying breaks emerging from therapist's proposals that exceeded the client's TZPD (i.e., therapeutic exchanges resulting from the therapist's challenging interventions and the client's intolerable risk responses) as they denote difficulties in the therapeutic work intended to encourage the client's gradual change. The findings showed that more important than maintaining or retreating from the previous action was how the therapist did so. When the therapist intervened by re-establishing a sense of continuity with the client's needs and experience, the therapist offered the client the time and opportunity to accept the challenges and to better tolerate innovations. Therefore, the therapist's ability to perceive their intervention as inappropriate or untimely (based on the client's response of invalidation) was critical for the responsive reestablishment of therapeutic collaboration breaks.

DIVERSITY AND CULTURAL IMPLICATIONS FOR THE TCM AND RESPONSIVENESS

The current and undeniably increasing centrality of the diversity and cultural topics on the global society demands from researchers and psychotherapists a growing awareness of their responsibilities as agents of appropriate actions promoting well-being and health. Therefore, (inter)cultural and demographic diversity issues are currently recognized as central in psychotherapy and specifically in the therapeutic relationship (Norcross & Wampold, 2019; Sue & Lam, 2002). As we wrote earlier, the therapist's responsiveness, by taking into account the client's TZPD, implies the consideration of both the immediate and global contexts of the therapeutic interaction. We acknowledge that demographic, historical, and cultural diversities are important to consider in both levels. In our view, the therapists attention to (inter)cultural and diversity issues is important not only when they negotiate with clients as to their TZPD (understanding of the problematic self-narratives and negotiation of the potential alternative self-narratives) but also in their management of the therapeutic interaction, moment by moment. However, so far, studies based on TCM have not given the necessary attention to the (inter)cultural context of therapeutic collaboration, such as considering issues of gender, ethnicity, or other diversity of population that calls for help in psychotherapy. We acknowledge that this is a relevant limitation that we will keep in mind in future studies. Moreover, our studies have been mostly with depression and anxiety disorders where it is clearer than other diagnoses what the problematic self-narratives consist of and how alternative meanings may be in the future. In other diagnoses, where the clarity of the problem is not so easy to grasp (e.g., personality disorders), and may be an important topic of negotiation between therapists and clients, are also needed to expand the application of TCM to other populations.

TRAINING IN THERAPEUTIC COLLABORATION MODEL AS A RESPONSIVE PROCESS

Studies referred previously on the TCM (Cardoso et al., 2020; Ferreira et al., 2015; A. P. Ribeiro et al., 2014, 2016; E. Ribeiro et al., 2013, 2014, 2016; E. Ribeiro, Silveira, et al., 2019) aimed to contribute to identify concrete guidelines about when, how, and why to implement specific interventions (Kramer & Stiles, 2015). Previous case studies, as well as the case of David, suggest that progress in therapy is characterized by the maintenance of the dyad's work within clients' TZPD, by progressively and carefully moving it into areas of unfamiliarity and increasing exposure to tolerable risk. This process presupposes that therapists must be able to pay attention to clients' responses to their interventions and to responsively balance both clients' needs for safety and their readiness to change.

The TCCS (E. Ribeiro et al., 2013; E. Ribeiro, Pinto, 2019) has been proved to be a useful tool for the comprehension of how therapeutic collaboration develops and contributes to clients' gradual change, thus making relevant the exploration of its potentialities for therapists' training and for their own monitoring of the intrasession interactive processes. It specifies markers of clients' responses of validation and invalidation that are interpreted as indicators of clients' experiences at a given point in therapy with regard to their TZPD. However, according the TCM, the client's TZPD is hypothetically and provisionally defined taking into account the idiosyncratic case formulation, the global context of therapy-specific goals, and the immediate context of the in-session sequences of therapeutic exchanges. Therefore, if the job of responsive therapists is to work within clients' TZPD, in addition to the specific therapy approach skills, therapists should be able to identify clients' needs and potentialities, being sensitive to their historical and cultural diversities, and revise their interventions with immediacy and in a flexible way. Accordingly, we speculate that formally training therapists on the TCM would help them to develop sensitivity to clients' emergent experiences and/or needs and to identify the opportunities to enhance responsiveness by adjusting their interventions to clients' TZPD limits. We assert that the TCM provides the therapist with a rationale to decide when and how to responsively support or challenge the client's perspective, to maintain or retreat from their interventions, whether to support (e.g., by questioning, reflecting, encouraging) or challenge (e.g., by externalizing, inviting to consider other hypothetical scenarios) clients' perspectives. In TCM terms, and in accordance with narrative principles, therapists' responsive interventions should be based on clients' responses of validation (e.g., affirming, giving information, elaborating therapists' proposal) or invalidation (e.g., disagreeing with therapist's proposal, persisting in their own perspectives), thereby recognizing clients' agency and knowing position in their collaboration.

CONCLUSION

Previous research indicates that therapist responsiveness, as conceptualized and illustrated in this chapter, is associated with good outcome. Therefore, the concept of TZPD (Leiman & Stiles, 2001) and the TCM (E. Ribeiro et al., 2013) is a valuable framework for monitoring and adjusting therapists' responsiveness. Future research on this topic could clarify whether this intuition has empirical support, by analyzing the impact of training therapists on the use of TCM in the therapeutic relationship and clinical outcomes of their cases. In addition, future studies focused on therapist's responsiveness as framed on TCM, taking into account the diversities and cultural characteristics from both therapists and clients, will further elaborate the TCM and enrich therapist training.

REFERENCES

Cardoso, C., Pinto, D., & Ribeiro, E. (2020). Therapist's actions after therapeutic collaboration breaks: A single case study. *Psychotherapy Research, 30*(4), 447–461. https://doi.org/10.1080/10503307.2019.1633483

Danziger, K. (1990). *Constructing the subject: Historical origins of psychological research.* Cambridge University Press. https://doi.org/10.1017/CBO9780511524059

Elkin, I., Falconnier, L., Smith, Y., Canada, K. E., Henderson, E., Brown, E. R., & McKay, B. M. (2014). Therapist responsiveness and patient engagement in therapy. *Psychotherapy Research, 24*(1), 52–66. https://doi.org/10.1080/10503307.2013.820855

Ferreira, A., Ribeiro, E., Pinto, D., Pereira, C., & Pinheiro, A. (2015). Colaboração terapêutica: Estudo comparativo de dois casos de um caso finalizado e de um caso de desistência [Therapeutic collaboration: A comparative study of two poor outcome cases—A completer and a dropout]. *Análise Psicológica, 33*(2), 165–177. https://doi.org/10.14417/ap.938

Frank, J. D., & Frank, J. B. (1991). *Persuasion and healing: A comparative study of Psychotherapy* (3rd ed.). Johns Hopkins University Press.

Freedman, J., & Combs, G. (1996). *Narrative therapy: The social construction of preferred realities.* W. W. Norton.

Gonçalves, M. M., Matos, M., & Santos, A. (2009). Narrative therapy and the nature of "innovative moments" in the construction of change. *Journal of Constructivist Psychology, 22*(1), 1–23. https://doi.org/10.1080/10720530802500748

Gonçalves, M. M., Ribeiro, A. P., Mendes, I., Alves, D., Silva, J., Rosa, C., Braga, C., Batista, J., Fernández-Navarro, P., & Oliveira, J. T. (2017). Three narrative-based coding systems: Innovative moments, ambivalence and ambivalence resolution. *Psychotherapy Research, 27*(3), 270–282. https://doi.org/10.1080/10503307.2016.1247216

Greenberg, L. S., & Goldman, R. N. (Eds.). (2019). *Clinical handbook of emotion-focused therapy.* American Psychological Association. https://doi.org/10.1037/0000112-000

Habermas, T., & Bluck, S. (2000). Getting a life: The emergence of the life story in adolescence. *Psychological Bulletin, 126*(5), 748–769. https://doi.org/10.1037/0033-2909.126.5.748

Hatcher, R. L. (1999). Therapists' views of treatment alliance and collaboration in therapy. *Psychotherapy Research, 9*(4), 405–423.

Hayes, S. C., Strosahl, K. D., & Wilson, K. G. (2009). *Acceptance and commitment therapy.* American Psychological Association.

Kazantzis, N., & Kellis, E. (2012). A special feature on collaboration in psychotherapy. *Journal of Clinical Psychology, 68*(2), 133–135. https://doi.org/10.1002/jclp.21837

Konopka, A., Hermans, H. J. M., & Gonçalves, M. M. (Eds.). (2019). *Handbook of dialogical self theory and psychotherapy: Bridging psychotherapeutic and cultural traditions.* Routledge.

Kramer, U., & Stiles, W. B. (2015). The responsiveness problem in psychotherapy: A review of proposed solutions. *Clinical Psychology: Science and Practice, 22*(3), 277–295. https://doi.org/10.1111/cpsp.12107

Leiman, M., & Stiles, W. B. (2001). Dialogical sequence analysis and the zone of proximal development as conceptual enhancements to the assimilation model: The case of Jan revisited. *Psychotherapy Research, 11*(3), 311–330. https://doi.org/10.1080/713663986

Madigan, S. (1998). Practice interpretations of Michel Foucault. In S. Madigan & I. Law (Eds.), *Praxis: Situating discourse, feminism & politics in narrative therapies* (pp. 15–34). Yaletown Family Therapy.

Madigan, S. (2010). *Narrative therapy over time* [DVD]. American Psychological Association.

McAdams, D. P. (2001). The psychology of life stories. *Review of General Psychology,* *5*(2), 100–122. https://doi.org/10.1037/1089-2680.5.2.100

McAdams, D. P. (2015). *The art and science of personality development.* Guilford Press.

McLean, K. C., Pasupathi, M., & Pals, J. L. (2007). Selves creating stories creating selves: A process model of self-development. *Personality and Social Psychology Review, 11*(3), 262–278. https://doi.org/10.1177/1088868307301034

McLeod, J. (2004). The significance of narrative and storytelling in postpsychological counseling and psychotherapy. In A. Lieblich, D. P. McAdams, & R. Josselson (Eds.), *The narrative study of lives. Healing plots: The narrative basis of psychotherapy* (pp. 11–27). American Psychological Association. https://doi.org/10.1037/10682-001

Muntigl, P. (2004). Ontogenesis in narrative therapy: A linguistic-semiotic examination of client change. *Family Process, 43*(1), 109–131. https://doi.org/10.1111/j.1545-5300.2004.04301009.x

Norcross, J. C. (2002). Empirically supported therapy relationship. In J. C. Norcross (Ed.), *Psychotherapy relationships that work: Therapist contributions and responsiveness to patients* (pp. 3–16). Oxford University Press.

Norcross, J. C., & Lambert, M. J. (2019). Evidence-based psychotherapy relationship: The third task force. In J. C. Norcross & M. J. Lambert (Eds.), *Psychotherapy relationships that work: Vol. 1. Evidence-based therapist contributions* (3rd ed., pp. 1–23). Oxford University Press.

Norcross, J. C., & Wampold, B. E. (2019). Evidence-based psychotherapy responsiveness: The third task force. In J. C. Norcross & B. E. Wampold (Eds.), *Psychotherapy relationships that work: Vol. 2. Evidence-based therapist responsiveness* (3rd ed., pp. 1–14). Oxford University Press.

Parry, A., & Doan, R. E. (1994). *Story re-visions: Narrative therapy in the postmodern world.* Guilford Press.

Pinto, D., Sousa, I., Pinheiro, A., Freitas, A. C., & Ribeiro, E. (2018). The therapeutic collaboration in dropout cases of narrative therapy: An exploratory study. *Revista de Psicoterapia, 29*(110), 167–184. https://doi.org/10.33898/rdp.v29i110.209

Ribeiro, A. P., Braga, C., Stiles, W. B., Teixeira, P., Gonçalves, M. M., & Ribeiro, E. (2016). Therapist interventions and client ambivalence in two cases of narrative therapy for depression. *Psychotherapy Research, 26*(6), 681–693. https://doi.org/10.1080/10503307.2016.1197439

Ribeiro, A. P., Ribeiro, E., Loura, J., Gonçalves, M. M., Stiles, W. B., Horvath, A. O., & Sousa, I. (2014). Therapeutic collaboration and resistance: Describing the nature and quality of the therapeutic relationship within ambivalence events using the Therapeutic Collaboration Coding System. *Psychotherapy Research, 24*(3), 346–359. https://doi.org/10.1080/10503307.2013.856042

Ribeiro, E., Cunha, C., Teixeira, A. S., Stiles, W. B., Pires, N., Santos, B., Basto, I., & Salgado, J. (2016). Therapeutic collaboration and the assimilation of problematic experiences in emotion-focused therapy for depression: Comparison of two cases. *Psychotherapy Research*, *26*(6), 665–680. https://doi.org/10.1080/10503307.2016.1208853

Ribeiro, E., Fernandes, C., Santos, B., Ribeiro, A., Coutinho, J., Angus, L., & Greenberg, L. (2014). The development of therapeutic collaboration in a good outcome case of person-centered therapy. *Person-Centered and Experiential Psychotherapies*, *13*(2), 150–168. https://doi.org/10.1080/14779757.2014.893250

Ribeiro, E., Pinto, D., Ribeiro, A. P., Gonçalves, M. M., Ferreira, A., Horvath, A. O., & Stiles, W. B. (2019). *The Therapeutic Collaboration Coding System (TCCS): Manual revised* [Unpublished manuscript]. School of Psychology, University of Minho, Braga, Portugal.

Ribeiro, E., Ribeiro, A. P., Gonçalves, M. M., Horvath, A. O., & Stiles, W. B. (2013). How collaboration in therapy becomes therapeutic: The therapeutic collaboration coding system. *Psychology and Psychotherapy*, *86*(3), 294–314. https://doi.org/10.1111/j.2044-8341.2012.02066.x

Ribeiro, E., Silveira, J., Azevedo, A., Senra, J., Ferreira, A., & Pinto, D. (2019). Colaboración terapéutica: Estudio comparativo de dos casos contrastantes con terapia constructivista [Therapeutic collaboration: A comparative study of two contrasting cases of constructivist therapy]. *Revista Argentina de Clínica Psicológica*, *28*(2), 127–139. https://doi.org/10.24205/03276716.2019.1104

Rorty, R. (1979). *Philosophy and mirror of nature*. Princeton University Press.

Sarbin, T. R. (Ed.). (1986). *Narrative psychology: The storied nature of human conduct*. Praeger.

Stiles, W. B. (2001). Assimilation of problematic experiences. *Psychotherapy: Theory, Research, Practice, Training*, *38*(4), 462–465. https://doi.org/10.1037/0033-3204.38.4.462

Stiles, W. B. (2007). Theory-building case studies of counselling and psychotherapy. *Counselling & Psychotherapy Research*, *7*(2), 122–127. https://doi.org/10.1080/14733140701356742

Stiles, W. B. (2009). Logical operations in theory-building case studies. *Pragmatic Case Studies in Psychotherapy: PCSP*, *2*(5), 9–22. https://doi.org/10.14713/pcsp.v5i3.973

Stiles, W. B. (2010). Theory-building case studies as practice-based evidence. In M. Barkham, G. E. Hardy, & J. Mellor-Clark (Eds.), *Developing and delivering practice-based evidence: A guide for the psychological therapies* (pp. 91–108). John Wiley & Sons. https://doi.org/10.1002/9780470687994.ch4

Stiles, W. B., Caro Gabalda, I., & Ribeiro, E. (2016). Exceeding the therapeutic zone of proximal development as a clinical error. *Psychotherapy*, *53*(3), 268–272. https://doi.org/10.1037/pst0000061

Stiles, W. B., Honos-Webb, L., & Surko, M. (1998). Responsiveness in psychotherapy. *Clinical Psychology: Science and Practice*, *5*(4), 439–458. https://doi.org/10.1111/j.1468-2850.1998.tb00166.x

Stiles, W. B., & Horvath, A. O. (2017). Appropriate responsiveness as a contribution to therapist effects. In L. G. Castonguay & C. E. Hill (Eds.), *How and why are some therapists better than others? Understanding therapist effects* (pp. 71–84). American Psychological Association. https://doi.org/10.1037/0000034-005

Sue, S., & Lam, A. G. (2002). Cultural and Demographic Diversity. In J. C. Norcross (Ed.), *Psychotherapy relationships that work: Therapist contributions and responsiveness to patients* (pp. 401–421). Oxford University Press.

Tryon, G. S., Birch, S. E., & Verkuilen, J. (2019). Goal consensus and collaboration. In J. C. Norcross & M. J. Lambert (Eds.), *Psychotherapy relationships that work: Evidence-based therapist contributions* (3rd ed., Vol. 1, pp. 167–204). Oxford University Press.

Tryon, G. S., & Winograd, G. (2002). Goal consensus and collaboration. In J. C. Norcross (Ed.), *Psychotherapy relationships that work: Therapist contributions and responsiveness to patients* (pp. 109–125). Oxford University Press.

Tryon, G. S., & Winograd, G. (2011). Goal consensus and collaboration. In J. C. Norcross (Ed.), *Psychotherapy relationships that work: Evidence-based responsiveness* (2nd ed., pp. 153–167). Oxford University Press. https://doi.org/10.1093/acprof:oso/9780199737208.003.0007

Vygotsky, L. S. (1978). *Mind in society: The development of higher psychological processes.* Harvard University Press.

White, M. (1994). Deconstruction and therapy. In D. Epston & M. White (Eds.), *Experience, contradiction, narrative and imagination* (2nd ed., pp. 109–152). Dulwich Centre Publications.

White, M. (2007). *Maps of narrative practice.* W. W. Norton.

White, M., & Epston, D. (1990). *Narrative means to therapeutic ends.* W. W. Norton.

Wilson, A., & Weinstein, L. (1996). The transference and the zone of proximal development. *Journal of the American Psychoanalytic Association, 44*(1), 167–200. https://doi.org/10.1177/000306519604400108

Zimmerman, J. L., & Dickerson, V. G. (1996). *If problems talked: Narrative therapy in action.* Guilford Press.

10

THERAPIST RESPONSIVENESS IN ATTACHMENT-BASED FAMILY THERAPY FOR SEXUAL AND GENDER MINORITY ADULTS AND THEIR NONACCEPTING PARENTS

GARY M. DIAMOND, ROTEM BORUCHOVITZ-ZAMIR, AND OFIR NIR-GOTTLIEB

This chapter describes the nature and importance of therapist responsiveness in attachment-based family therapy (ABFT) for sexual and gender minority young adults and their nonaccepting parents (G. M. Diamond et al., 2019). ABFT is a family-based, manualized, experiential, and emotion- and relationship-focused treatment designed for families in which parents have difficulty accepting their adult child's sexual orientation or gender identity.

Families come to us for a number of reasons. In some cases, it is the young adult who initiates treatment. They may harbor unresolved anger and hurt about how their parents reacted to their coming out years ago or because their parents are still ashamed and disappointed by them. Others come because they feel guilty about causing their parents pain and are worried about their parents' emotional and physical welfare. These young adults want to be not only heard and validated but also accepted and connected. In other cases, it is parents who initiate the therapy. Some come because, even after years, they remain stuck in their fear, shame, and grief and are looking for a way out. Others come because their relationship with their adult child has become increasingly distant or conflictual and they are afraid to lose their bond with their child.

https://doi.org/10.1037/0000240-011
The Responsive Psychotherapist: Attuning to Clients in the Moment, J. C. Watson and H. Wiseman (Editors)

This chapter first presents a brief overview of ABFT. Then, we use clinical vignettes to illustrate how therapists respond appropriately (Hatcher, 2015; Kramer & Stiles, 2015; see also Chapter 1, this volume) to common clinical challenges.[1] We present results from research on family therapy in general, and ABFT in particular, related to therapist responsiveness. Finally, we describe how we train and supervise therapists to apply ABFT in a responsive manner.

According to Stiles (Chapter 1, this volume), appropriate responsiveness refers to the therapist using the most sensitive and effective interventions in the context of a given treatment task, the client's characteristics (e.g., flexibility, worldview), and the client's immediate, emerging behavior (e.g., defensiveness, level of emotional arousal). In the context of ABFT, as in all systemic therapies, choosing the most appropriate response is further complicated by the fact that the therapist needs to simultaneously attend and respond to multiple family members' needs and emerging behaviors as well as the influence of each family member's behavior on other family members. For example, this complexity is immediately evident at the start of ABFT, when family members often present with different and competing definitions of the problem at hand and ideas about how to solve the problem and who needs to do the changing. The therapist is faced with the challenge of making sure that each family member feels heard but then must also shift to helping them develop a shared, mutually agreed upon, higher order goal (e.g., repairing relational bonds) that resonates for all family members (Friedlander et al., 2011; Shelef et al., 2005). Thus, what may be an appropriate therapist response in the first part of the first session (e.g., exploring what is hard for a parent in terms of their accepting their child's sexual orientation) is not appropriate in the second part of the same session, when the task at hand is to focus on how the parent's difficulty accepting their child's identity is affecting their child and the relationship (e.g., "How has your unwillingness to meet your son's partner affected your son and your relationship with him?").

The complexity involved in responding appropriately when working with multiple family members is also evident when conducting in-session enactments (i.e., spontaneous or planned interactions between family members). During such enactments, when family members are talking directly to each other, appropriate therapist responses are dependent on many factors, including the level of emotional arousal each family member is experiencing, how open each family member is to hearing and processing what others are saying, and whether the content being discussed touches on important, core relational

---

[1]The identities of the clients in the case examples throughout this chapter have been disguised either by changing identifying information or using composites.

themes. Thus, when family members are connecting with deep vulnerable emotions, they are compassionate toward one another, and the conversation is productive, the therapist will use explorative and deepening interventions. In contrast, if family members become defensive, dysregulated, or attack one another, the appropriate therapist response is to block such behaviors, de-escalate the situation, sooth family members' concerns, and refocus the conversation onto core underlying themes, vulnerable emotions, and unmet needs (Davis & Butler, 2004; G. M. Diamond et al., 2019).

BRIEF OVERVIEW OF ATTACHMENT-BASED FAMILY THERAPY

ABFT (G. M. Diamond et al., 2012; G. S. Diamond et al., 2014) is rooted in structural family therapy (Minuchin, 1977), multidimensional family therapy (Liddle, 2002), and emotion-focused therapy and theory (Greenberg, 2011, 2012; Greenberg et al., 2010; Johnson & Greenberg, 1995). The first stage of the treatment involves eliciting and amplifying the frustration and pain family members are suffering because of the rupture in their relationships and establishing relationship building as the primary treatment goal. The second stage involves preparing for and conducting conjoint in-session corrective attachment/identity episodes (i.e., enactments) designed to productively process past hurts and create more open, loving, mutually accepting and validating, and healthy relationships. Results from a pilot open clinical trial showed pre- to posttreatment decreases in attachment anxiety and avoidance among depressed and suicidal lesbian, gay, and bisexual (LGB) adolescents (G. M. Diamond et al., 2012). Preliminary results from a current 5-year open clinical trial suggest that ABFT is associated with significant increases in adult children's perceptions of their parents' acceptance and significant decreases in their perceptions of their parents' rejection, from pre- to posttreatment (G. M. Diamond, 2018).

The treatment, which typically ranges from 18 to 26 weeks in duration, comprises five tasks. At the start of therapy, the therapist meets together with the young adult and their parents.

Task 1: Establish Relationship Building as the Main Treatment Goal

The first task of treatment is to define relationship building as the primary goal of treatment. During this initial session, the therapist develops an initial therapeutic bond with family members; gets a general sense of the contours of their lives (e.g., work, school, hobbies, friendships, romantic relationships, extended family network); explores the rupture in the young adult–parent relationship due to parental nonacceptance; amplifies family members' sense of loss and pain associated with the relational rupture; offers therapy as an opportunity to (re)establish more open, empathic, loving, respectful, and mutually validating relationships; establishes relationship building as a shared goal; and instills hope.

Task 2: Build a Working Alliance Between the Therapist and the Young Adult

Once family members are "signed on" to work on their relationships, the therapist meets with the young adult alone for a number of sessions. This second task of treatment, building a working alliance with the young adult, involves hearing more about the details of the young adult's life, including their experience of their parents' nonacceptance; helping the young adult to access and more fully connect to their hurt, assertive anger, and unmet attachment/identity needs (e.g., the need to be loved, need to be validated) associated with their parents' nonacceptance; and preparing the young adult to communicate such emotions and needs directly to their parents during subsequent conjoint corrective attachment/identity episodes.

Task 3: Build a Working Alliance Between the Therapist and the Parents

In the third task of the treatment, the therapist meets for a number of sessions alone with parents to develop a working alliance. This task involves hearing more about the details of each parent's life, including their experience of having a sexual or gender minority child; helping parents to connect to their shame, fear, grief, and anger associated with their child's minority identity; exploring how these feelings and inability to accept their child have negatively affected their child and their relationship with them; amplifying their sense of loss, pain, and regret; offering therapy as an opportunity to hear and support their child in way they have not been able to do before; and preparing parents to listen to their young adult in an empathic, nondefensive, open manner during subsequent conjoint corrective attachment/identity episodes.

Task 4: Create Change Through Dialogue Between Young Adults and Parents

The fourth task, conjoint corrective attachment/identity episodes, is considered the primary change mechanism in the treatment. Such episodes are in-session conversations (i.e., enactments) between young adults and their parents, during which the young adult shares previously unspoken thoughts and emotions (e.g., loss, hurt, fear, assertive anger) and unmet attachment and identity needs (e.g., the need to be cared for, to be validated, and to feel a sense of connectedness and belongingness) associated with their parents' nonacceptance. Simultaneously, parents are helped to respond in an open, empathic, validating, and nondefensive manner. As a result, the young adult feels heard, often for the first time. This process leads to a reduction in frustration, hurt, and loneliness and to an increase in safety, intimacy, and connection. Such corrective attachment/identity experiences are thought to transform interactional patterns, young adults' experience of their relationships with their parents (e.g., feel more cared about, accepted, connected, safer in the relationship), and internal working models (i.e., representations of self and parent).

Task 5: Collaborative Problem-Solving

After family members' anger, resentment, fear, and grief have subsided and a new sense of closeness, security, and mutual commitment has emerged, family members are able to engage in the fifth and final task of treatment: collaborative problem-solving. During this task, family members openly and productively discuss topics that were previously impossible to talk about because of the tension in the relationship and collaboratively resolve differences. For example, family members may talk, for the first time, about their child's plans to get married or have children, or they may work as a team to determine how and when to come out to grandparents. Whereas at the start of the treatment such issues were avoided or quickly escalated into conflict, now such conversations are collaborative and constructive.

EXAMPLES OF THERAPIST RESPONSIVENESS TO COMMON CLINICAL CHALLENGES

In this section, we present a number of examples illustrating common challenges in ABFT. We also discuss how therapists respond appropriately in the context of the specific treatment task at hand.

Shifting From Maladaptive Blaming to Empathy in Task 1

The first example, which occurred halfway through a first session while working on Task 1, illustrates a therapist's responsiveness as she worked to shift family members' focus away from maladaptive blaming and onto the young adult's vulnerable emotions. After listening to the adult daughter angrily criticize her father for his attacking, frightening response to her coming out to him 2 years prior, the therapist attempted to elicit more vulnerable, unspoken aspects of the daughter's experience: "I can hear how angry you are at your father about the way he responded. I wonder if, in that moment, you also felt hurt or scared?" After taking a breath, the daughter looked downward and began to cry. Then, turning to her father, she said softly, "I felt so humiliated. Like you thought I was crazy or that something was wrong with me. It was scary because I had never seen you like that. I didn't know what was going to happen. I just felt completely alone. I needed you to hug me and tell me that you still loved me and that everything was going to be all right." These moments, when young adults are vulnerable in the presence of their parents, are both heart-wrenching and sacred. Often, this is the first time that parents have witnessed their child's unadulterated pain. Despite the therapist's impulse to comfort the young adult and reassure parents, the appropriate therapist response is to let such moments linger. Indeed, the young adult's pain and unmet needs are the raison d'etre and fuel for the treatment, and the more powerfully they are felt, the more motivated parents are to respond with empathy, curiosity, and compassion.

In some cases, however, witnessing their child's pain elicits defensive responses by parents. They may feel guilty, blamed, inept, or helpless. As a result, they may begin to dispute the details of the child's narrative (e.g., "That's not true. I didn't say she could never come to the house. I said that I wanted her to leave at that moment"), explain why they could not have reacted better in the moment (e.g., "What did you expect? You dropped it on me like a bomb! It was the end of the day; I was exhausted; it was the worst timing possible"), invalidate their child's identity (e.g., "It just doesn't make sense—you have had boyfriend after boyfriend"), or blame their young adult for overreacting (e.g., "I don't know why you are blowing things out of proportion. With you, everything becomes a drama"). When parents become defensive, the appropriate therapist response is to simultaneously soothe the parent so that they do not feel judged or guilty; validate the young adult's narrative so that they do not feel dismissed, abandoned, or pathologized; and then redirect the focus of the conversation back to the young adult's subjective, vulnerable experience. For example, in this same segment, the therapist responded by saying, "Mr. K., clearly you love your daughter and want the best for her. No one reacts optimally when they are exhausted and things are popped on them at the end of a long day. Your daughter's disclosure likely hit you like a ton of bricks. I want to hear all about that, and what it has been like for you since, when we meet alone in later sessions. But right now, in this moment, what is it like for you to hear her say how scared and alone she felt, to see her tears?" The father, turning to his daughter, replied, "It hurts to see her like that. She's my daughter."

Relationship Building as the Main Goal in Task 1

The next example, taken from later in the same session, illustrates how therapists respond appropriately as they work to establish relationship building as the first and primary goal of treatment (i.e., Task 1). After the young adult's pain and vulnerability are manifested in the room, the therapist presents therapy as an opportunity for parents to more fully hear their child's vulnerable emotions and unmet attachment and identity needs and thus develop more open, honest relationships. However, while relationship building is why family members have come to therapy, and this goal resonates at some level, family members are wary or even petrified. It is not by chance that years have gone by without having such conversations.

Some young adults are afraid that if they share how they are really feeling, their parents will be overwhelmed or will attack or dismiss them. They do not necessarily believe that their parents have the motivation or capacity to hear them or to change and are afraid of being disappointed. In this example, the therapist turns to the daughter and speaks to both her fear and her deep-seated desire to be heard and connected:

> I see and hear how hurt you were by your dad's response when you came out and how unsure you are about where dad stands right now. On one hand he says he is in a different spot, more accepting and open to hearing how you feel, but on the other hand you are afraid to rock the boat and perhaps lose what you have been able to build so far. If, however, you felt surer about the strength of the relationship, and safe to say more about how you really feel inside to your dad so that he could understand, would that be meaningful to you?

To this, the daughter responded, "I am not sure. There were times when I thought he understood, and then suddenly he would get angry and turn on me. With Mom, it's a different story. It always ends up being all about her. She basically falls apart and then I need to take care of her."

In such instances, the appropriate therapist response is to simultaneously validate the young adult's past disappointments, fear, and healthy skepticism about the future; exude competence and instill hope; set realistic expectations by acknowledging that the young adult's parents may not be able to respond perfectly, at least not at first; commit to protecting the young adult from attacks, invalidation, and abandonment in the therapy room; and remind the young adult how much they long for things to be different. In this example, the therapist responded in a way that attended to all five of these dimensions:

> Lisa, I know that you have tried to tell your parents how you feel in the past and have been frustrated. My job is to help them listen better. I have worked with lots of parents and almost all of them have been able to listen and understand

at least a little better over time. If I don't think your mom and dad are ready, we won't move forward with the sessions together. It's a step-by-step process. But if I could help them better hear how you feel and what you need, and for it to really sink in, would that be meaningful for you?

Almost always, the young adult is willing to endorse this goal, even if they are still cautious or ambivalent.

Parents, on the other hand, may have different concerns. Some feel like they are continuously "walking on eggshells," afraid that anything they say will quickly escalate into conflict and mutual blaming. Others are convinced that their child is not really interested in engaging in sustained, open, meaningful conversations with them: "Every time I try to talk to her about this, she walks away." In such instances, the appropriate therapist response is to remind parents of their deep-seated desire to be emotionally present for their child, validate and normalize parents' fears, exude competence and instill hope, and set realistic expectations. In the following example from the second segment, the therapist responded by saying,

> Mr. and Mrs. K, you clearly love your daughter and want to be there for her. I know that, in the past, such conversations haven't gone well. I am going to help you have a different kind of conversation, during which you will be able to ask Lisa questions and she will be able to respond without attacking you or withdrawing. That is my job, to help prepare her to respond differently. It will be a process. But, if Lisa is eventually able to share with you some of the things that have hurt her and made her angry, and do it in an open, heartfelt, respectful manner, is that something you would want?

In almost all cases, the answer is "Yes, that is what we came here for."

Responding Appropriately to Parents' Feeling and Concerns in Task 3

The third example, taken from another case, takes place during the last stage of Task 3, when the therapist meets alone with parents to prepare them for subsequent conjoint corrective attachment/identity episodes. The segment illustrates how therapists respond appropriately to parents' concerns about being coerced into changing their beliefs or accommodating to things that they feel are intolerable. In this instance, the father said,

> I love my son and would do anything for him, but I have my religious beliefs. I see it [homosexuality] as being unnatural and wrong. I don't want him to get the message that I agree or approve. I understand that it is frustrating for him, but my position is not going to change. He can come over to the house for dinner and talk about other things.

This particular example illustrates parents' common misconception that being empathic and validating their child's experience (e.g., frustration, loneliness, longing to be accepted) is equivalent to agreement, approval, or having to acquiesce to all their child's requests. Just because a parent feels their child's pain does not necessarily mean that they can, or have to, solve it. Sometimes, just being there empathically is all that parents are able to do in that moment. Teasing apart these important but different parental functions (i.e., empathic listening, validation, support, and boundary setting) creates an opening for movement and change.

In such instances, the appropriate therapist response is to simultaneously acknowledge the parent's honesty; communicate respect for parents' religious beliefs and customs; highlight the father's recognition that his position is causing his son great pain; amplify the emotional price the young adult is paying (e.g., isolation, grief, hopelessness) and the negative impact on their relationship; distinguish between empathizing with his son's experience of feeling rejected and approving of homosexuality or agreeing to do things that feel intolerable; reassure him that he will not be asked to do things that feel intolerable; and offer therapy as an opportunity to be there for his son emotionally, in a manner different than ever before. In this particular case, the therapist responded by saying,

> Mr. S., I appreciate you being straight and clear. I understand that, in your house, homosexuality is not acceptable or talked about. I also see how hard it is for you. You love your son; you don't want to lose him or for him to feel bad. I, like you, also see how much pain he is in, feeling like he cannot be open at home and, therefore, disconnected from you and the family. I think that, more than anything, he wants to at least be able to tell you how it feels to be in the closet in his own home and to have to keep this secret from his sisters. You don't have to necessarily do anything different. But just being there to listen, understand, and care will make him feel less alone.

Responsiveness in Conjoint Corrective Attachment/Identity Episodes (Task 4)

The fourth and final example, taken from the middle of a Task 4 session from a different case, illustrates therapist responsiveness in the context of a conjoint corrective attachment/identity episode. Such episodes are characterized by highly aroused, emotionally laden conversations between family members about heretofore avoided and painful topics. During such conversations, the therapist's role is primarily to track and monitor, only intervening when necessary. However, because of the intensity and fear intrinsic to such conversations, there are times when parents or their child needs support and redirection. In some instances, parents may begin to explain how their child feels rather than ask their child how they actually feel. In other instances, parents may be inclined to jump to problem-solving before fully hearing how their child feels or what they need. In yet other instances, parents may become overwhelmed emotionally upon hearing the full extent of their child's pain or frustration for the first time. Adult children, for their part, may be hesitant to divulge vulnerable feelings or may react reflexively and angrily when parents momentarily respond in an unattuned manner.

In this example, the father began the session by telling his daughter that he knew how she felt when her girlfriend broke up with her and she had nobody to go to for support. He explained that he himself had gone through a similar experience. In response to the father's explanations, the therapist quickly intervened by suggesting that he had an opportunity, in the here and now, to find out from his daughter how she actually felt at the time: "Mr. R, it is great that you can connect to Shari through your own, similar experiences. However, right now you have the opportunity to hear how *she* experienced this break-up, what it was like for *her*." The father responded by asking his daughter, "How did you feel?" Noting the change in father's stance, the daughter began to share previously avoided, painful aspects of her experience: "It was horrible. I found out from a friend who saw her with somebody else. I felt like the world had fallen apart." The daughter then began to sob.

As the intensity of her daughter's expressed pain increased, the mother began asking her about how she had coped with her loss. While born of good intentions, the mother's question distracted from the more difficult and scary, but essential, task at hand: being emotionally present with their daughter in her fear, loss, and grief, even in retrospect. In this instance, the therapist responded by saying, "Mrs. R., what is going on inside of you as you hear Shari talk about feeling so alone and humiliated?" "It is heartbreaking," the mother responded, "I wish it never happened to her." To this, the therapist responded,

> Today, right now, you have a chance to be with your daughter and hear what that was like for her, so that she doesn't have to carry it around alone anymore. See if you can find out more about what that whole episode was like for her.

As can be seen in this example, the therapist's appropriate response in the context of this particular task is not to explore the thoughts and emotions fueling parents' avoidant, defensive responses or to allow the conversation to drift to important but secondary topics such as how the adolescent has coped, but rather to soothe parents and redirect them to focus on the adolescent's experience so as to create a new, corrective experience.

INTERSECTIONALITY AND RESPONSIVENESS

ABFT was developed to treat what might be considered a very specific clinical population: LGBT adult children and their nonaccepting parents. However, we have found tremendous variability among our clients and unique clinical challenges related to their particular sexual/gender identities, cultural/ethnic backgrounds, and degree of religiosity. In regard to sexual orientation, for example, parents of bisexual children sometimes hold the belief that their child can choose to be attracted to other-gender individuals and, therefore, expect them to do so for their own sake and for the sake of the family. They may view bisexuality, in contrast to a lesbian or gay identity, as less valid, essential, or fixed. Such beliefs and attitudes can cause resentment and power struggles and may impair the acceptance process. In such instances, one appropriate therapist response is to invite parents to be more curious and ask their child about their experience of being bisexual, including falling in love and choosing a partner, rather than making assumptions. Another example is the difficulty parents of transgender or genderqueer clients often have when trying to imagine and make sense of their child's gender identity. In response, therapists help the parents invite their children to share their experience of gender. Such conversations can facilitate parents' identification with, and empathy toward, their child. As an aside, conversations about gender identity can be complicated. In today's culture, people do not yet have sufficient language to describe their experience of gender—the essence of being male, female, or both—above and beyond describing gender-typical or atypical interests and behaviors (e.g., playing sports, wanting to wear a dress), gender roles (e.g., being assertive), sexual orientation, and other proxies.

ABFT therapists also need to be sensitive to families' cultural beliefs about identity. The tension between self-actualization and self-expression and conforming to family and/or community needs and rules exists in all families (Minuchin, 1977). In families with sexual-minority and gender-minority individuals, this balance is often strained. In families from communal cultures who place a premium on family togetherness and conformity, the adult child's inherent needs to openly and authentically express their sexual orientation or gender identity is often seen as secondary to the welfare of the family as a whole. In such families, for example, parents may take the position that their child should come to family events without their partner in order not to upset members of the extended family, even if that causes their child distress. Again, the appropriate therapist response in such instances is not to judge or even challenge parents' values but, instead, to invite them to engage further and explore the full extent of how their position and demands affect their child and their relationship with their child. Often, during such conversations, parents recognize that their emphases on the appearance of family cohesion and pseudorelationships and their desire to avoid discomfort and tension come at the expense of, rather than promoting, strong, meaningful family relationships.

ABFT therapists are also responsive to family members' religious beliefs. Many parents tell us that their child's sexual identity is not in accord with biblical writings. With such families, we first validate their concerns. Then, we remind them of no less important competing biblical values, such as the importance of family togetherness; accepting others; living an honest, open life; not lying or misrepresenting oneself to others; not insulting or shaming others; and not living alone without a partner. For some parents, such conversations are a first step in reconciling their religious beliefs with their deep-seated desire to be psychologically and emotionally available for their child. We may also inquire regarding the attitudes of their own religious leaders (e.g., rabbi, imam, pastor) toward LGBT individuals and make them aware of religious leaders and communities with LGBT supportive/affirming stances.

RESEARCH ON RESPONSIVENESS IN ATTACHMENT-BASED FAMILY THERAPY

Over the years, family therapy research has focused on how therapists can be responsive to families' unique characteristics when engaging them in treatment or forming a therapeutic alliance and how to adapt family treatments so that they are more culturally sensitive. Perhaps the most systematic program of research on responsive engagement comes from Santisteban, Szapocznik, and colleagues at the University of Miami (Coatsworth et al., 2001; Santisteban et al., 1996; Szapocznik et al., 1988). In their work engaging Hispanic families with youth with conduct problems in brief strategic family therapy (BSFT), they developed strategic structural-systems engagement—a procedure for analyzing the resistance profile for a given family (e.g., overly powerful adolescent, ambivalent mother) and then selecting which family member to approach and how. Across a number of randomized clinical trials, these researchers found that BSFT was consistently superior to comparison/control conditions in terms of engaging and retaining such families in treatment.

In regard to responding to initial adolescent resistance and forming therapeutic alliances, findings from one study of adolescents receiving multidimensional family therapy (G. M. Diamond et al., 1999) suggest that when therapists attended to the adolescents' experiences, presented themselves as the adolescents' ally, and helped the adolescents formulate personally meaningful goals, their initially poor alliances with the adolescents improved. In another study of resistant at-risk adolescents participating in family therapy, Higham et al. (2012) found that certain therapist behaviors were associated with adolescents' shifts to positive engagement in treatment. These interventions were structuring conversations, fostering autonomy, building systemic awareness, rolling with resistance, and working to understand the adolescent's subjective experience. Such alliance building is important in light of substantial research showing the link between the strength of the alliance and treatment engagement and outcome in family therapy (Friedlander, Escudero, et al., 2011; Robbins et al., 2006; Shelef et al., 2005).

Finally, there is consensus regarding the need to develop culturally informed family-based treatments as well as to adapt existing family-based treatments so that they are responsive to the needs of, and effective with, minority populations (Zane et al., 2016), including sexual and gender minority individuals (Pachankis & Safren, 2019). In the first phase of a treatment development study adapting attachment-based family therapy for depressed and suicidal LGB adolescents, G. M. Diamond and colleagues (2012) found that treatment needed to (a) include more individual time working with parents to process their disappointments, pain, anger, and fears related to their adolescents' minority sexual orientation; (b) address the meaning, implications, and process of parental acceptance; and (c) heighten parents' awareness of subtle yet potent invalidating responses to their adolescents' sexual orientation (i.e., microaggressions). In the second phase, they found that the adapted treatment was acceptable to both the adolescents and their parents and evidenced preliminary evidence of its efficacy, including decreases in depressive symptoms, suicidal ideation, attachment anxiety, and attachment avoidance (G. M. Diamond et al., 2012).

With that said, more research is needed. In particular, it would be important to empirically examine the effectiveness of various engagement strategies in ABFT. We have found that some parents are resistant even to coming for an initial screening. They are afraid that the therapy will be too emotionally overwhelming, are too ashamed, are afraid that they will be railroaded into accepting their child's identity by a pro-LGBT therapist, and so on. In such cases, we typically meet with the adult child alone to help them craft an appeal to their parents that comes from the heart—something like "Mom, Dad, it is no secret that things are tense between us. I know that this is hard for you. It is also hard for me. But I love you, and our relationship is important to me. I want to find a way to talk this through so that, over time, we do not grow apart. Would you at least be willing to talk to the person who runs the project or come to a first meeting to meet them? If, afterwards, you don't want to continue, that is up to you but at least please come once." Sometimes these appeals are more individualized to attend to a specific parental concern. In some instances, we help the adult child craft a letter to give or leave for their parents. In other instances, they prefer to work on articulating exactly what they want to say to their parents in a face-to-face meeting. Future research has the potential to illuminate whether variations of this engagement procedure are effective.

In addition, more research is needed to uncover and describe the moment-by-moment processes by which therapists help parents to grieve and to let go of their heteronormative dreams and work through their fear and shame. For example, we are currently using task-analytic methodologies (Greenberg & Foerster, 1996) to flesh out clinical maps of sequences of therapist interventions and client performance states that reflect such working through. Moment-by-moment clinical maps are invaluable both for model development and for training therapists to use the model.

TRAINING AND SUPERVISING THERAPISTS TO BE RESPONSIVE

Training therapists to become competent in ABFT is no small feat. ABFT requires therapists to elicit and contain strong, painful emotions; monitor and manage multiple therapeutic alliances; be experience near; and monitor their own responses. These demands require that one be aware of their own biases. For example, sometimes ABFT therapists find themselves over-identifying with the adult child, becoming frustrated with or even angry at a parent for not being able to accept their child's identity and causing them pain. In such moments, the supervisor's job is to help the therapist explore their frustration and compassionately connect more with the parent's fear of losing control while thinking about what will help the parent feel safe enough to move forward in the process. ABFT therapists must also be continuously cognizant of the immediate treatment task at hand, where they are timewise in a given session, how each family member is responding, the point they are hoping to reach by the end of the session, and the steps on the way. In fact, if one were to push the "pause button" and ask an ABFT therapist why they just responded in the manner that they did (e.g., remained silent and allowed family members to continue speaking to one another; blocked a family member's explanation about how they coped in a certain situation and, instead, redirected them to explore how they felt in the here and now; stopped to soothe a parent), they should be able to say based on the goals and tasks at hand, the immediate content, process, and affect in the room, and the next step required to help family members move forward. Therapists are working intentionally at every moment.

Fortunately, the rationale of the treatment, structure, goals, and specific steps of each task are articulated in detail in the therapy manual (G. M. Diamond et al., 2019). Moreover, as the result of years of treatment development work and training, the manual includes descriptions of common negative client resistances and optimal therapist responses, such that moment-to-moment responsiveness is built into the model and training. All ABFT therapists participate in an initial intensive 3-day workshop that includes learning the tasks and steps, watching exemplary segments from actual cases that demonstrate the successful traversing of each task, and simulations. Therapists then watch all of the sessions of at least three archived good cases so that they can see how the treatment unfolds over time and how expert ABFT therapists operate. Finally, therapists sit in the room with an expert ABFT therapist as cotherapists for at least one case.

Upon being trained, our therapists receive weekly videotape supervision. Videotape supervision is invaluable because it allows the therapist and supervisor to evaluate the appropriateness of the therapist's actual responses, including content, tone, and timing. Therapists will usually bring preselected segments of tape or, less frequently, randomly pick a spot to begin watching. While watching the tape, the therapist and supervisor pay attention to the process, content, and affective tone. In some cases, therapists recognize that they did not sufficiently elicit or amplify vulnerable, painful emotions. In other instances, therapist can see that their alliance with a particular family member has become strained. In yet other instances, the therapist may realize that they are too central in the process, perhaps talking too much rather than having family members speak to one another. Videotape supervision allows the therapist to observe their responses and retrospectively reevaluate their appropriateness in a less stressful, more objective context. Outside of the immediate relational field between them and family members, and without the need to monitor and respond online, therapists are able to gain a bit of distance as they observe their responses. The utility of videotape supervision in family therapy has been extolled elsewhere (Liddle et al., 1997; Wetchler et al., 1989). It is worth noting, however, that in the beginning, videotape supervision can be particularly threatening or anxiety producing and, as such, must be conducted in the context of a safe, open, and strong therapist–supervisor relationship. Our experience has led us to believe that ongoing, regular videotape supervision is not only invaluable but essential during at least the first years of training in ABFT.

CONCLUDING THOUGHTS

ABFT is a manualized, focused, experiential, emotion- and relationship-focused therapy designed specifically for sexual and gender minority adults and their nonaccepting parents. The model is the result of more than 2 decades of intensive treatment development research, including intensive analyses of the moment-to-moment processes reflecting each task. Consequently, the manual and training are extremely specific and detailed and include the discussion of common client resistances and behaviors, along with effective therapist responses. As such, ABFT is inherently responsive at the most micro level.

The therapists who currently deliver ABFT have received intensive, costly training and ongoing supervision in the context of clinical trials and represent the "gold standard." As dissemination efforts expand, we will face many of the known challenges of exporting a research-based model to community clinics and private practitioners. We hope such efforts will be accompanied by adherence/competence, effectiveness, and further task-analytic treatment development research.

REFERENCES

Coatsworth, J. D., Santisteban, D. A., McBride, C. K., & Szapocznik, J. (2001). Brief strategic family therapy versus community control: Engagement, retention, and an exploration of the moderating role of adolescent symptom severity. *Family Process, 40*(3), 313–332. https://doi.org/10.1111/j.1545-5300.2001.4030100313.x

Davis, S. D., & Butler, M. H. (2004). Enacting relationships in marriage and family therapy: A conceptual and operational definition of an enactment. *Journal of Marital and Family Therapy, 30*(3), 319–333. https://doi.org/10.1111/j.1752-0606.2004.tb01243.x

Diamond, G. M. (2018, July 22). *Relationship-focused therapy for sexual and gender minority young adults and their non-accepting parents* [Paper presentation]. International Conference of the Society for Psychotherapy Research, Toronto, Canada.

Diamond, G. M., Boruchovitz-Zamir, R., Gat, I., & Nir-Gottlieb, O. (2019). Relationship-focused therapy for sexual minority individuals and their parents. In J. Pachankis & S. Safren (Eds.), *Handbook of evidence-based mental health practice with sexual and gender minorities* (pp. 430–456). Oxford University Press.

Diamond, G. M., Diamond, G. S., Levy, S., Closs, C., Ladipo, T., & Siqueland, L. (2012). Attachment-based family therapy for suicidal lesbian, gay, and bisexual adolescents: A treatment development study and open trial with preliminary findings. *Psychotherapy, 49*(1), 62–71. https://doi.org/10.1037/a0026247

Diamond, G. M., Liddle, H. A., Hogue, A., & Dakof, G. (1999). Alliance-building interventions with adolescents in family therapy: A process study. *Psychotherapy: Theory, Research, & Practice, 36*(4), 355–368. https://doi.org/10.1037/h0087729

Diamond, G. S., Diamond, G. M., & Levy, S. L. (2014). *Attachment-based family therapy for depressed adolescents*. American Psychological Association. https://doi.org/10.1037/14296-000

Friedlander, M. L., Escudero, V., Heatherington, L., & Diamond, G. M. (2011). Alliance in couple and family therapy. *Psychotherapy, 48*(1), 25–33. https://doi.org/10.1037/a0022060

Greenberg, L. S. (2011). *Emotion-focused therapy*. American Psychological Association.

Greenberg, L. S. (2012). Emotions, the great captains of our lives: Their role in the process of change in psychotherapy. *American Psychologist, 67*(8), 697–707. https://doi.org/10.1037/a0029858

Greenberg, L. S., & Foerster, F. S. (1996). Task analysis exemplified: The process of resolving unfinished business. *Journal of Consulting and Clinical Psychology, 64*(3), 439–446. https://doi.org/10.1037/0022-006X.64.3.439

Greenberg, L., Warwar, S., & Malcolm, W. (2010). Emotion-focused couples therapy and the facilitation of forgiveness. *Journal of Marital and Family Therapy, 36*(1), 28–42. https://doi.org/10.1111/j.1752-0606.2009.00185.x

Hatcher, R. L. (2015). Interpersonal competencies: Responsiveness, technique, and training in psychotherapy. *American Psychologist, 70*(8), 747–757. https://doi.org/10.1037/a0039803

Higham, J., Friedlander, M., Escudero, V., & Diamond, G. M. (2012). Engaging reluctant adolescents in family therapy: An exploratory change process study. *The American Journal of Family Therapy, 34*(1), 24–52. https://doi.org/10.1111/j.1467-6427.2011.00571.x

Johnson, S. M., & Greenberg, L. S. (1995). The emotionally focused approach to problems in adult attachment. In N. S. Jacobson & A. S. Gurman (Eds.), *Clinical handbook of couple therapy* (pp. 121–141). Guilford Press.

Kramer, U., & Stiles, W. B. (2015). The responsiveness problem in psychotherapy: A review of proposed solutions. *Clinical Psychology: Science and Practice, 22*(3), 277–295. https://doi.org/10.1111/cpsp.12107

Liddle, H. A. (2002). *Multidimensional family therapy for adolescent cannabis users, Cannabis Youth Treatment (CYT) series* (Vol. 5). Center for Substance Abuse Treatment, Substance Abuse and Mental Health Services Administration.

Liddle, H. A., Becker, D., & Diamond, G. M. (1997). Family therapy supervision. In C. E. Watkins, Jr., (Ed.), *Handbook of psychotherapy supervision* (pp. 400–418). John Wiley & Sons.

Minuchin, S. (1977). *Families and family therapy*. Routledge.

Pachankis, J., & Safren, S. (Eds.). (2019). *Handbook of evidence-based mental health practice with sexual and gender minorities*. Oxford University Press. https://doi.org/10.1093/med-psych/9780190669300.001.0001

Robbins, M. S., Liddle, H. A., Turner, C. W., Dakof, G. A., Alexander, J. F., & Kogan, S. M. (2006). Adolescent and parent therapeutic alliances as predictors of dropout in multidimensional family therapy. *Journal of Family Psychology, 20*(1), 108–116. https://doi.org/10.1037/0893-3200.20.1.108

Santisteban, D. A., Szapocznik, J., Perez-Vidal, A., Kurtines, W. M., Murray, E. J., & LaPerriere, A. (1996). Efficacy of intervention for engaging youth and families into treatment and some variables that may contribute to differential effectiveness. *Journal of Family Psychology, 10*(1), 35–44. https://doi.org/10.1037/0893-3200.10.1.35

Shelef, K., Diamond, G. M., Diamond, G. S., & Liddle, H. A. (2005). Adolescent and parent alliance and treatment outcome in multidimensional family therapy. *Journal of Consulting and Clinical Psychology, 73*(4), 689–698. https://doi.org/10.1037/0022-006X.73.4.689

Szapocznik, J., Perez-Vidal, A., Brickman, A. L., Foote, F. H., Santisteban, D., Hervis, O., & Kurtines, W. M. (1988). Engaging adolescent drug abusers and their families in treatment: A strategic structural systems approach. *Journal of Consulting and Clinical Psychology, 56*(4), 552–557. https://doi.org/10.1037/0022-006X.56.4.552

Wetchler, J. L., Piercey, F. P., & Sprenkle, D. H. (1989). Supervisors' and supervisees' perceptions of the effectiveness of family therapy supervisory techniques. *The American Journal of Family Therapy, 17*(1), 35–47. https://doi.org/10.1080/01926188908250750

Zane, N., Bernal, G., & Leong, F. T. L. (Eds.). (2016). *Cultural, racial, and ethnic psychology book series. Evidence-based psychological practice with ethnic minorities: Culturally informed research and clinical strategies*. American Psychological Association.

11

THERAPIST RESPONSIVENESS IN TREATMENTS FOR PERSONALITY DISORDERS

UELI KRAMER

Therapist responsiveness may be both understood as an obstacle for psychotherapy researchers and as an opportunity for clinicians. For psychotherapy researchers, therapist responsiveness represents an almost insurmountable obstacle standing in the way of clean and neat research conclusions: The therapist, like any other human being, is affected by emerging contexts, such as specific client behaviors (Stiles, 2009; Stiles et al., 1998). For psychotherapists, therapist responsiveness may be the "glue" that makes their relational and technical interventions work for a particular client: It is doing the right thing at the right time (Kramer & Stiles, 2015; Stiles & Horvath, 2017).

In this chapter, I argue that treatments for clients with personality disorders (PDs) represent a particularly fruitful context to (a) demonstrate responsiveness effects; (b) find a context-appropriate definition of therapist responsiveness; (c) show which interventions work with which client

Parts of this research were supported by the Swiss National Science Foundation (SNSF) Grants 100019_152685 and 100014_134562/1. Special thanks to Cédric Berthelin, Franz Caspar, Ines Culina, Martin Debbané, Irene Elkin, Elsa Fiscalini, Florence Lepdor, and Chantal Martin Soelch for their support and their collaboration in the empirical parts of this chapter. I thank Sandra (a pseudonym) for providing her data for publication.

https://doi.org/10.1037/0000240-012
The Responsive Psychotherapist: Attuning to Clients in the Moment, J. C. Watson and H. Wiseman (Editors)

behavior; and, finally, (d) help clinicians make productive, or appropriate, use of opportunities that arise in the therapy process. In the first section, I discuss PDs and explain why these disorders may represent a paradigmatic context to study appropriate therapist responsiveness, then move to three different operationalizations of therapist responsiveness: (a) generic responsiveness, (b) disorder-specific responsiveness, and (c) individualized responsiveness. Each is illustrated and discussed by using a particular study focusing on clients with PDs.

In the second section of the chapter, I illustrate therapist responsiveness with a clinical example from early in therapy. I discuss considerations about how to take account of diversity in the study of responsiveness with clients with PDs, and I make some recommendations for training and practice.

WHY IS RESPONSIVENESS SO IMPORTANT IN THE TREATMENT OF CLIENTS WITH PERSONALITY DISORDERS?

Personality disorders may be understood as disturbances of the individual's interpersonal, regulatory, and identity functional domains (American Psychiatric Association, 2013; Livesley, 2017; Livesley et al., 2016; Zanarini & Frankenburg, 2007). As a consequence of these dysfunctions, clients with PDs may present interpersonal dysfunction, which may appear in the here and now of the therapeutic interaction and affect the course of therapy (Kramer, 2019b; Kramer & Levy, 2017; McMain et al., 2015). In session, clients with PDs may adopt an external focus; this may mean that they present a particular aspect of themselves and neglect the presentation of certain others (e.g., they may not present with central or fragile processes and contents), in order to evoke a particular reaction or feeling in the interaction partner. For example, a client may present as particularly weak in order for the other to feel guilty if they do not take care of the client immediately, or in order to increase the likelihood that they will take on tasks the client aims to delegate (see Pos & Greenberg, 2012; Sachse, 2020). A client with a PD may ask for extraordinary treatment in order to avoid making a full commitment to psychotherapy. For example, they may ask the therapist to be more present, offer longer sessions, or organize extra sessions. Clients with a PD may at times use border-crossing behaviors, such as aggressive or sexually connoted behaviors, which may have the function of (a) testing the stability of the therapeutic relationship (Weiss, 1993) and/or (b) deterring attention from the core content of therapeutic work (because it seems too hard for the client to focus on this content; Sachse, 2020). Clients with a PD, in particular, borderline personality disorder (BPD), may present with self-harming behaviors or suicidal behaviors with an instrumental or interpersonally functional component. Some clients, for example, may self-harm to seek attention from the other, seek comfort, or make sure that the other is permanently available.

These psychopathological presentations of clients with PDs may have an impact on the course of therapy, in particular, therapist responsiveness, and may represent risks for the collaborative process. As a response to the client's adopting an external focus—meaning behaving in ways that are oriented toward producing a specific effect on the other—and presenting as particularly weak and in need, the therapist may take on the client's tasks, which may hinder the client's growth toward responsible action. As a response to the client requiring special treatment (e.g., evening sessions), the therapist may offer sessions beyond regular office hours, which may prove problematic to the necessary limit-setting and ending of the sessions. As a response to client border-crossing behaviors, such as aggressive behaviors, the therapist may react with hostility using a personally dismissive voice or express contempt nonverbally to the client (instead of addressing it verbally), either of which may prove problematic for further collaboration. As a response to the client engaging in self-harming behaviors aiming to gain attention from the therapist, the latter may offer extra time after a session to take care of the client's sense of woundedness, which may prove problematic with the treatment aim of reducing the frequency of the client's self-harming behaviors. With such interactions in mind, certain psychotherapists may even decide not to take on these clients in order to avoid potential problems.

These examples show that a fine line is to be drawn between appropriate and less appropriate therapist responsiveness in the process of facing interpersonally constraining behaviors on the client's part. These examples illustrate how central appropriate therapist responsiveness is for the treatment of clients with PDs, and the understanding of therapist responsiveness in this paradigmatic context might inform the generic understanding of the underlying mechanisms (Kramer, 2019b). I would assume that while responsiveness is certainly ubiquitous in psychotherapy facing all types of clients, psychotherapy for clients with PDs may represent a particular challenge to clinicians because of stronger effects related to responsiveness (as compared to other clients). Clients with PDs may pose an extra responsiveness challenge to clinicians who treat them in psychotherapy; psychotherapy researchers must address this challenge when studying treatments for clients with PDs. The question may be, as formulated by van Kessel and Lietaer (1998) when they ask, in the context of client-centered and interpersonal therapies, "How does the therapist steer clear of following the client's preferred style of interaction in a complementary way?" (p. 159). This question may be interpreted as pointing toward any good form of therapy, and *a fortiori* toward the notion of therapist competence.

THE DIFFERENCE BETWEEN THERAPIST COMPETENCE AND THERAPIST RESPONSIVENESS

While the concepts of therapist competence and responsiveness overlap—both focus on what the therapist may do in terms of the "right thing at the right time"—these concepts also differ in a number of aspects. As argued by Stiles (2013), therapist competence may be understood as an "evaluative" variable indicating the global quality of the client–therapist interaction (and, in particular, the therapist contribution to that interaction). Therapist responsiveness operates on a different level: It *describes* the therapist interpersonal behavior—moment-by-moment, session-by-session, and over the course of the entire therapy—in response to the client behaviors. As such, responsiveness may be a core principle that contributes to therapist competence and may be understood as one of the primary principles of change in therapy for clients with PDs. It may also explain why some treatments with these clients do not work. While the study of therapist competence may be an attempt to solve and control effects related to responsiveness in psychotherapy research (Kramer & Stiles, 2015), it remains an open empirical question whether therapist competence with a specific therapeutic approach captures the more descriptive interaction-based principle of responsiveness.

THREE OPERATIONALIZATIONS OF THERAPIST RESPONSIVENESS IN ACTION

Therapist responsiveness may be examined by focusing on the behaviors used by the therapist when being responsive ("responsive with") and may be examined by focusing on the client and context markers to which the therapist responds ("responsive to"). In the following subsections, I focus mostly on the latter and differentiate between three degrees of granularity of the "responsive to" conceptualization. The therapist can be responsive to any client behavior (generic responsiveness), to processes supposedly underlying the disorder (disorder-specific responsiveness), and to idiosyncratic behaviors as formulated for an individual client (individualized responsiveness).

Generic Responsiveness

Generic therapist responsiveness describes the degree to which the therapist is (a) attentive to the patient; (b) acknowledging and attempting to understand the patient's current concerns; (c) clearly interested in and responding to the patient's communication, both in terms of content and feelings; and (d) caring, affirming, and respectful toward the patient (Elkin et al., 2014).

Generic responsiveness thus encompasses a number of appropriate therapist reactions to client behaviors that are meant to cut across therapy approaches and client contexts (e.g., therapist empathy, attentiveness, positive therapeutic atmosphere, along with the negative therapist behavior, inversely coded). On the basis of this conceptualization, Elkin et al. (2014) developed an observer-rated measure (Elkin & Smith, 2007) aiming to capture these generic responsiveness processes. The scale encompasses three levels of assessment: (a) assessment every 5 minutes, (b) averaged scores across all the 5-minute excerpts of a session, and (c) global ratings of a session of appropriate responsiveness. Elkin showed acceptable coefficients of internal and external validity, as well as interrater reliability, of the scale in the context of treatment for depression. In particular, the subscale positive therapeutic atmosphere (i.e., caring and compassionate, respectful, compatible level of discourse, and appropriate emotional quality and intensity) assessed at the first two sessions of therapy predicted client engagement and (inversely) dropout in psychotherapy. The global (summary) item of responsiveness was also a strong predictor of engagement and dropout (but therapist empathy and attentiveness were not). So far, it is unclear whether this generic operationalization of therapist responsiveness applies to treatments for PDs.

Disorder-Specific Responsiveness

Appropriate disorder-specific therapist responsiveness captures therapist reactions and interventions thought to focus on the underlying disorder-specific psychological processes. As such, it has been argued that epistemic trust and mentalization are lacking in PDs, in particular, BPD (Fonagy et al., 2017). To address this problem, specific mentalization-fostering therapist interventions, in the context of mentalization-based therapy (MBT)—an evidence-based treatment for PDs (Bateman & Fonagy, 2006, 2009)—may be implemented. They include addressing the client's pretend mode, focusing on interpersonal affects, and discussing the therapeutic relationship. As such, they may represent central building blocks of disorder-specific responsiveness facing clients with PDs. The scale used to operationalize responsiveness in this context describes therapist competence in the quality of mentalization-fostering processes (Karterud et al., 2013). Even though this measure was not explicitly developed as a measure of responsiveness, but rather as an assessment of adherence and competence in the context of MBT, it may be used in this particular context. Therapist competence goes beyond the mere adherence to a protocol: It encompasses the timing, quality, and appropriateness of a specific intervention. As such, the competence may address some of the problems posed by responsiveness (Kramer & Stiles, 2015). Karterud et al. (2013) showed good validity coefficients for most items of the scale from both an adherence and a competence perspective. Competent delivery of mentalization-fostering interventions predicted a better quality of in-session reflective functioning in clients with BPD (Möller et al., 2017), particularly when therapists focused on increasing the client's curiosity about their own (and others') mental states. So far, this scale, developed in the context of MBT, has not been applied to different therapy contexts with clients presenting with a PD, where interpersonal and mentalization deficits may be equally important to consider and to address therapeutically.

Individualized Responsiveness

Individualized therapist responsiveness describes therapist reactions, behaviors, and interventions as they ensue from an individualized case formulation that may or may not be independent of a specific therapy approach. Case formulation serves the overarching goal of tailoring psychotherapy to the individual client and fostering the therapeutic relationship in a manner that is unique to each individual (Kramer, 2019a). In order to do this, an idiographic model of understanding may be formulated; one method particularly adapted to clients with PDs is Plan Analysis[1] (Caspar, 2007, 2019). Plan Analysis is a method of case formulation that adopts an instrumental perspective on behaviors and experiences; the latter are explained with hypothetical links to Plans and motives. Beyond being useful in the clinical context as a research tool, Plan Analysis has been shown to have good interrater reliability, and the ensuing motive-oriented therapeutic relationship (MOTR; Caspar, 2019; Grawe, 1992) may be reliably rated in the therapy session. MOTR encompasses therapist behaviors and interventions that foster direct therapeutic work with the behavior-underlying acceptable Plans and motives, rather than therapists responding to the presenting behaviors and experiences per se. In the example elaborated below (see Figure 11.1), the acceptable Plans and motives are written in bold characters to highlight their acceptability within the therapeutic relationship and offer direct avenues of intervention in terms of individualized appropriate responsiveness. It is assumed that when the therapist focuses on the motives underlying the behavior, and holds back from

---

[1]"Plan" is written with a capital P to underline the difference with meaning in common language: "Plans" in Plan Analysis may not necessarily be conscious or rational.

FIGURE 11.1. Parts of Sandra's Plan Analysis

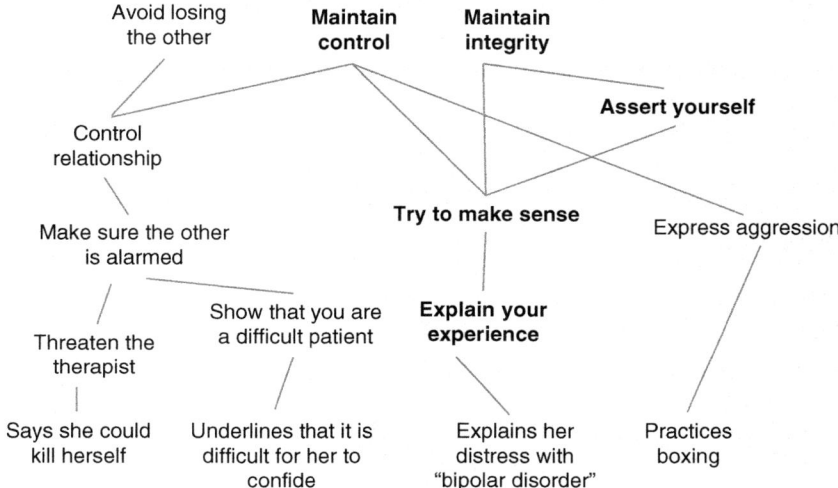

Note. Bold entries indicate the acceptable Plans and motives to highlight their acceptability within the therapeutic relationship and offer direct avenues of intervention in terms of individualized appropriate responsiveness.

responding to certain more problematic Plans and behaviors, the motivational basis for the latter is taken away, and, thus, the intensity and frequency of these behaviors should lessen and the collaboration should increase (Caspar, 2019; Grawe, 1992).

Clinical experience with this formulation method, as do research data, tend to confirm these assumptions. In a study of interpersonal therapy for depression, the verbal and nonverbal components of therapist MOTR were reliably differentiated and rated with regard to the individual client's activated Plans (Caspar et al., 2005). It was found that the nonverbal component of MOTR (i.e., the *manner* in which the therapist focused on the individual client's motives) was related to symptom change, but the verbal component of MOTR (i.e., the actual content the therapist expresses to focus on the individual client's motives) was not (for a clinical example, see Kramer, Berthoud, et al., 2014). A second study confirmed this link between nonverbal MOTR (assessed at the first session of treatment) and outcome in a small sample of brief psychodynamic psychotherapy for PDs, while the verbal component of therapist MOTR did not correlate with outcome in this study (Kramer et al., 2011). So far, it is unclear whether these effects hold in larger samples with clients presenting with BPD.

IMPACT OF THERAPIST RESPONSIVENESS ON THE THERAPEUTIC ALLIANCE AND OUTCOMES IN BPD

In this section, I discuss three studies carried out with the three operational-izations of therapist responsiveness. Because of lack of space, methodological aspects are not discussed in detail and only some of the results are presented. The focus is on the links between therapist responsiveness (generic, disorder-specific, and individualized) and (a) the session-by-session progression of the therapeutic alliance and (b) symptom change at the end of brief treatment for BPD. All three studies draw on a larger data set testing the effects of the MOTR in the first 4 months of psychiatric treatment for BPD (for the treatment, see Charbon et al., 2019; Gunderson & Links, 2014). A controlled outcome study (Kramer, Kolly, et al., 2014) showed significant pre–post changes for this psychiatric treatment for $N = 85$ clients with BPD, with slight advantages favoring clients who received the individualized (MOTR) treatment as compared to the standard (general psychiatric) treatment.

Empirical Demonstrations

Reanalyses of specific subsamples included responsiveness measured using observer-rated measures at the first session (for generic and disorder-specific responsiveness) and at a random session during the therapy process (for indi-vidualized responsiveness, with the case formulation based on the first ses-sion). The therapeutic alliance was measured after each session both client and therapist using the self-reported Working Alliance Inventory-12 (WAI; Horvath & Greenberg, 1989), and outcome was measured after the Sessions 1 and 10 of therapy (at the last session of the 4-month long intervention) using client self-reported OQ-45.2 (Lambert et al., 2004).

Generic Responsiveness

Generic responsiveness, as defined by Elkin et al. (2014), was examined with regard to its links with the progression of the therapeutic alliance (client and therapist perspectives) and outcome (symptom change after a brief psychi-atric treatment). The global (summary) item of generic responsiveness was used. Results, presented in Table 11.1, suggest that while there was no link between generic responsiveness and outcomes (Fiscalini, 2019), a differen-tiated picture was drawn for the therapeutic alliance. The session-by-session progression of the therapeutic alliance rated by the therapist was affected by the level of the global measure of generic responsiveness at Session 1, whereas the session-by-session progression of the therapeutic alliance rated by the clients remained unaffected by therapist responsiveness (Culina, 2019).

TABLE 11.1. Three Operationalizations of Responsiveness and Their Links With the Progression of the Therapeutic Alliance and With Outcome in Brief Treatment for Borderline Personality Disorder

Responsiveness operationalization	Progression of the therapeutic alliance		Outcome
	Client-rated	Therapist-rated	
Generic ($n = 59$)[a,b]	$C = 0.32, p = .40$	**$C = 0.91, p = .01$**	rs between $-.22$ and $.05$ (ns)
Disorder-specific ($n = 49$)[c,d]	$F = 0.14, p = .71$	$F = 0.15, p = .70$	$r = .00$ (ns)
Individualized ($n = 56$)			
Verbal	$C = 0.08, p = .82$	**$C = 1.57, p = .00+$**	$B = 14.56, p = .11$
Nonverbal	$C = 0.05, p = .88$	**$C = 0.96, p = .00+$**	**$B = 20.30, p = .02$**

Note. C = coefficient of hierarchical linear modeling; p = p value; r = Pearson's correlation coefficient; F = F-statistics; ns = nonsignificant; B = standardized β coefficient of linear regression analysis. Statistically significant effects are presented in bold. [a]Data from Culina (2019). [b]Data from Fiscalini (2019). [c]Data from Berthelin (2018). [d]Data from Lepdor (2018).

Precisely, generic responsiveness in the first session was linked with increasingly stronger therapist-rated alliances.

Thus, the global quality of the interaction—defined as appropriate responsiveness from the very first session of psychotherapy—affects the therapist's, but not the client's, perceptions of the alliance over time. The therapeutic alliance may be understood as a global indicator of "good" or "good enough" collaboration and bonding between the therapist and client. It is possible that the therapist may not only rate the alliance as a function of the momentary assessment, but also in terms of the underlying theory and their own clinical experience (Horvath, 2000). Therapists doing "the right thing at the right time" very early in treatment facing clients with PDs may be able to, based on theory and their experience, assess the collaborative process as a generic, emergent property of the therapy. We may speculate that therapists' assessment and case formulation when facing clients with PDs may influence this process.

Disorder-Specific Responsiveness

Disorder-specific therapist responsiveness as defined by Karterud et al. (2013) as competent delivery of mentalization-fostering interventions was examined with regard to its links with the progression of the therapeutic alliance (client and therapist perspectives) and outcome (symptom change after a brief psychiatric treatment). The summary score of MBT competence was used. Results, presented in Table 11.1, suggest that there was no link between MBT competence and alliance progression or outcome (Berthelin, 2018; Lepdor, 2018).

We may conclude that disorder-specific responsiveness, in the form of competent delivery of evidence-based treatment in the very beginning of therapy for BPD, may be relevant for a particular therapy context (Möller et al., 2017), but it remains unclear whether it is essential for other therapy contexts, even for the same psychological disorders. This may put into question a disorder-specific approach to therapist responsiveness. While several treatments for BPD, including MBT, have been developed based on "specific" theorization of BPD-underlying processes, they are increasingly being used for a broader range of disorders because the processes seem to fit to broader client populations. Similarly, our results do not confirm the relevance of a BPD-specific conception of responsiveness. We also have to admit that it remains unclear whether therapist responsiveness can really be operationalized as therapist competence, both in terms of mentalization and in general. Such global evaluation of competency in psychotherapy may obstruct a more descriptive approach to the interaction process. This methodological problem may have played a role in our results (for a fuller discussion of this problem, see Stiles, 2013, and Chapter 1 of this volume).

Individualized Responsiveness
Individualized responsiveness as defined by Caspar (2019) was examined with regard to its links with the progression of the therapeutic alliance from both client and therapist perspectives and outcome (symptom change after a brief psychiatric treatment). Verbal and nonverbal components of the individualized MOTR were differentiated. Results suggest that the verbal component of MOTR was linked with the progression of the therapeutic alliance rated by the therapist, but not with the client's rating or with outcome (see Table 11.1). The nonverbal component of MOTR was linked, once again, with the progression in the therapists' ratings of the alliance (but not the clients'), and the more the therapist was nonverbally responsive to the client with BPD, the better the outcome at the end of the brief treatment.

We may conclude that the individualized MOTR, in particular, its nonverbal component, has both an impact on the quality of the collaborative process and symptom change in treatments for BPD. As such, it confirms earlier work of the centrality of the nonverbal aspects of responsiveness when working with clients with major depression and PDs (Caspar et al., 2005; Kramer et al., 2011). The individualization of the therapeutic relationship in the context of PDs was discussed as having the potential to "wash out" otherwise strong predictors of outcome (Kramer & Stiles, 2015). This means that we assume that in standard (less individualized) treatments, intake predictors are linked with outcome measured at the end of treatment, while these effects will be weakened ("washed out") through the responsive component. In a series of studies, our group has empirically demonstrated this effect of responsiveness for four predictors of symptom reduction in the context of treatment for BPD: (a) symptom level at intake (Kramer et al., 2017), (b) in-session frequency of cognitive biases (Keller et al., 2018), (c) in-session interpersonal agreeableness (Zufferey et al., 2019), and (d) in-session social interaction patterns (Signer et al., 2019).

One cautionary note is that the direct comparison between the three different operationalizations of therapist responsiveness may be criticized, as the data used for all three empirical demonstrations were drawn from a study where the effects of MOTR in brief treatment for BPD was tested. Therefore, it is not possible to rule out that the design may have introduced a bias favoring the individualized operationalization of responsiveness. Initially, the study was not designed to assess generic or disorder-specific responsiveness.

CLINICAL ILLUSTRATION OF INDIVIDUALIZED THERAPIST RESPONSIVENESS AT THE BEGINNING OF BPD TREATMENT

Sandra,[2] 29 years old, consults a psychotherapist for problems related to impulsivity, suicidal thoughts and impulses, loneliness, and lack of perspective. Sandra's clinical presentation is consistent with the diagnosis of BPD, as evidenced by a standardized semistructured interview. The client mentions that she has had several previous intimate relationships that all ended in stormy ways. Currently, Sandra does not have a partner, as she is still strongly affected by the last relationship that her boyfriend ended a year before. At the beginning of treatment, Sandra does not have a job. The client has just been released from a 2-week inpatient stay in a psychiatric hospital, where the bipolar disorder was discussed with her, but without certainty. Despite this uncertainty, Sandra seems to accept this diagnosis, but also feels somewhat unhappy with it, as she shares with her current therapist. The current therapist invests several of the initial sessions to assess in detail what the actual problems are. In this context, diagnosis of BPD is discussed as correct; the affective instability observed in the psychiatric hospital was attributable to her affective reactions to the interpersonal triggers (i.e., of rejection) in her intimate and professional life.

---

[2]The identity(ies) of the client(s) in this chapter's case example(s) has/have been disguised to protect client confidentiality.

The individualized conceptualization to guide therapist responsiveness holds that an idiographic formulation must be made before the therapist can select a specific verbal and nonverbal set of motive-oriented interventions (Caspar, 2019). In the present case, the therapist used Plan Analysis to formulate Sandra's case. The principles of how to develop a case formulation are explained elsewhere (Caspar, 2019). I focus on the relationship implications of the Plan analytic formulation, as they played out early in this treatment (Session 4). Figure 11.1 proposes a part of the Plan Analysis for Sandra, which was elaborated by the therapist based on the information collected after the first session. Plan Analysis depicts the client's individual experiences and behaviors (see the bottom of the graphical representation in Figure 11.1 [e.g., "explains her distress with 'bipolar disorder'"]). The therapist must then develop hypotheses for possible underlying Plans and motives, explaining these observed behaviors and experiences. For example, the behavior "explains her distress with 'bipolar disorder'" may serve the lower-level Plan of "explain your experience" (as shown with the direct instrumental linkage), which again may be underpinned by a higher-level, more general, purpose or Plan ("Try to make sense"). The latter may be explained by the very general motives of "maintain control," "maintain integrity," and "assert yourself" (by convention, all Plans are written as imperatives toward the self). In addition, the formulation shows that Sandra expresses that she "could kill herself," which may serve in this specific case the purpose (i.e., motive or Plan) to "threaten the therapist." The goal of this Plan may ultimately be to help her control the therapeutic relationship—avoid being left alone—and maintain control in her life in general. By explaining her distress with a biological (and thus ego-external) explanation that she suffers from "bipolar disorder" may serve to explain her disruptive experience (e.g., the Plan "symbolize what is happening" [not shown in the figure]) to her and help her to make sense of it, which serve the purpose, as explained above, to assert herself, maintain her integrity, and maintain control.

A therapist using the MOTR may retain all items in bold in Figure 11.1 to develop a complementary intervention to the client's Plans. This means that this therapist may express compassion for the client trying to make sense out of her hitherto inexplicable experience, or her efforts to try to find a good explanation. In contrast, the therapist should *not* act in complementary ways to the sub-Plan "show that you are a particular patient," as this may increase the likelihood that this Plan will be used more often to serve the upper Plan "make sure the other is alarmed," which may prove problematic for the collaborative process.

In the following excerpt from Session 4, the therapist was implementing a complementary response to the Plans "Explain your experience" and "Try to make sense." Such an intervention was chosen to lessen the intensity and frequency of a behavior like sticking to her initial explanation in the context of a "bipolar disorder." It is hypothesized that this latter client behavior, if not addressed using an MOTR intervention, may become problematic, preventing the client from full engagement in psychotherapy focusing on her core problems. The therapist's responsiveness to Sandra's underlying motives are presented in bold.

SANDRA: I have a lot of girlfriends. My feeling is that they move much quicker through life than me. I kind of stay where I am . . .

THERAPIST: Mmhm.

SANDRA: I had a boyfriend during six years; now we are separated for one year, and I am still struggling with it.

THERAPIST: Mmhm.

SANDRA: This means that I am unfit to move forward in my life. Is it my character? Or maybe my illness, bipolar disorder . . . maybe.

THERAPIST: **These are a lot of questions, yes, you are asking. Why is this? Where does it come from? . . . You really want to know and you really want to solve these problems.**

SANDRA: Exactly.

THERAPIST: **I see you really want to answer some of these questions. You really want to make sense of what you are going through. I want to tell you that you are at the right place here to ask these questions.**

SANDRA: Yes, I really want to make sense. Know who I really am.

This brief excerpt from session 4 demonstrates that therapist responsiveness to the individual's underlying motives is already possible as part of a discussion of diagnosis and presenting problems. In fact, it might be at this early stage of therapy that the client's commitment and engagement in therapy are being formed, and the therapist may orient their own behaviors and intervention proactively toward an individualized responsive approach to treatment.

Later in treatment, Sandra nonverbally dismissed the therapist's effort to help her structure her day and find a new job; she expressed self-contempt over her failure and uttered that she may have been "better off dead." From a case formulation perspective, the therapist understood that in this specific moment, the Plan "show that you are a difficult patient" or "make sure the other is alarmed" is activated. In order to intervene effectively using individualized responsiveness, the therapist may here consider what the purpose of these activated Plans is: according to Figure 11.1, it may serve the client to control the relationship, and more generally "avoid losing the other" and "maintain control." A complementary therapist behavior, one that is oriented explicitly toward the underlying motives, takes into account these purposeful motives and tries to satisfy them within the therapeutic relationship. In order to do that, the therapist may say,

> I can see the struggle you are in now to find meaning in your life [general empathic stance], and I want to tell you that you decide the rhythm with which you move forward in this task [oriented toward the individual's motive "maintain control"]; whatever happens during therapy, you can count on me and the resources we have here to support you in your search for meaning [oriented toward the individual's motives "avoid losing the other" and "try to make sense"].

Individualized responsiveness appears as an integrative, clinically meaningful, and empirically supported principle of change when interactions become particularly challenging, and specific problems related to a personality disorder threaten to affect the psychotherapy process and outcome.

DIVERSITY AND THERAPIST RESPONSIVENESS

While on a conceptual level, PDs as potential client features are responsive to their cultural context (Mulder, 2018), I would argue that the principle of therapist responsiveness cuts across culture. Rather, the specific client behaviors and therapist behaviors that constitute the nuts and bolts of responsiveness in the treatment of PDs may vary as a function of cultural context. For example, a therapist may want to diagnose a client with dependent personality disorder in a given culture based on the client's unassertive, self-effacing, and particularly shy presentation. A therapist in a different culture may understand such behavior as part of courtesy and politeness viewed as normal interaction and behavior in that specific context (Mulder, 2018).

Client expressiveness may evoke different therapist and contextual responses as a function of the acculturation of both interaction partners. The strength of family ties and social cohesiveness has been discussed as important cultural moderators of development of a diagnosis of PD (Paris & Lis, 2012). For example, in India, the mean age of first consultation for clients presenting with any PDs was 29 years, which contrasts with the child and adolescent psychotherapy and early detection programs for personality difficulties found in other countries (Narayanan & Rao, 2018). This was interpreted as a consequence of particularly strong social and family ties that may inhibit some of the PD features during early adulthood. Such late clinical development of the actual disorder may both be linked with better treatment outcomes (i.e., the family ties may act as a resource for treatment) and poorer treatment outcomes (i.e., the time before treatment begins may contribute to the pervasiveness of the pathological pattern over time, making it more resistant to change).

IMPLICATIONS FOR PRACTICE AND TRAINING IN THERAPY FOR PERSONALITY DISORDERS

Gunderson (2016) argued that while the specific evidence-based psychotherapies for BPD are the gold standard of clinical intervention, training therapists in one or more of these psychotherapy models is a lengthy, expensive, and cumbersome process. The result is nonoptimal service to the general population in terms of BPD treatment. Based on this argument, he developed a good enough, easily learnable, and easy to disseminate psychiatric treatment, called "good psychiatric management" (Gunderson & Links, 2014), which condenses the essential "good enough" therapist attitudes and interventions to help solve the core problems of these clients. Similar considerations may be made concerning psychotherapies for other PDs (Livesley et al., 2016).

Therapist responsiveness, conceptualized as a central component explicating change in psychotherapy that continues throughout therapy from the very first contact when working with clients with PDs, should be taken into account by therapists in their training. Clinicians from different therapy approaches may learn how to identify interpersonally constraining client behaviors and how to formulate a case according to their intervention theory (Kramer, 2019a). As shown in this chapter, Plan Analysis is one formulation method among others fostering responsive interventions. Before learning effective (and somewhat complex) psychotherapy techniques, training in case formulation and responsiveness, integrated into a series of good-enough interventions, may be a cost-effective strategy and help increase the effectiveness of the interventions delivered by trainees.

CONCLUSION

Therapist responsiveness represents an opportunity in clinical work with PDs but also creates problems in research designs. It may help for therapists to differentiate conceptualizations of appropriate responsiveness as a function of the granularity of client behavior. A generic conceptualization may be complemented by a disorder-specific one and by an individualized approach to appropriate therapist responsiveness. While they all show potential for increasing the effectiveness of therapy and offer rigorous assessments, the nonverbal aspect of an individualized appropriate therapist responsiveness, based on case formulations, stands out as a particularly promising intervention tool. Training psychotherapists to respond in warm, welcoming, prizing, and committed ways may be helpful for some clients with a PD, while others may only develop the required deep trust in the therapeutic relationship when the therapist proposes an individually tailored psychotherapy relationship by responding nonverbally with what may be "the right thing at the right time."

Future work in the field of responsiveness in the treatment of PDs includes a more systematic study of responsiveness in other PD categories than BPD, as well as more controlled trials and case studies. In addition, it may be necessary to study less appropriate therapist responsiveness (Stiles et al., 1998), such as therapist reassurance of the client's problematic in-session behaviors, therapist overt and covert criticism of client behavior and the effects of these behaviors on process and outcome.

REFERENCES

American Psychiatric Association. (2013). *Diagnostic and Statistical Manual of Mental Disorders* (5th ed.). https://doi.org/10.1176/appi.books.9780890425596

Bateman, A. W., & Fonagy, P. (2006). *Mentalization-based treatment for borderline personality disorder: A practical guide*. Oxford University Press. https://doi.org/10.1093/med/9780198570905.001.0001

Bateman, A. W., & Fonagy, P. (2009). Randomized controlled trial of outpatient mentalization-based treatment for borderline personality disorder versus structured clinical management. *The American Journal of Psychiatry, 166*(12), 1355–1364. https://doi.org/10.1176/appi.ajp.2009.09040539

Berthelin, C. (2018). *Analyse de la mentalisation chez les thérapeutes neophytes: La relation avec l'alliance et le changement thérapeutique.* [Analysis of mentalization in neophyte therapists: The relationship with alliance and therapeutic change] [Unpublished manuscript]. Department of Psychology, University of Geneva.

Caspar, F. (2007). Plan Analysis. In T. Eells (Ed.), *Handbook of psychotherapy case formulations* (2nd ed., pp. 251–289). Guilford Press.

Caspar, F. (2019). Plan Analysis and the motive-oriented therapeutic relationship. In U. Kramer (Ed.), *Case formulation for personality disorders: Tailoring psychotherapy to the individual client* (pp. 265–290). Academic Press. https://doi.org/10.1016/B978-0-12-813521-1.00014-X

Caspar, F., Grossmann, C., Unmüssig, C., & Schramm, E. (2005). Complementary therapeutic relationship: Therapist behavior, interpersonal patterns, and therapeutic effects. *Psychotherapy Research, 15*(1–2), 91–102. https://doi.org/10.1080/10503300512331327074

Charbon, P., Kramer, U., Droz, J., & Kolly, S. (2019). Implementation of good psychiatric management in 10 sessions. In L. W. Choi-Kain & J. G. Gunderson (Eds.), *Applications of good psychiatric management for borderline personality disorders: A practical guide* (pp. 233–252). American Psychiatric Publishing.

Culina, I. (2019). *L'impact de la responsiveness sur l'alliance thérapeutique dans un traitement bref du trouble de la personnalité borderline.* [The impact of responsiveness on the therapeutic alliance in a brief treatment of borderline personality disorder] [Unpublished manuscript]. Department of Psychology, University of Fribourg.

Elkin, I., Falconnier, L., Smith, Y., Canada, K. E., Henderson, E., Brown, E. R., & McKay, B. M. (2014). Therapist responsiveness and patient engagement in therapy. *Psychotherapy Research, 24*(1), 52–66. https://doi.org/10.1080/10503307.2013.820855

Elkin, I., & Smith, Y. (2007). *Therapist responsiveness study rating scale* [Unpublished manuscript]. School of Social Service Administration. University of Chicago.

Fiscalini, E. (2019). *Est-ce qu'un degré élevé de responsiveness adequate est susceptible d'améliorer les symptômes du trouble de la personnalité borderline?* [Is a high degree of adequate responsiveness likely to improve symptoms of borderline personality disorder?] [Unpublished manuscript]. Department of Psychology, University of Fribourg.

Fonagy, P., Luyten, P., Allison, E., & Campbell, C. (2017). What we have changed our minds about: Part 1. Borderline personality disorder as a limitation of resilience. *Borderline Personality Disorder and Emotion Dysregulation, 4,* Article 11. https://doi.org/10.1186/s40479-017-0061-9

Grawe, K. (1992). Komplementäre Beziehungsgestaltung als Mittel zur Herstellung einer guten Therapiebeziehung [Complementary therapeutic relationship as a mean for the establishment of a good therapeutic relationship]. In J. Margraf & J. C. Brengelmann (Eds.), *Die Therapeut-Patient-Beziehung in der Verhaltenstherapie* (pp. 215–244). Röttger-Verlag.

Gunderson, J. G. (2016). The emergence of a generalist model to meet public health needs for patients with borderline personality disorder. *The American Journal of Psychiatry, 173*(5), 452–458. https://doi.org/10.1176/appi.ajp.2015.15070885

Gunderson, J. G., & Links, P. S. (2014). *Handbook of good psychiatric management for borderline personality disorder.* American Psychiatric Publishing.

Horvath, A. O. (2000). The therapeutic relationship: From transference to alliance. *Journal of Clinical Psychology, 56*(2), 163–173. https://doi.org/10.1002/(SICI)1097-4679(200002)56:2<163::AID-JCLP3>3.0.CO;2-D

Horvath, A. O., & Greenberg, L. S. (1989). Development and validation of the Working Alliance Inventory. *Journal of Counseling Psychology, 36*(2), 223–233. https://doi.org/10.1037/0022-0167.36.2.223

Karterud, S., Pedersen, G., Engen, M., Johansen, M. S., Johansson, P. N., Schlüter, C., Urnes, O., Wilberg, T., & Bateman, A. W. (2013). The MBT Adherence and Competence Scale (MBT-ACS): Development, structure and reliability. *Psychotherapy Research, 23*(6), 705–717. https://doi.org/10.1080/10503307.2012.708795

Keller, S., Stelmaszczyk, K., Kolly, S., de Roten, Y., Despland, J.-N., Caspar, F., Drapeau, M., & Kramer, U. (2018). Change in biased thinking in a treatment based on the motive-oriented therapeutic relationship for borderline personality disorder. *Journal of Personality Disorders, 32*(Suppl.), 75–92. https://doi.org/10.1521/pedi.2018.32.supp.75

Kramer, U. (2019a). *Case formulation for personality disorders: Tailoring psychotherapy to the individual client*. Academic Press.

Kramer, U. (2019b). Personality, personality disorders, and the process of change. *Psychotherapy Research, 29*(3), 324–336. https://doi.org/10.1080/10503307.2017.1377358

Kramer, U., Berthoud, L., Keller, S., & Caspar, F. (2014). Motive-oriented psychotherapeutic relationship facing a patient presenting with narcissistic personality disorder: A case study. *Journal of Contemporary Psychotherapy, 44*(2), 71–82. https://doi.org/10.1007/s10879-013-9249-5

Kramer, U., Keller, S., Caspar, F., de Roten, Y., Despland, J.-N., & Kolly, S. (2017). Early change in coping strategies in responsive treatments for borderline personality disorder: A mediation analysis. *Journal of Consulting and Clinical Psychology, 85*(5), 530–535. https://doi.org/10.1037/ccp0000196

Kramer, U., Kolly, S., Berthoud, L., Keller, S., Preisig, M., Caspar, F., Berger, T., de Roten, Y., Marquet, P., & Despland, J.-N. (2014). Effects of motive-oriented therapeutic relationship in a ten-session general psychiatric treatment of borderline personality disorder: A randomized controlled trial. *Psychotherapy and Psychosomatics, 83*(3), 176–186. https://doi.org/10.1159/000358528

Kramer, U., & Levy, K. N. (2017). *Therapist responsiveness in treatments for personality disorders: A challenge and a principle of change* [Conference presentation]. 23rd Annual Meeting of the Society for the Exploration of Psychotherapy Integration (SEPI), Denver, CO.

Kramer, U., Rosciano, A., Pavlovic, M., Berthoud, L., Despland, J.-N., de Roten, Y., & Caspar, F. (2011). Motive-oriented therapeutic relationship in brief psychodynamic intervention for patients with depression and personality disorders. *Journal of Clinical Psychology, 67*(10), 1017–1027. https://doi.org/10.1002/jclp.20806

Kramer, U., & Stiles, W. B. (2015). The responsiveness problem in psychotherapy: A review of proposed solutions. *Clinical Psychology: Science and Practice, 22*(3), 277–295. https://doi.org/10.1111/cpsp.12107

Lambert, M. J., Morton, J. J., Hatfield, D., Harmon, C., Hamilton, S., Reid, R. C., Shimokowa, K., Christoperson, C., & Burlingame, G. M. (2004). *Administration and scoring manual for the Outcome Questionnaire-45*. American Professional Credentialing Services.

Lepdor, F. (2018). *Qualité des interventions basées sur la mentalisation et trouble de la personnalité borderline* [Quality of mentalization-based interventions and borderline personality disorder] [Unpublished manuscript]. Department of Psychology, University of Lausanne.

Livesley, W. J. (2017). *Integrated modular treatment for borderline personality disorder: A practical guide to combining effective treatment methods*. Cambridge University Press. https://doi.org/10.1017/9781107298613

Livesley, W. J., Dimaggio, G., & Clarkin, J. F. (2016). *Integrated treatment for personality disorder: A modular approach*. Guilford Press.

McMain, S., Boritz, T. Z., & Leybman, M. J. (2015). Common strategies for cultivating a positive relationship in the treatment of borderline personality disorder. *Journal of Psychotherapy Integration, 25*(1), 20–29. https://doi.org/10.1037/a0038768

Möller, C., Karlgren, L., Sandell, A., Falkenström, F., & Philips, B. (2017). Mentalization-based therapy adherence and competence stimulates in-session mentalization in psychotherapy for borderline personality disorder with co-morbid substance dependence. *Psychotherapy Research, 27*(6), 749–765. https://doi.org/10.1080/10503307.2016.1158433

Mulder, R. T. (2018). Cultural aspects of personality disorder. In W. J. Livesley & R. Larstone (Eds.), *Handbook of personality disorders: Theory, research, and treatment* (2nd ed., pp. 88–100). Guilford Press.

Narayanan, G., & Rao, K. (2018). Personality disorders in the Indian culture: Reconsidering self-perceptions, traditional society and values. *Psychological Studies, 63*(1), 32–41. https://doi.org/10.1007/s12646-017-0437-3

Paris, J., & Lis, E. (2012). Can sociocultural and historical mechanisms influence the development of borderline personality disorder? *Transcultural Psychiatry, 50*(1), 140–151. https://doi.org/10.1177/1363461512468105

Pos, A. E., & Greenberg, L. S. (2012). Organizing awareness and increasing emotion regulation: Revising chair work in emotion-focused therapy for borderline personality disorder. *Journal of Personality Disorders, 26*(1), 84–107. https://doi.org/10.1521/pedi.2012.26.1.84

Sachse, R. (2020). *Personality disorders: A clarification-oriented psychotherapy treatment model*. Hogrefe.

Signer, S., Estermann Jansen, R., Sachse, R., Caspar, F., & Kramer, U. (2019). Social interaction patterns, therapist responsiveness, and outcome in treatments for borderline personality disorder. *Psychology and Psychotherapy: Theory, Research and Practice, 93*(4), 705–722. https://doi.org/10.1111/papt.12254

Stiles, W. B. (2009). Responsiveness as an obstacle for psychotherapy outcome research: It's worse than you think. *Clinical Psychology: Science and Practice, 16*(1), 86–91. https://doi.org/10.1111/j.1468-2850.2009.01148.x

Stiles, W. B. (2013). The variables problem and progress in psychotherapy research. *Psychotherapy, 50*(1), 33–41. https://doi.org/10.1037/a0030569

Stiles, W. B., Honos-Webb, L., & Surko, M. (1998). Responsiveness in psychotherapy. *Clinical Psychology: Science and Practice, 5*(4), 439–458. https://doi.org/10.1111/j.1468-2850.1998.tb00166.x

Stiles, W. B., & Horvath, A. O. (2017). Appropriate responsiveness as a contribution to therapist effects. In L. G. Castonguay & C. E. Hill (Eds.), *How and why are some therapists better than others? Understanding therapist effects* (pp. 71–84). American Psychological Association. https://doi.org/10.1037/0000034-005

van Kessel, W., & Lietaer, G. (1998). Interpersonal process. In L. S. Greenberg, J. C. Watson, & G. Lietaer (Eds.), *Handbook of experiential psychotherapy* (pp. 155–177). Guilford Press.

Weiss, J. (1993). *How psychotherapy works: Process and technique*. Guilford Press.

Zanarini, M. C., & Frankenburg, F. R. (2007). The essential nature of borderline psychopathology. *Journal of Personality Disorders, 21*(5), 518–535. https://doi.org/10.1521/pedi.2007.21.5.518

Zufferey, P., Caspar, F., & Kramer, U. (2019). The role of interactional agreeableness in responsive treatments for patients with borderline personality disorder. *Journal of Personality Disorders, 33*(5), 691–706. https://doi.org/10.1521/pedi_2019_33_367

12

ENHANCING THERAPIST RESPONSIVENESS IN DIALECTICAL BEHAVIOR THERAPY

JAMIE D. BEDICS AND HOLLY J. McKINLEY

Dialectical behavior therapy (DBT; Linehan, 1993) is a cognitive behavior therapy initially developed for the treatment of suicidal behavior and later expanded for the treatment of borderline personality disorder (BPD) with co-occurring Axis I disorders. The initial success of DBT, along with its flexibility in methods of delivery, has led to its adaption across numerous clinical settings and diagnostic groups (Lynch et al., 2007). Despite this evolution in application, the theoretical principles that organize and guide DBT have remained largely unmodified from the original treatment manual (Linehan, 1993).

The goal of this chapter is to highlight several core theoretical principles underlying DBT that allow for therapist responsivity to be most effective. The first part of the chapter discusses responsivity in the overall framework of delivering DBT (i.e., defining treatment goals and modules of interventions). The second part reviews the relevant principles guiding effective responsivity within one mode of DBT: outpatient individual psychotherapy. Future directions with respect to clinical training and research on responsivity in DBT are provided.

https://doi.org/10.1037/0000240-013
The Responsive Psychotherapist: Attuning to Clients in the Moment, J. C. Watson and H. Wiseman (Editors)

DBT AS A RESPONSIVE FRAMEWORK FOR TREATMENT

In the process of developing DBT, Linehan realized the complexity and severity of the cases being treated required a clear framework for organizing treatment goals and for selecting appropriate interventions (Linehan & Wilks, 2015). In the absence of such direction, therapists were vulnerable to responding to clients' multiple, and often life-threatening, problematic behaviors in ways that were either overly accommodating or overly proscriptive. Linehan (1993) saw this type of flexibility as a common source of therapeutic errors leading to both ineffective treatment and eventual therapist burnout. As part of the solution, the principles of hierarchy and modularity were incorporated into DBT to direct therapist responsivity in structuring the overall framework of the treatment (Linehan & Wilks, 2015).

The Four Stages of DBT

The hierarchical approach taken in DBT allows therapists to organize and prioritize treatment goals based on the degree to which clients' behaviors are life-threatening, complex, severe, pervasive, and disabling (Linehan & Wilks, 2015). On the basis of these factors, Linehan defined four hierarchical stages of treatment: (a) Stage 1 where behavioral dyscontrol (e.g., life-threatening behavior, behavior interfering with therapy) and skills deficits are present and client stabilization is a priority, (b) Stage 2 where client stabilization is evident and the emphasis is on emotional experiencing and processing, (c) Stage 3 where the emphasis is on the reduction of everyday problems in living, and (d) Stage 4 where the emphasis is on an increase in a sense of fulfillment and joy in life. Although DBT was originally developed for clients in Stage 1, where life-threatening behavior is present, research has begun to explore the effectiveness of treatments following the successful completion of Stage 1 (e.g., Comtois et al., 2010).

The staged hierarchy allows therapists to meet clients "where they are at" by defining the priorities and focus of attention for every individual session of therapy. Such a perspective is consistent with a responsive *aptitude-treatment-interaction* approach to treatment assignment (Stiles et al., 1998). The clearest examples of this process in DBT, and as described in the second section of this chapter, are the prioritized targets within Stage 1 of treatment where the presence of any life-threatening behavior (e.g., nonsuicidal self-injury, increased suicide ideation) takes precedence over other topics discussed in session. Such clarity in the priority of treatment goals allows for flexibility in the topics discussed while also providing a sense of continuity across sessions and between therapist–client dyads. Last, stage-based targets can act as clear directional markers or anchors from which therapists can assess moments when the focus of attention during an individual session goes too far astray from the priorities defined by the treatment.

The Four Modes of Standard DBT

Whereas the principle of hierarchy allows therapists to flexibly define *what* is focused on during therapy, the principle of modularity allows DBT therapists to responsively address *how* therapy is conducted through adding or removing interventions based on clients' needs. As a comprehensive treatment, DBT consists of four major modes, or modules, of intervention: individual therapy, as-needed telephone consultation, group skills training, and therapist participation on a consultation team (Linehan, 1993). Together, these four modes serve to address five functions typical of comprehensive treatments: an increase in clients' motivation to change, an increase in clients' capacity to act with skillful behavior, an increase in the generalization of skillful behavior to clients' everyday lives, an increase in therapists' motivation and enhancement of skill, and the provision of some sense of structure and cohesion to the various intervention strategies through case management. At Stage 1 of DBT, each of these five functions was seen as necessary for effective treatment. Consequently, Stage 1 DBT was developed with the expectation that all four major modules would be delivered (Linehan & Wilks, 2015). This original implementation of DBT is referred to as standard DBT (S-DBT) and is delivered on an outpatient basis for the period of 1 year. S-DBT for clients entering Stage 1 is the version of DBT that has received the largest base of replicated empirical support through randomized controlled trials (RCTs; see, e.g., Linehan et al., 1991, 2006, 2015; McMain et al., 2009; Verheul et al., 2003).

Responsive Modifications to Standard DBT

Although S-DBT is considered the gold standard of treatment delivery for Stage 1 clients, DBT's modularity allows for responsive modifications to the delivery of DBT in two ways (Linehan & Wilks, 2015). First, therapists can modify S-DBT by removing one of the four major modules of interventions. Therapists might consider doing so when clients are, for example, entering treatment at Stage 2 or higher or when particular functions provided by the four standard modes of DBT are not seen as necessary given the needs of the specific client population. Of the various methods of modifying S-DBT, the delivery of DBT group skills training as a stand-alone intervention for problems related to emotion dysregulation appears to be the most common (see

Linehan, 2015, for a review). Despite the prevalence of such a major adaption, there has only been one controlled study examining the efficacy of DBT skills training as a stand-alone treatment compared with S-DBT for Stage 1 clients (Linehan et al., 2015). In this study, the efficacy of DBT skills training was compared with S-DBT and a third condition consisting of individual DBT therapy, as-needed telephone consultation, and therapist participation on a consultation team with no skills training. The treatment was provided for a period of 1 year, and all treatment arms were trained in a DBT-based crisis management protocol (Linehan et al., 2012). Overall, the findings showed reductions in suicidal behavior across groups with no significant differences between the three components. Although preliminary and not statistically powered to test for equivalence, these results showed that two variations in S-DBT, skills training only and individual therapy with team consultation and telephone coaching, were effective in reducing suicidal behavior for clients entering treatment at Stage 1 and meeting diagnostic criteria for BPD.

A second approach for the responsive adaption of S-DBT is based on the inherent modularity within each of the four major modes of DBT themselves (Linehan & Wilks, 2015). For example, the individual therapy component of DBT consists of multiple strategies of interventions (e.g., dialectics, problem-solving, validation) that therapists can modify depending on the complexity of clients' presenting problems. One study, for example, added an exposure therapy protocol to the individual module of S-DBT as a method of improved treatment for posttraumatic stress disorder (PTSD) during Stage 1 (Harned et al., 2014). In another adaptation of S-DBT for Stage 1 clients, researchers added strategies tailored to treat drug abstinence in a sample of participants meeting diagnostic criteria for a substance use disorder (Linehan et al., 1999).

Similar to the individual therapy component of S-DBT, the DBT skills training module also contains an inherent modularity consisting of the four core skills modules of mindfulness, interpersonal effectiveness, emotion regulation, and distress tolerance (Linehan, 2015). A typical method of adapting DBT skills training, as a stand-alone intervention, has been to add to or subtract from these four modules to suit the needs of specific client populations. A review of the literature examining the research on DBT skills training confirmed significant variation in methods of delivery (Valentine et al., 2015; see also Valentine et al., 2020, for a more recent review). Results from this review showed that 10 of the 17 studies examining DBT skills included the four modules typical of DBT skills training in S-DBT and six of the 17 studies added additional modules of intervention (Valentine et al., 2015). The same review found the number of hours of DBT skills training classes delivered to clients ranged between 17.5 and 47 hours compared with the recommended dose of 130 hours for Stage 1 S-DBT.

The variation seen in delivering modified versions of S-DBT and DBT skills group training as a stand-alone intervention is consistent with the responsive nature of the framework of DBT that seeks to "do what works" given clients' needs based on their stage. At the same time, a certain degree of caution is required in the adaptation of methods of delivering DBT. S-DBT, and all its constituent parts, was developed to match the interpersonal, emotional, and cognitive challenges faced by Stage 1 clients meeting diagnostic criteria for BPD. Certain treatment modifications to S-DBT, such as the added protocol-based interventions for PTSD (Harned et al., 2014) and substance use (Linehan et al., 1999, 2002), are clearly in alignment with the overarching theoretical framework from which DBT was originally derived. Such adaptations are also supported by the empirical literature (Harned et al., 2009). In contrast, the extent to which the various adaptations of DBT skills training conditions fit into the larger DBT framework is often less clear. Instead, the most often cited rational for the use of DBT skills is their general ability to address "emotion dysregulation" across diagnostic populations and separate from the particular cognitive, affective, and behavioral experiences of clients' meeting diagnostic criteria for BPD (Valentine et al., 2020).

Summary and Recommendations for Responsive Treatment

The principles of hierarchy and modularity allow clinicians and researchers to create a responsive treatment framework for delivering DBT based on client needs or the needs of the treatment setting. S-DBT is the gold standard in treatment delivery for Stage 1 clients and is the evidence base most commonly referred to when citing the success of DBT. There are, however, many types of "DBT" that can be delivered in the community and studied in a research setting. DBT can be scaled down for simpler clinical presentations (e.g., DBT skills training only) or scaled up for more complex presentations (e.g., the addition of exposure interventions for specific anxiety disorders to S-DBT).

The high degree of flexibility in the delivery of DBT requires care and caution in its dissemination in the community. Clinically, therapists should do their best to be clear and transparent in communicating the type of DBT they are delivering (e.g., S-DBT, DBT skills training only, presence or absence of team consultation). Therapists also have the responsibility of staying abreast of the research base that most closely approximates the methods of DBT they are delivering. A DBT therapist might inform their clients of the type of DBT available to them in the following way:

> I want to take the time to tell you a little bit about DBT. There are actually many types of DBT that a person can receive. At our clinic we provide DBT skills training. DBT skills training can be compared with "standard DBT," which includes individual therapy, telephone coaching, therapists' participation on a

team consultation, and the skills training class. Standard DBT lasts for 1 year, and the majority of evidence that people think of when referring to DBT comes from research on standard DBT. Standard DBT was also developed for adults with recent suicidal behavior who met criteria for what's called borderline personality disorder. As you are hoping to work on anger, I can tell you that one study of DBT skills only, similar to the group we offer, has shown reductions in anger following 13 weeks of 2-hour-a-week DBT skills training for clients who met diagnostic criteria for borderline personality disorder. Although our treatment lasts 16 weeks, and you do not meet criteria for borderline personality disorder, my best guess is that the skills provided in our DBT skills training class will also provide you with the necessary tools to more effectively manage your experience of anger.

Such transparency seeks to provide prospective clients with the best available information regarding the effectiveness of the treatment being delivered while also not being overly exclusive in limiting the opportunity of clients to receive the benefit of the skills. Equally as important is the simple fact that such a statement has the effect of maintaining the integrity of the treatment by acknowledging the gold standard of DBT (i.e., S-DBT) while at the same time not diminishing the value of modifications.

Last, and with respect to research, when summarizing the empirical evidence surrounding DBT and its adaptations, greater attention can be paid to the heterogeneity in methods of treatment delivery. The current dominance of meta-analytic thinking that seeks to estimate a population parameter of overall effect size regardless of research methodology is not without its limitations (Nelson et al., 2018). Such limitations are further exaggerated when the existing evidence base consists mostly of pilot work with small sample sizes where positive results (i.e., statistical significance and effect sizes) are likely exaggerated and nonsignificant effects are often dismissed as attributable to low power. Finally, meta-analyses simply do not replace the scientific principle of replication (Stanley et al., 2018). Future pilot studies would be greatly improved if researchers planned repeated experiments as a method of assessing the stability and replicability of their findings.

RESPONSIVITY DURING OUTPATIENT INDIVIDUAL THERAPY IN S-DBT

The DBT framework provides the overarching structure of treatment and represents the initial steps that allow for effective therapist responsivity within each major module in S-DBT. The goal of this section is to highlight principles in DBT that allow for effective responsivity during an individual session of Stage 1 S-DBT. In this section, responsivity in DBT is discussed as it occurs in the moment-to-moment interaction between therapist and client as it emerges in context of the larger treatment goals (Stiles et al., 1998). The first part of this section discusses the influence of Stage 1 goals on in-session therapist responsivity. These are referred to as the *structural strategies* in DBT (Linehan, 1993). The second part of this section surveys therapist responsivity within the four core interventions typical of S-DBT, including dialectics, problem-solving and validation, stylistic strategies, and strategies of case management.

Structural Strategies: Defining the Direction of Individual Sessions in S-DBT

The stage-defined behavioral targets, or goals of therapy, in S-DBT are central in defining the priorities and direction for each individual therapy session. There are three broad classifications of behavioral targets in Stage 1 of S-DBT, including an increase in dialectical behavioral patterns, attention to primary behavioral targets (i.e., a decrease in life-threatening behavior, therapy-interfering behavior, quality-of-life-interfering behavior, and an increase in behavioral skills), and the ability to address secondary behavioral targets as they relate to the primary behavioral targets (Linehan, 1993). In addition to representing major categories of outcome in S-DBT, the behavioral targets serve as key markers in determining the responsiveness of therapists to clients' behavior during each individual session of S-DBT. The goal of this section is to briefly describe each of the three behavioral targets while highlighting the therapist's use of these targets as markers for responsivity during an individual psychotherapy session in S-DBT.

Increasing Dialectical Behavioral Patterns: Finding Balance in the Moment
In S-DBT, the goal of increasing dialectical behavioral patterns occurs throughout the treatment and is targeted in every session of individual psychotherapy (Linehan, 1993). An increase in dialectical behavioral patterns refers to the clients' ability to think dialectically as well as the clients' ability to apply dialectical principles to their everyday lives. Such dialectical principles include a belief that truth is neither absolute nor relative, that change is constant, and that a more complete understanding of the world is the result of a continually evolving process of acknowledging and reconciling multiple, often opposing, polarities or points of view (Linehan & Schmidt, 1995).

Up until the release of the second edition of the DBT skills manual (Linehan, 2015), the goal of increasing dialectical behavioral patterns was not explicitly taught to clients. Instead, dialectics was largely taught from and modeled on the responsiveness of the therapist to the topics reviewed as they arose in session. During an individual session of S-DBT, the goal of increasing dialectical behavioral patterns remains largely a responsive one. As therapists and clients proceed from topic to topic, therapists actively search for opportunities to reinforce dialectical thinking with statements such as "What is being left out?" or "What are we missing?" Therapists also highlight multiple perspectives in the client's language while searching for a synthesis inclusive of diverging points of view with statements such as "both . . . and." A responsive therapist in DBT is one that maintains a practical knowledge of dialectics applicable to everyday life while continually assessing for its relevance in session.

Primary Behavioral Targets: Creating a Responsive Session Agenda

The primary behavioral targets define the focus and priority for every individual session in Stage 1 of outpatient S-DBT (Linehan, 1993). The primary targets include (a) a decrease in suicidal behavior, including suicide attempts, communication about suicide, suicide planning, nonsuicidal self-injury, and suicide ideation; (b) a decrease in therapy-interfering behavior, including any behavior on the part of the client and therapist that would interfere with the client's ability to receive the treatment or the therapists' ability to deliver the treatment; (c) a decrease in behavior that interferes with the clients' quality of life, which can include additional mental health diagnoses (e.g., panic attacks, depression) or life circumstances (e.g., unemployment); and (d) an increase in behavioral skills where therapists seek to encourage existing or newly acquired behavioral skills. Together, these four targets comprise a treatment hierarchy with the priority of importance arranged in descending order from suicidal behavior to behavioral skills. In contrast to the goal of increasing dialectical behavior patterns, the primary behavioral targets, and the treatment hierarchy they comprise, are explicitly discussed and agreed upon at the onset of S-DBT.

A primary source of in-session therapist responsivity in Stage 1 S-DBT is centered on the treatment hierarchy. During every individual session, the treatment hierarchy requires the therapist to balance the immediate needs of the client with the priorities defined by the hierarchy. In doing so, the hierarchy defines the order in which topics are addressed in each session. In DBT this responsive strategy for assessment and intervention is a structural strategy referred to as *targeting* and is required in S-DBT (Linehan, 1993).

The standard method for the assessment of primary targeted behavior in S-DBT is the DBT diary card. The DBT diary card consists of client's daily self-reported ratings of targeted behavior (e.g., suicide attempts, suicidal thoughts/urges, urges to quit therapy, use of behavioral skills) for the prior week leading up to the current session. Similar to a weathervane showing the direction of the wind, the DBT diary card is an essential tool in determining the course and direction for each individual session in S-DBT. Based on the diary card, along with any additional information offered by the client and therapist, the order with which the therapist attends to and applies treatment strategies will depend on the highest priority target reported during the prior week. An example dialogue can demonstrate these points:

THERAPIST: I see you brought your diary card. Great. (*Therapist accepts diary card from client and begins to read out loud.*) I see you had higher ratings of sadness on Saturday. That was unusual relative to the rest of week. Anxiety also peaked on that day and, oh, I see you had high urges, 4/5, to self-harm but you did not act on that urge. Is that right?

PATIENT: Yeah.

THERAPIST: Saturday seemed like a challenging day?

PATIENT: Yeah. I was pretty lonely that day, and during those times I see everything that's wrong with my life and the sadness was just too much.

THERAPIST: It sounds like a painful moment. Thoughts that everything is wrong along with feelings of sadness. Probably a day worth understanding more?

PATIENT: I guess. (*Said with some uncertainty and hesitation.*)

THERAPIST: Yes, I 100% agree. Okay, that will be number one on our agenda today. What else did you have on your mind to talk about today?

PATIENT: I really wanted to talk about my job today. I'm worried about my next few shifts as I'll be on my own.

THERAPIST: Okay. That sounds really good to me. We want to prepare for that the best we can. I'm glad you brought it up. Let's start with Saturday and go from there.

This dialogue is a typical example of the beginning few minutes of every session of Stage 1 S-DBT. Although not explicitly described, it is clear that the therapist has the treatment hierarchy in mind and is using the diary as means to collaboratively develop the day's agenda. The therapist is both flexible and open and at the same time firm in their position by organizing the agenda according to the treatment hierarchy.

Secondary Behavioral Targets: Responding to Client Characteristics

The secondary behavioral targets in S-DBT are targets of interventions based on six general response patterns (i.e., thoughts, feelings, and behaviors) thought to be typical of individuals meeting diagnostic criteria for BPD (Linehan, 1993). These response patterns are referred to as *dialectical dilemmas* and are organized according to three dimensions, each consisting of two opposing poles. The dialectical dilemmas are as follows: (a) emotional vulnerability versus self-invalidation, (b) active passivity versus apparent competence, and (c) unrelenting crises versus inhibited grieving. The essential point in considering the dialectical dilemmas is that each pole represents a collection of behaviors (thoughts, emotions, actions) that are so painful for clients that they find themselves vacillating between the poles' dimensions. The dialectical dilemmas become secondary targets of treatment only when their presence plays a role in the maintenance of the primary targeted problems.

For example, emotional vulnerability versus self-invalidation was described by Linehan (1993) as the core dialectical dilemma resulting in the development of DBT. On the pole of emotional vulnerability, clients have the experience of being more emotionally sensitive and reactive while also perceiving themselves as such. On this pole, people in their lives, including therapists, can be criticized or blamed for failing to understand them and failing to provide them with the assistance they need. In such a position, therapists are pulled toward offering acceptance-based strategies such as validation that may prove inadequate compared to a responsive approach that would seek to both validate and continue to push for change. In contrast, self-invalidation can be described as times when clients inhibit their emotional experience, mistrust themselves, and see themselves as fatally flawed. Any blame or attack will be directed toward themselves rather than others. In this position, therapists are pulled to offer change-based strategies, such as problem-solving, while failing to appreciate the role of acceptance and tolerance as a natural, responsive balance to the dilemma. The critical point with respect to responsivity in DBT and the dialectical dilemmas is to highlight the necessity of therapists' awareness of the *person* of the client informed by theory. A responsive DBT therapist maintains an awareness of these dilemmas and continually assesses for their relevance as a means of better understanding, communicating, and treating the primary targets.

Summary of Responsivity and the Behavioral Targets in DBT

The topics covered in an individual therapy session in S-DBT will reflect a blend of the immediate needs of the client along with the goals and priorities defined by the treatment stage. Therapists are responsive in structuring each therapy session based on the topics most relevant to the client and address them in order of importance consistent with the stage-appropriate treatment hierarchy (i.e., primary behavioral targets). Regardless of the session topic, therapists apply a dialectical philosophy to their in-session assessment and model dialectical thinking by highlighting polarities, modeling the search for a synthesis in opposing positions, and modeling change as a natural process. Last, in addressing the primary targets, therapists consider the relevance of secondary targets (i.e., the dialectical dilemmas) and provide a balanced response (i.e., change vs. acceptance) predicated on the needs of the client. Taken together, although each session of individual S-DBT will be unique with respect to content and topics covered, DBT sessions are recognizable based on an ongoing dialectical assessment, the use of the Stage 1 treatment hierarchy and targeting strategies, and responsivity based on client behavioral patterns (i.e., dialectical dilemmas).

Intervening With Responsivity in S-DBT

A major source of responsivity in DBT lies in the selection and delivery of the core DBT treatment strategies. The DBT manual describes four major categories of treatment interventions from which therapists can select: dialectical strategies, the core strategies of problem-solving and validation, stylistic strategies, and case management strategies (Linehan, 1993). These four categories contain a variety of techniques and protocols from which a therapist can choose to address the behavioral targets. The following section provides a brief summary of each of the four major categories while highlighting principles within each that allow for effective therapist responsivity.

Dialectical Treatment Strategies: Creating Balance in the Moment

Consistent with the goal of increasing dialectical behavioral patterns, the dialectical treatment strategies not only serve the purpose of reinforcing and modeling dialectical thinking but also provide a framework for balancing treatment interventions based on the core dialectic in DBT of acceptance versus change. In applying dialectics, therapists consider the degree to which the solutions provided balance acceptance (e.g., validation) versus change (e.g., problem-solving), the extent to which they are supportive (i.e., nurturing) versus confrontational (i.e., demanding), and the degree to which they are open to the opinions of the client (i.e., flexible) versus confident in their own positions (i.e., stability; Linehan, 1993). Consider the therapist's remarks in the following example in which a client and a therapist spent a portion of the session problem-solving following a challenging week:

> The week has been a particularly challenging one, and I hear you wanting to move forward and get through the moment. That makes sense to me. We've done some good problem-solving to get you "back in the saddle" so to speak. At the same time, now that I think about it, I wonder what we can do that would allow some recognition that, yes, you are back on the horse but *without* a

saddle. Any bump on the road in this upcoming week will be felt that much more intensely. Does that make sense? Let's consider how to accept the moment more fully and appreciate the impact of the week.

In these remarks, the therapist demonstrates an awareness that the majority of the session was focused on problem-solving. In this case, the client might have been especially motivated to move forward and "not look back," which would have put the client in the dialectical dilemma of self-invalidation and not acknowledging their own emotional vulnerability. An empathetic, but ill-guided, therapist might follow suit with strategies focused on change without recognition of the heightened vulnerability from the prior week's events. A responsive therapist in DBT would seek to balance the natural dialectic that arises in each session (i.e., balance acceptance and change) and will approach each opposing solution wholeheartedly and with conviction. Such a strategy is antithetical to the notion that would consider a dialectical synthesis to be equivalent to "watering down" a solution or finding some "shade of gray" or compromise between the two positions. Finally, in the preceding dialogue, the use of a simple metaphor emphasizes the fundamental dialectic in a novel, slightly off-kilter way consistent with dialectical strategies in DBT.

Empirical evidence in support of the importance of dialectics in DBT is shown in one study examining the therapeutic relationship in DBT (Bedics et al., 2012a). The results show that clients' self-reported perceptions of DBT therapists as simultaneously acting with autonomy (i.e., being supportive) and control (i.e., focused on change) were most effective in reducing nonsuicidal self-injury (NSSI). In contrast, the same dialectic was associated with increased NSSI in the active control condition of nonbehavioral experts. These results suggest that therapists' attention to the responsive nature of their interpersonal style might improve outcomes related to NSSI.

Validation and Problem-Solving: Moving Forward With Understanding
In addition to the dialectical strategies, validation and problem-solving represent the core strategies of S-DBT (Linehan, 1993). Linehan described the core skill of validation as highlighting the inherent wisdom in the clients' perspective, whereas problem-solving highlights the wisdom of the therapist and treatment. Similar to most strategies in DBT, validation and problem-solving each comprise multiple strategies. Therapists rely on context and timing for the selection of these techniques. DBT therapists seek to strike a balance between validation and problem-solving in every interaction.

Validation. Linehan (1997) described six validation strategies available to therapists: *paying attention and expressing interest, accurate reflecting, expressing the unverbalized* (e.g., emotions, thoughts), *validating the causes, acknowledging the valid given current events,* and *expressing belief in the client.* The effectiveness of validation relies on not only what type of validation is delivered but also when it is delivered. Therapists can apply validation to improve clients' understanding of themselves, repair the therapeutic relationship, or encourage effective behavior. In all of these cases the main responsive function of validation is positive reinforcement. In contrast, the withdrawal of validation occurs primarily in the presence of unwanted behavior, such as the occurrence of self-harm or therapy-interfering behavior. In this situation, the withdrawal of validation could serve the responsive function of extinction.

Two studies attempted to unpack the contingent link between therapist validation and positive outcome during an RCT of DBT. In the first study, researchers found that DBT clients perceived their therapist as acting toward them with greater affirmation and warmth in assessment periods immediately following those in which clients rated themselves as having a more positive self-concept (Bedics et al., 2012a). Interestingly, the opposite was true in the control condition where nonbehavioral therapists were perceived as acting more warmly following periods when clients reported a less positive self-concept. In a complementary study from the same trial, but from the therapists' perspective, results showed DBT therapists perceived themselves as acting with greater affiliation toward clients whom they perceived as reporting a more positive self-concept in the prior week (Bedics et al., 2012b). These results suggest timing may be a critical factor for the use of affirmation in the therapeutic relationship in DBT as therapists seek to contingently affirm positive gains.

Problem-solving. DBT therapists maintain the perspective that problematic behaviors, such as the primary targets in the treatment hierarchy, are best conceptualized as attempted solutions to problems (Linehan, 1993). The dilemma for the client is that their solutions, in the long run, have been ineffective. The goal of DBT is to provide clients with more effective solutions through the use of the four change strategies that compose the problem-solving module. These are *contingency management, cognitive modification, exposure therapy,* and *skills training.* Responsivity in problem-solving largely centers on ongoing behavioral assessment. In the moment, DBT therapists will continually ask themselves, "What is getting in the way of the client reaching their goal?" Contingency management is most helpful when the clients find themselves in life circumstances that do not reinforce or motivate positive change. In other circumstances clients might be experiencing emotions too intensively or maladaptive thoughts could block them from pursuing their goal. In these moments exposure therapy and cognitive modification would be the most appropriate, respectively. Last, it might simply be the case that clients do not have the prerequisite skill to achieve their goal. In those instances, skills training would be most appropriate.

Stylistic Strategies: Adjusting Your Style to Fit the Moment
The stylistic strategies in DBT reflect the therapist's overall attitude and style of communicating with the client as they deliver the treatment interventions. DBT therapists can choose from two sets of stylistic strategies: *reciprocal communication strategies* and *irreverent communication strategies* (Linehan, 1993). In delivering the reciprocal strategies, therapists attend to and listen to their clients' concerns (i.e., are responsive), share their own opinions and experiences (i.e., self-discloses), demonstrate a baseline of affiliation and warmth (i.e., warm engagement), and strive to act in a manner that is natural and typical of the therapists' personality styles beyond the defined role of therapist (i.e., genuineness; Linehan, 1993). The goal of the reciprocal strategies is to reduce the power differential that naturally exists within the therapeutic relationship by increasing therapist vulnerability. In contrast, the irreverent style can be confrontational and, at minimum, is a style of interacting that is very matter-of-fact.

The effectiveness of the communication style relies on purpose and timing. A therapist who is overly reciprocal can move at a pace that is too slow and risk overfragilizing the client. The therapist who overuses irreverence can be seen as harsh or mean spirited. An example of irreverence can be found in the statement demonstrating the treatment agenda noted earlier. In that example, the therapist recognized the client was not interested in discussing the day of the week when self-harm urges were more heightened. The therapist, irreverently, ignored the client's lack of enthusiasm and pressed ahead with the agenda. These, often playful, moments in the therapeutic relationship are typical of irreverent responding. What could have been a long, laborious conversation about the importance of self-harm and the treatment hierarchy was quickly surpassed and resolved. The therapist also followed the irreverence by taking seriously and validating the clients' immediate concerns and by doing so effectively balanced the change strategy (i.e., irreverence) with acceptance (i.e., validation and reciprocal responsiveness).

Case Management Strategies: Balancing Consultation With Intervention
In addition to in-session decisions regarding responsiveness to client behavior, DBT calls for decisions regarding how and when to interact with the client's environment. This category of responsiveness encompasses three case management strategies: *consultation to the patient, environmental intervention,* and *consultation team* (Linehan, 1993). Case management within DBT is unique

in that the focus of the therapist's attention is to act as consultant to the client rather than directly intervening in the client's relationships. However, at times the situation may call for intervention directly by the therapist, resulting in the choice of environmental intervention strategies. Treating the therapist mirrors consultation to the client strategies in that the job of the DBT consultation team is to apply DBT to the therapist, thus supporting the therapist while maintaining their effectiveness.

Consultation to the patient strategies: Letting the patient drive. "Consultation to the client or patient" strategies serve to assist the client in interacting effectively with the environment rather than intervening with the environment on the client's behalf (Linehan, 1993). In employing this strategy, the therapist is attuned to the presence of a core dialectical dilemma faced by clients diagnosed with BPD, that of active passivity versus apparent competence. Active passivity represents the tendency of the client to approach problems in the environment with helplessness, while pulling for—or at times demanding that—the environment (e.g., the therapist) solve problems for the client. Conversely, the therapist must be aware of the client's tendency to appear competent in some contexts but be unable to apply the same observed competence in other contexts. Awareness of these characteristics and how they appear in the client's experience provides the basis for selection of the strategy of consultation to the client.

Environmental intervention strategies: When the therapist takes the wheel. Although the preference in DBT is to act as consultant to the client, the therapist may at times determine that the situation is crucial enough and/or the client's own capacity for intervening in the situation is limited enough that it is necessary for the therapist to select environmental intervention strategies (Linehan, 1993). Selection of these strategies represents simultaneous therapist attunement to the client's context, problems, and capabilities. In terms of context, for example, the client may be facing a situation in which the environment (e.g., other medical professionals, insurance companies) requires direct intervention by another professional. Furthermore, DBT is unique among many therapies in that it does not restrict intervention to the therapy room. Given a particular client's context, the therapist may elect to enter the client's environment in order to assist with certain activities. For example, clients with a lack of supportive others in their lives (as is frequently the case with DBT clients) may need assistance navigating a particularly complicated public agency or may need to be accompanied on a task about which they are severely phobic. Again, the therapist selects such strategies based on knowledge of the particular client's context, paying special attention to how that context intersects with the client's presenting problems.

Consultation to the therapist: Guiding the therapist. The consultation team can be seen as essential in enhancing optimal responsiveness by helping the DBT therapist maintain the flexibility required to respond appropriately and effectively over the course of the treatment. Primarily, this mode of S-DBT assists the therapist in maintaining a dialectical balance throughout the course of therapy, thus avoiding extreme, rigid, and polarized points of view that can develop in working with a challenging population (Linehan, 1993). Conducting effective DBT means responding in ways that may be aversive to the client (e.g., focusing on suicide) or aversive to the therapist (e.g., withdrawing warmth when the client engages in suicidal behaviors). One purpose of the team is to validate the therapist's struggles, cheerlead the therapist, and thus assist the therapist in maintaining the level and type of responsiveness required in order to effectively treat the client. Additionally, input from all team members provides diverse data about a client's interactions, thus assisting the individual therapist in applying treatment strategies that are most effective, rather than simply rooted in the individual therapist's unexamined response. Maintaining optimal responsiveness is particularly challenging when the therapist is under extreme stress, experiencing high burnout, or being reinforced for ineffective behaviors (e.g., being shaped by the client in ways that reduce optimal responsiveness). All of the above are likely to occur in working with complex cases. Thus, the consultation team serves to treat the therapist in such a way that he or she can maintain the frame of responding effectively as dictated by DBT principles and appropriate responsiveness to client characteristics.

CLINICAL TRAINING IN DBT RESPONSIVITY

Clinicians can begin delivering an effectively responsive DBT intervention by first demonstrating clarity regarding the framework from which they are delivering DBT. As described previously, a clear framework sets out the treatment goals and methods of delivery that define the parameters for effective in-session responsivity. Nearly all the concepts taken in this chapter showcase in-session responsivity in S-DBT and have been drawn from the original treatment manual (Linehan, 1993). A simple recommendation for practitioners to enhance their responsivity is to continually improve their familiarity with the core text. Each chapter in the text includes tables that provide the "dos" and "don'ts" of DBT that speak to principles reviewed in this chapter. The tables provide a comprehensive guide to the essential qualities necessary to optimize an individual session of S-DBT.

The current gold standard for the evaluation of an individual S-DBT session is provided as part of acquiring DBT certification offered by the DBT-Linehan Board of Certification (see https://dbt-lbc.org/). Critical to the certification process is the assessment and evaluation of session adherence. DBT adherence ratings (Linehan & Korslund, 2003) provide overall and subscale ratings of the quality of treatment delivered in a session of DBT. The feedback can be invaluable in highlighting areas of strength and weakness during an individual session while also providing a clinician with an overall sense of what is needed for a session to meet adherence in DBT. It is important, however, to remember that adherence is not a stable trait or disposition that a person acquires even after certification. Adherence, instead, is best conceptualized as a "verb" rather than a "noun" with natural variability and fluctuations across sessions and clients.

FUTURE DIRECTIONS IN RESEARCH ON RESPONSIVITY IN DBT

Current research on DBT has yet to unpack many of the responsive processes thought to, at least partly, underlie the treatment's effectiveness. The majority of research in DBT can, broadly speaking, be classified as ballistic in nature (Stiles et al., 1998). Although many of the RCTs of DBT include ratings of adherence, they have traditionally spoken only to the global quality of the sessions and have not been correlated with outcome in a systematic fashion. Given the considerable variation in intervention modalities that can be delivered, future research would benefit by attempting to examine this variability as it relates to outcome.

Although research has begun to examine the relevance of timing during DBT in response to primary targeted behavior (e.g., Bedics et al., 2012a, 2012b), this research has yet to explore the microprocesses that occur within each individual session. For example, a clear line of future research based on prior work would be to focus on in-session therapist behavior during the discussion of primary treatment targets. The relative balance of problem-solving versus validation strategies, for example, during these conversations along with their association with long-term outcome would be a meaningful contribution to the literature. Finally, the extent to which these processes vary by characteristics of the client has yet to be fully explored. Future work could explore how, for example, therapist responsiveness is moderated by the presence or absence of client dialectical dilemmas. Similarly, research has only recently begun to examine the role of cultural diversity in the delivery of DBT. In one study, the authors worked with tribal leaders in an American Indian/Native Alaskan population using mindfulness as the core, integrative concept bridging DBT with traditional spiritual activities (Beckstead et al., 2015). The result of this integration was a responsive protocol for the treatment of adolescents diagnosed with substance abuse disorders. Although preliminary, results showed 96% of participants to report clinically significant improvement during treatment. The extent to which cultural and historical factors result in unique dialectical balances or affect the delivery of specific treatment interventions is an important area of future work.

CONCLUSION

DBT is inherently a responsive treatment from the development of treatment goals to the selection and delivery of interventions. Although S-DBT for the treatment of Stage 1 clients remains the gold standard of delivering DBT, DBT can be scaled down or up to meet the needs of clients based on the principles of stage hierarchy and modularity. In-session responsivity in S-DBT relies on understanding behavioral characteristics, or dialectical dilemmas, in clients diagnosed with BPD; therapeutic principles from dialectical philosophy and behavioral assessment; and modularity.

REFERENCES

Beckstead, D. J., Lambert, M. J., DuBose, A. P., & Linehan, M. (2015). Dialectical behavior therapy with American Indian/Alaska Native adolescents diagnosed with substance use disorders: Combining an evidence based treatment with cultural, traditional, and spiritual beliefs. *Addictive Behaviors, 51*, 84–87. https://doi.org/10.1016/j.addbeh.2015.07.018

Bedics, J. D., Atkins, D. C., Comtois, K. A., & Linehan, M. M. (2012a). Treatment differences in the therapeutic relationship and introject during a 2-year randomized controlled trial of dialectical behavior therapy versus nonbehavioral psychotherapy experts for borderline personality disorder. *Journal of Consulting and Clinical Psychology, 80*(1), 66–77. https://doi.org/10.1037/a0026113

Bedics, J. D., Atkins, D. C., Comtois, K. A., & Linehan, M. M. (2012b). Weekly therapist ratings of the therapeutic relationship and patient introject during the course of dialectical behavioral therapy for the treatment of borderline personality disorder. *Psychotherapy, 49*(2), 231–240. https://doi.org/10.1037/a0028254

Comtois, K. A., Kerbrat, A. H., Atkins, D. C., Harned, M. S., & Elwood, L. (2010). Recovery from disability for individuals with borderline personality disorder: A feasibility trial of DBT-ACES. *Psychiatric Services, 61*(11), 1106–1111. https://doi.org/10.1176/ps.2010.61.11.1106

Harned, M. S., Chapman, A. L., Dexter-Mazza, E. T., Murray, A., Comtois, K. A., & Linehan, M. M. (2009). Treating co-occurring Axis I disorders in recurrently suicidal women with borderline personality disorder: A 2-year randomized trial of dialectical behavior therapy versus community treatment by experts. *Personality Disorders, S*(1), 35–45. https://doi.org/10.1037/1949-2715.S.1.35

Harned, M. S., Korslund, K. E., & Linehan, M. M. (2014). A pilot randomized controlled trial of Dialectical Behavior Therapy with and without the Dialectical Behavior Therapy Prolonged Exposure protocol for suicidal and self-injuring women with borderline personality disorder and PTSD. *Behaviour Research and Therapy, 55,* 7–17. https://doi.org/10.1016/j.brat.2014.01.008

Linehan, M. (1993). *Cognitive-behavioral treatment of borderline personality disorder.* Guilford Press.

Linehan, M. M. (1997). Validation and psychotherapy. In A. C. Bohart & L. S. Greenberg (Eds.), *Empathy reconsidered: New directions in psychotherapy* (pp. 353–392). American Psychological Association. https://doi.org/10.1037/10226-016

Linehan, M. M. (2015). *DBT® skills training manual* (2nd ed.). Guilford Press.

Linehan, M. M., Armstrong, H. E., Suarez, A., Allmon, D., & Heard, H. L. (1991). Cognitive-behavioral treatment of chronically parasuicidal borderline patients. *Archives of General Psychiatry, 48*(12), 1060–1064. https://doi.org/10.1001/archpsyc.1991.01810360024003

Linehan, M. M., Comtois, K. A., Murray, A. M., Brown, M. Z., Gallop, R. J., Heard, H. L., Korslund, K. E., Tutek, D. A., Reynolds, S. K., & Lindenboim, N. (2006). Two-year randomized controlled trial and follow-up of dialectical behavior therapy vs therapy by experts for suicidal behaviors and borderline personality disorder. *Archives of General Psychiatry, 63*(7), 757–766. https://doi.org/10.1001/archpsyc.63.7.757

Linehan, M. M., Comtois, K. A., & Ward-Ciesielski, E. F. (2012). Assessing and managing risk with suicidal individuals. *Cognitive and Behavioral Practice, 19*(2), 218–232. https://doi.org/10.1016/j.cbpra.2010.11.008

Linehan, M. M., Dimeff, L. A., Reynolds, S. K., Comtois, K. A., Welch, S. S., Heagerty, P., & Kivlahan, D. R. (2002). Dialectical behavior therapy versus comprehensive validation therapy plus 12-step for the treatment of opioid dependent women meeting criteria for borderline personality disorder. *Drug and Alcohol Dependence, 67*(1), 13–26. https://doi.org/10.1016/S0376-8716(02)00011-X

Linehan, M. M., & Korslund, K. E. (2003). *University of Washington Adherence Scale* [Unpublished manuscript]. Department of Psychology, University of Washington, Seattle.

Linehan, M. M., Korslund, K. E., Harned, M. S., Gallop, R. J., Lungu, A., Neacsiu, A. D., McDavid, J., Comtois, K. A., & Murray-Gregory, A. M. (2015). Dialectical behavior therapy for high suicide risk in individuals with borderline personality disorder: A randomized clinical trial and component analysis. *JAMA Psychiatry, 72*(5), 475–482. https://doi.org/10.1001/jamapsychiatry.2014.3039

Linehan, M. M., & Schmidt, H., III. (1995). The dialectics of effective treatment of borderline personality disorder. In W. T. O'Donohue & L. Krasner (Eds.), *Theories of behavior therapy: Exploring behavior change* (pp. 553–584). American Psychological Association. https://doi.org/10.1037/10169-020

Linehan, M. M., Schmidt, H., III, Dimeff, L. A., Craft, J. C., Kanter, J., & Comtois, K. A. (1999). Dialectical behavior therapy for patients with borderline personality disorder and drug-dependence. *The American Journal on Addictions, 8*(4), 279–292. https://doi.org/10.1080/105504999305686

Linehan, M. M., & Wilks, C. R. (2015). The course and evolution of dialectical behavior therapy. *American Journal of Psychotherapy, 69*(2), 97–110. https://doi.org/10.1176/appi.psychotherapy.2015.69.2.97

Lynch, T. R., Trost, W. T., Salsman, N., & Linehan, M. M. (2007). Dialectical behavior therapy for borderline personality disorder. *Annual Review of Clinical Psychology, 3*(1), 181–205. https://doi.org/10.1146/annurev.clinpsy.2.022305.095229

McMain, S. F., Links, P. S., Gnam, W. H., Guimond, T., Cardish, R. J., Korman, L., & Streiner, D. L. (2009). A randomized trial of dialectical behavior therapy versus general psychiatric management for borderline personality disorder. *The American Journal of Psychiatry, 166*(12), 1365–1374. https://doi.org/10.1176/appi.ajp.2009.09010039

Nelson, L. D., Simmons, J., & Simonsohn, U. (2018). Psychology's Renaissance. *Annual Review of Psychology, 69*(1), 511–534. https://doi.org/10.1146/annurev-psych-122216-011836

Stanley, T. D., Carter, E. C., & Doucouliagos, H. (2018). What meta-analyses reveal about the replicability of psychological research. *Psychological Bulletin, 144*(12), 1325–1346. https://doi.org/10.1037/bul0000169

Stiles, W. B., Honos-Webb, L., & Surko, M. (1998). Responsiveness in psychotherapy. *Clinical Psychology: Science and Practice, 5*(4), 439–458. https://doi.org/10.1111/j.1468-2850.1998.tb00166.x

Valentine, S. E., Bankoff, S. M., Poulin, R. M., Reidler, E. B., & Pantalone, D. W. (2015). The use of dialectical behavior therapy skills training as stand-alone treatment: A systematic review of the treatment outcome literature. *Journal of Clinical Psychology, 71*(1), 1–20. https://doi.org/10.1002/jclp.22114

Valentine, S. E., Smith, A. M., & Stewart, K. (2020). A review of the empirical evidence of DBT skills training as a stand-alone intervention. In J. D. Bedics (Ed.), *The handbook of dialectical behavior therapy: Theory, research, and evaluation* (pp. 325–358). Academic Press. https://doi.org/10.1016/B978-0-12-816384-9.00015-4

Verheul, R., Van Den Bosch, L. M. C., Koeter, M. W. J., De Ridder, M. A. J., Stijnen, T., & Van Den Brink, W. (2003). Dialectical behaviour therapy for women with borderline personality disorder: 12-month, randomised clinical trial in The Netherlands. *The British Journal of Psychiatry, 182*(2), 135–140. https://doi.org/10.1192/bjp.182.2.135

13 RESPONSIVENESS IN INTEGRATIVE THERAPIES

JAMES F. BOSWELL, BRITTANY R. KING,
CARLY M. SCHWARTZMAN, RACHEL H. WASSERMAN,
AND MICHAEL J. CONSTANTINO

Responsivity is the *raison d'être* of integrative psychotherapies, which cannot be defined by a single model or a static set of prescribed interventions. There are multiple models and pathways to integrative practice and a given course of psychotherapy can become a de facto integrative one at any given moment, even with clinicians who would not identify themselves as integrative practitioners (Goldfried et al., 1998).

Given that it is not tied to any particular theoretical orientation, integrative therapists can easily adopt Stiles's working definition of responsiveness (1998, 2009), which states that therapists and clients use emerging information and context to modify their behavior in therapy. Such modifications represent *appropriate* responsiveness when they optimize therapy outcome. In addition, responsiveness occurs on a continuum of time scales, including moments within a session or patient-centered treatment selection at the earliest stages of a course of therapy (Beutler & Harwood, 2000). Interestingly, these different time scales map onto different pathways to integrative practice.

https://doi.org/10.1037/0000240-014
The Responsive Psychotherapist: Attuning to Clients in the Moment, J. C. Watson and H. Wiseman (Editors)

In this chapter, we outline how responsiveness has been the leitmotif of integrative therapy for nearly a century. Given the diversity of existing integrative approaches and their constant evolution, we begin by providing some historical context and identifying how different types and levels of responsiveness map onto general pathways to integrative practice. We then present two complementary metaframeworks that can inform responsive integrative practice, irrespective of one's preferred method of integration. Next, we offer clinical examples of responsiveness in integrative therapies. Finally, we address the intersection of responsiveness and diversity considerations, and we propose implications for training to maximize clinicians' responsiveness in integrative psychotherapies. Throughout the chapter, we integrate relevant research examples.

PATHWAYS OF INTEGRATION AS CONTEXTS FOR RESPONSIVITY

Responsiveness buttresses the history of psychotherapy integration. Neo-Freudians adapted psychoanalysis based on accumulating clinical observation and recognition that the existing state of psychoanalytic practice was insufficient for many cases (Boswell & Goldfried, 2010; Boswell, Sharpless, Greenberg, et al., 2010). Even Freud himself recognized the limitations of his initial conceptions (see Liff, 1992). In the first half of the 20th century, the rise of behaviorism and evidence from learning research led scholars to attempt to reconcile (i.e., integrate) psychodynamic and behavioral models of functioning and intervention (Hull, 1939). Around the same time, scholars began to articulate the role of common factors in accounting for psychotherapy outcomes (Rosenzweig, 1936; Watson et al., 1940). Disillusionment with the prevailing models of psychoanalysis and behaviorism led to Rogers's (1951) paradigm-shifting client-centered psychotherapy, which prized relational attunement and itself has evolved into contemporary experiential therapies based on accumulating theory and observation (Greenberg, 1995). Subsequently, the so-called cognitive revolution created acrimony among behaviorists for many years, prior to its formal integration as cognitive behavioral therapy (CBT) that is well known today (see Beck, 1991). Recent years have witnessed yet another shift with integrative underpinnings, as so-called third wave CBT approaches more formally incorporate concepts and strategies that are exogenous to traditional CBT or have at least been historically underemphasized (Prochaska & Norcross, 2014).

This overly simplistic summary is our attempt to convey that (a) the evolution of psychotherapies is steeped in the spirit of integration, and (b) the "impulse" to integrate has invariably been driven by the need to be responsive to emerging evidence, theory, and context. Although we view the evolution of psychotherapy as being driven by a recognition of the need for theoretical and technical assimilation and accommodation, the "integrative movement" as it exists today is a relatively recent phenomenon (Norcross & Goldfried, 2005).

At a more practical level, the development of integrative therapies has been multidetermined, stemming from a recognition that many clients do not respond to frontline treatments, as well as extant outcome research on "pure form" psychotherapies pointing to considerable room for improvement (Lambert, 2013). In addition, some clients decline and/or drop out of single-model treatments, suggesting that adaptations may be necessary to make these treatments more palatable. Clinicians and researchers recognize the limits of a particular theoretical model and its associated techniques when applied to particular types of clients and contexts (Goldfried et al., 2014). As such, the importance of responsiveness has been a consistent thread in the psychotherapy integration movement, yet the nature of responsiveness has varied at least partly as a function of the type of integration.

Four Pathways to Psychotherapy Integration

We distinguish among four routes, or pathways, to psychotherapy integration: theoretical integration, technical eclecticism, assimilative integration, and common factors.

Theoretical Integration

One pathway to psychotherapy integration is *theoretical* integration, in which a clear overarching theory drives the choice of techniques. The theory is not necessarily derived primarily from a single type of mainstream psychotherapy; it may be developed from an amalgam of two or more theories, developed anew, or imported from a relevant field (e.g., social-ecological). As noted, the choice of techniques is guided by the theory and may include techniques from one or more systems of psychotherapy. This approach arguably represents a more *macro* structure to support responsiveness vis-à-vis integration. For example, Wachtel's (2014) cyclical psychodynamics model prospectively integrates psychodynamic, CBT, systemic, and experiential perspectives into an overarching model. Ostensibly, such integration accounts for more within- and between-client complexity, setting the stage for clinicians to have a broader, yet cohesive, framework for understanding the nature of the client's problem, as well as the unfolding process within and between sessions. Dialectical behavior therapy (DBT; Linehan, 2015) for borderline personality disorder is the most studied and empirically supported integrative therapy for a particular disorder, often connected to the theoretical integration pathway. In addition to its dialectic frame (Heard & Linehan, 2019), DBT integrates interventions such as mindfulness, acceptance, and focusing on dialectical processes into more traditional CBT interventions, such as problem-solving (Linehan, 2015). This integration can facilitate responsiveness, as described in Chapter 12 of this volume. Yet, the "how to" of responsiveness can be unclear even with approaches that are naturally integrative.

Technical Eclecticism

A second pathway to integrative practice is *technical eclecticism*, which involves the use of empirically derived methods drawn from different schools of therapy without necessarily subscribing to their underlying theoretical foundations. However, such eclecticism should not be confused with haphazardness, as prevailing models involve a systematic approach in choosing methods and tailoring them to individual clients. Such tailoring can inform decisions regarding the initial course of action with a given client, as well as the selection of interventions over the course of therapy.

For example, systematic treatment selection (STS; Beutler et al., 2005) uses research findings to determine which clients are most likely to benefit (or not) from particular interventions. This integrative approach is defined by responsiveness insofar as a therapist's methods and relational stances will change client to client. Routine assessment is the linchpin to informing both intervention selection and interpersonal style. STS was originally based on a comprehensive review of the research literature and then subjected to several randomized controlled trials (RCTs) to validate matching scenarios. Clients are matched with a particular approach by virtue of their transdiagnostic characteristics, such as functional impairment, readiness for change, reactance level, social support, and coping style (Beutler et al., 2005). For example, based on a depressed client's written and/or verbal self-report, the observed degree of reactance would steer the therapist to adopt either a directive or more insight-oriented approach, given that a recent meta-analysis found that clients higher in reactance had better outcomes when their therapist adopted a less directive approach, whereas clients lower in reactance had better outcomes when their therapist adopted a more directive approach

(Beutler et al., 2018). Although reactance is considered to be more traitlike and distinguishable from within-session resistance, knowledge of a client's trait reactance can and should raise a therapist's antennae for markers of resistance as a function of perceived threats to autonomy. Related to this, STS incorporates stages of change theory (Prochaska & Norcross, 2002) to determine if and when to introduce more action-oriented work based on a given client's motivation and readiness to change (Beutler & Harwood, 2000). A particular benefit of technical eclecticism is that it offers a decision-making framework to support global technical and relational responsiveness. The relevance of distinguishing between technical and relational responsiveness could be argued. For our purposes, the distinction simply demarcates a flexibility regarding the type of intervention to be delivered in a particular instance (e.g., "Would it be more helpful to introduce relaxation training before exposure or should we proceed with exposure?") or the decision to adopt a particular relational stance (e.g., be more or less directive).

Assimilative Integration

A third integrative pathway is labeled *assimilative* integration, defined as "the incorporation of attitudes, perspectives, or techniques from an auxiliary therapy into a therapist's primary, grounding approach" (Messer, 2001, p. 1). Assimilative integration consists of a "home" theoretical orientation explicitly augmented by specific concepts and/or techniques from one or more exogenous systems. Assimilation can occur at different times, much like our working definition of responsiveness itself. For example, basic and applied research on the nature and treatment of generalized anxiety disorder (GAD) led Newman et al. (2011) to prospectively integrate interpersonal and emotional processing (IEP) interventions into an existing, empirically supported CBT approach. A CBT clinician can select this augmented CBT model prior to working with primary GAD clients. Alternatively, a clinician can pursue a CBT plan, while integrating exogenous techniques and concepts in response to within-session markers. For example, Westra and colleagues (2016) trained CBT clinicians to shift to motivational interviewing (MI) strategies in response to markers of client change ambivalence or treatment resistance. Relative to standard CBT, participants receiving MI-CBT experienced significantly greater reductions in worry severity across a 12-month follow-up.

The distinction between the Newman et al. (2011) and Westra et al. (2016) designs warrants additional consideration. Both trials adopted an additive design, yet with different features. In Newman et al., participants were randomized to receive either 50 min of CBT plus 50 minutes of IEP or 50 minutes of CBT plus 50 minutes of supportive listening (SL). In Westra et al., a freestanding MI module was added to CBT, *and* therapists in the MI-CBT condition were trained to shift to MI to address moments of client resistance, thus representing a more seamless assimilative approach anchored in momentary responsiveness. Importantly, Newman et al. failed to find a significant between-condition outcome difference at posttreatment or 6-month follow-up. This finding is relatively consistent with the results of a meta-analysis of component control treatment studies (Bell et al., 2013), which found no statistically significant difference between full treatments and dismantled treatments, as well as a small effect slightly favoring treatments with an added component compared with the standard treatment. In the context of RCTs, between-subject analyses mask important intra- and interindividual variability in process and outcome (Fisher & Boswell, 2016). Although responsiveness is by no means eliminated in RCTs, it is potentially attenuated when a protocol therapist is expected to follow a set of carefully prescribed interventions, while avoiding the introduction of "off model" techniques.

The results of Westra et al. (2016) demonstrate how between-treatment differences can begin to emerge when marker-driven responsiveness is explicitly integrated into a home orientation. As they say, it is the "feature rather than a bug." In contrast, the traditional application of protocols in RCTs focuses more on faithful adherence to a sequence of prescribed interventions. Westra et al.'s results also demonstrate that clinicians can be trained to detect important process markers and behave responsively upon detection. Although studies have shown that technical flexibility within a course of therapy can be associated with better outcome (Katz et al., 2019), there are also empirical examples of the pitfalls of apparent flexibility. For example, Boswell, Castonguay, and Wasserman (2010) found that clients of "high common factor" therapists (i.e., therapists who reported focusing more on common factors than the average therapist in the sample), who were participating in treatments that focused more heavily on common factors than the average client's treatment in that therapist's caseload, rated sessions with higher than average CBT intervention use significantly less helpful and less positively impactful. The use of CBT interventions per se was not problematic; rather, it was the increased use of CBT interventions on the part of historically nondirective therapists who were delivering relatively nondirective treatments, potentially illustrating the negative effects of breaking an established treatment frame (i.e., *inappropriate* responsiveness).

Encouragingly, it appears that therapists can be trained to become more appropriately responsive when departing from a baseline model.

Common Factors

Common factors are often labeled as a fourth route to integrative therapy and have been offered as an explanation for the apparent lack of difference in outcomes between additive and dismantled treatments, whereby the researchers were attempting to causally isolate theory-specific change mechanisms (Ahn & Wampold, 2001). At a basic level, heeding the importance of common factors in psychotherapy is foundational to responsivity. We, however, struggle with viewing common factors as a unique, standalone integrative pathway, as common factors themselves are divorced from explicit strategies that harness and enhance common factors for therapeutic benefit. In addition, certain therapy approaches may emphasize particular common factors over others (Weinberger, 1995). For example, certain therapy models are explicitly relational (thereby, ostensibly capitalizing on the importance of the alliance as the "flagship" common factor), whereas CBT approaches more often appeal to outcome evidence and the therapist as expert when providing a rationale, potentially harnessing expectancy and credibility effects more so than alternative approaches. Interestingly, our recent meta-analysis of the expectancy-outcome association did not find a moderating effect of treatment orientation, specifically, yet we did find a stronger expectancy-outcome association in studies where therapists used either a treatment manual or a mixture of manualized and nonmanualized treatment compared to no manual (Constantino et al., 2018).

Key Considerations Regarding the Four Pathways

Integrative pathways are not mutually exclusive. For example, technical eclecticism is not purely atheoretical. The STS is, after all, *systematic*; decision making is based on theory and evidence-informed matching assumptions. Further, different approaches to integrative therapy may, at least conceptually, appeal to certain types of responsiveness, yet there is likely to be substantial heterogeneity in practice within and between clients. Assimilative integrationists have the capacity and wherewithal to depart from a home model if deemed useful for a given case, but this is unlikely to be necessary for all cases; staying the course could be considered appropriate responsiveness with such clients. Given this complexity, we believe the "how to" of responsive practice in integrative therapies may require a metaframework to guide decision making. We next outline two complementary metaframeworks, prior to offering clinical examples.

METAFRAMEWORKS TO FACILITATE RESPONSIVE INTEGRATION

Depending on the level of analysis, metaframeworks could be considered integrative pathways themselves or guides for integrative practice. Two such frameworks are common principles of change (Goldfried, 1980) and context responsive psychotherapy integration (CRPI; Constantino et al., 2013).

Common Principles of Change

Stemming from the work of Frank (1961; among others, e.g., Garfield, 1980), Goldfried (1980) articulated a common principles approach that seeks to elucidate the core ingredients that different therapies have in common. Although factors that are considered to be unique to a specific therapy are still considered important, it is the commonalities across approaches that are thought to be most important in accounting for treatment outcomes.

The principles of change framework should be distinguished from what are labeled common factors. Although common factors represent important elements of psychotherapy that cut across orientations and diagnostic categories, change principles focus on common clinical *strategies* and putative mechanisms of action to guide clinician behavior. The distinction is illustrated in the following quote:

> I would suggest, however, that the possibility of finding meaningful consensus exists at a level of abstraction somewhere between theory and technique which, for want of a better term, we might call "clinical strategies." Where these strategies to have a clear empirical foundation, it might be more appropriate to call them "principles" of change. In essence, such strategies function as clinical heuristics that implicitly guide efforts during the course of therapy. (Goldfried, 1980, p. 994)

Goldfried (1980) argued that such strategies exist at an intermediate level of abstraction, between model-unique theory (e.g., psychodynamic) and associated techniques (e.g., transference interpretation). One of the first examples offered by Goldfried was providing the client with new, corrective experiences. Theory regarding the nature of the experience(s) to be corrected, as well as how to facilitate this corrective experience (i.e., what the therapist does to facilitate the change process), exist at the higher and lower levels of abstraction, respectively (see Castonguay & Hill, 2012). In an intensive case analysis involving a client in the aforementioned Newman et al. (2011) GAD trial, Castonguay et al. (2012) explored the corrective experience of a responder case, across both CBT and IEP treatment segments. Among the reported results, they found that observed corrective experiences in both segments were characterized by the client deliberately and consciously engaging in responses that were different from those that were typically triggered by previously feared situations; further, these atypical reactions were explicitly experienced as a disconfirmation of previous negative expectations.

Interestingly, the nature of the corrective experiences were more intrapersonal in CBT and interpersonal/relational in IEP. Although perhaps not explicitly framed this way, the facilitation of a corrective relational experience was an important aim of the IEP segment, and the therapist's ability to remain attuned and appropriately responsive appeared paramount. Not unlike many clients with GAD, the client in question engaged in a fair amount of experiential avoidance and was prone to intellectualizing. Consistent with the manual, the therapist attempted to explore the client's experience, including in the moment with the therapist. The client struggled to engage in this type of work and eventually expressed frustration with the tasks of the therapy. The therapist identified this as a marker of an alliance rupture (Eubanks et al., 2018; see also Chapter 4, this volume). In IEP, metacommunication was a prescribed/allowed repair strategy, and this was implemented along with an apparent attempt to adjust her style. A version of this process occurred in additional episodes in the therapy, and the client appeared more willing to deepen his experience, self-disclose, and join in the metacommunication as therapy progressed. In fact, he independently employed a similar strategy of metacommunication with his partner with great success. Using a valued principles of change (corrective relational experience) as a guidepost, the therapist was able to attend to markers and respond flexibly and make adjustments to keep the client engaged in the work.

Context Responsive Psychotherapy Integration

A more recently developed, complementary framework is CRPI (Constantino et al., 2013). This framework supports the use of pandiagnostic and pantheoretical strategies that can be employed in response to the identification of specific and commonly occurring treatment markers. These markers can include client characteristics as well as within-treatment (e.g., session) processes. Context responsive integration is not a standalone orientation or manualized approach; rather, it is an *if–then* framework supporting evidence-based clinical responsiveness in the form of matching therapist decision making and strategy to therapy contexts and clients' needs (Constantino et al., 2019). Such a framework has the potential to reduce errors in decision making when confronted with difficult, yet fairly common, clinical scenarios that are less clearly addressed by a single (or one's preferred) treatment model.

While arguing that the framework should constantly evolve with the evidence base, Constantino et al. (2013) identified five candidate context-responsive markers and evidence-based responsive modules: (a) low outcome expectations, which reflect a lack of confidence in treatment's efficacy, may mark the need to explicitly address and persuade treatment beliefs; (b) change ambivalence may mark the need for clinicians to employ MI strategies; (c) self-strivings, such as a client's need for self-verification, even if in contrast with treatment aims, may call for attending to and affirming the self in order to avoid incongruence in the therapeutic process and subsequent negative relational consequences; (d) alliance ruptures may precipitate the need for explicit repair strategies; and (e) outcomes monitoring, which emphasizes the importance of tracking client progress, may mark the need to respond to deterioration or lack of expected clinical change.

A prime example of the CRPI framework is found in the previously mentioned Westra et al. (2016) RCT, where clinicians were trained to attend to markers of change ambivalence or treatment resistance. When such markers were detected, CBT clinicians shifted into less directive MI strategies. The previously mentioned principles of change case example by Castonguay et al. (2012) on corrective experiences also illustrates the complementarity between principle-focused and CRPI frameworks, in that the therapist was trained to identify and respond to markers of alliance rupture. Once identified, the therapist shifted into rupture-repair strategies. The rupture-repair process itself was considered to be a facilitator of the valued corrective relational experience process. Stated differently, a principles of change approach assumes that there are multiple roads to Rome. However, one is unlikely to arrive in Rome without first identifying Rome as the destination and keeping that specific destination in awareness when faced with bumps and forks in the road. How to respond to the bumps and the forks to most efficiently and safely reach Rome is a related yet different empirical question. Now enter CRPI, which is focused on teaching the traveler to (a) attend to the landmarks, bumps, and forks; and (b) effectively respond to these markers. The usefulness of these metaframeworks as guides to promoting responsivity in integrative therapy is relatively clear given their pantheoretical and pandiagnostic focus.

CLINICAL ILLUSTRATIONS

Case Example 1: Combining the Principles of Change and CRPI Metaframeworks

Our first clinical illustration[1] showcases the intersection of the CRPI and principles of change metaframeworks in responsive integrative psychotherapy. The client presented for treatment with primary complaints of anxiety and panic symptoms. The therapist identifies as an assimilative integrationist who primarily works from a psychodynamic orientation. The therapist also has training in and experiences with employing different therapy models, including CBT. On the basis of a comprehensive initial assessment, the client and the therapist agreed that panic-related difficulties were most concerning and impairing. The therapist explained that there were multiple options for addressing her concerns or different angles to approaching the problem. More concretely, the therapist provided descriptions and rationales for panic-focused psychodynamic psychotherapy (Busch & Milrod, 2013) and a CBT approach (Barlow et al., 2011). After discussion, the client expressed a preference for panic-focused psychodynamic therapy, and this approach was adopted. Subsequently, the client regularly attended and participated in sessions. She expressed finding therapy helpful and achieving some useful insights. Nevertheless, her panic symptoms were worsening. She reported experiencing more panic attacks in more situations (i.e., stimulus generalization), which was leading to increases in behavioral avoidance and social isolation.

PATIENT: I feel like I'm slowly starting to avoid everything. I avoid driving now because of the panic. I'm starting to worry about how to get to work.

THERAPIST: It sounds like you are experiencing the panic symptoms in more contexts, and it's starting to have more impact on your day-to-day life. I understand that's concerning.

PATIENT: Don't get me wrong. I understand what we've been doing, and I'm still on board. But this aspect is only getting worse and starting to have a major impact. I'm at a loss.

THERAPIST: Are your panic experiences still pretty consistent? I mean, are you noticing the same sensations that we've talked about in these different situations, they're just generalizing?

---

[1] The identities of the clients in the case examples throughout this chapter have been disguised either by changing identifying information or using composites.

PATIENT: Yes. I feel like I can't breathe, my heart starts racing, my chest feels tight, and I get dizzy to the point of feeling like I'm going to pass out. Getting to the point of not wanting to walk up stairs so my heart doesn't start racing.

THERAPIST: Do you remember in one of our initial sessions, when I talked about the panic cycle and different approaches to addressing panic?

PATIENT: Yes, I still think about the fear of fear point. I'm really sensitized to these feelings.

THERAPIST: Right, and there are ways to become less sensitized to those feelings. I think it might be useful to integrate some strategies to more directly address that and give you more options to regulate in these situations. Do you want to revisit what those strategies might look like and consider doing some of that work in addition to what we've been doing?

PATIENT: Absolutely. That sounds good.

The client and therapist then discussed the rationale, tasks, and goals of interoceptive exposures, which primarily focused on hyperventilation exercises given the nature of the client's panic symptoms. From a change principles perspective, both psychodynamic and CBT models for panic are interested in promoting new understanding, more adaptive regulation, and corrective learning opportunities. Both approaches in this instance were relatively structured and directive. Explicitly appealing to the principle of facilitating more adaptive regulation provided a pathway to shift between the psychodynamic and CBT-oriented models. In addition, the client already had some familiarity with an alternative, because the therapist collaboratively discussed available treatment options and was responsive to the client's preferences. From a CRPI perspective, multiple markers could be identified. The client appeared to be communicating a potential alliance rupture in relation to the tasks of the treatment, as well as communicating a perceived deterioration in her condition. Although not based on a standardized progress assessment tool, this represents useful and important progress-outcome feedback. Rather than try to convince the client that she simply needed to stick with the current plan or minimize the concern ("these things often get worse before they get better"), the therapist invited the client to discuss the option of integrating something new and, at least momentarily, depart from their current course.

Case Example 2: Assimilative Integration With CBT and Emotion-Focused Therapy

Our second example illustrates a different instance of responsive assimilative integration. The client presented for psychotherapy with a primary complaint of social anxiety. The therapist identifies as an assimilative integrationist who primarily works from a CBT orientation. The therapist also has training in and experiences with employing different therapy models, including emotion-focused therapy (EFT). After discussing treatment options and eliciting client preferences, a manualized CBT approach was adopted (Hope et al., 2010). As such, early work was primarily monitoring and cognitive-focused. Prior to the beginning of each session, the client was asked to complete a general measure of anxiety symptoms and functioning. Although the client regularly attended sessions and was compliant with the treatment plan, the therapist noticed little change on the anxiety self-report measure. Prior to discussing the client's scores/feedback on the self-report measure, the client and therapist reviewed a homework assignment at the start of the session. As part of the assignment, the client recorded an "anxious-self-coping-self dialogue," which is designed to help clients notice and articulate anxious thoughts and beliefs and practice responding to those thoughts/beliefs with a more "objective," alternative perspective (a method of cognitive appraisal-reappraisal).

PATIENT: I did the homework that we talked about last week. It was difficult at first but got easier once I got going. I guess it's easy because my mind just works that way.

THERAPIST: Yes, I see that you've recorded a lot here! Can you say more about what this was like for you, what you noticed?

PATIENT: Well, I wanted to get it done, and get it done right. I was like that in school too. If I get an assignment, I'm going to finish it. It's not that hard to come up with alternative responses, as you can see. I can see, logically, that my initial anxious-self response is pretty biased, but . . . (*hesitates, looks pensive*)

THERAPIST: I think this is important; please, take your time.

PATIENT: I just don't see how talking myself out of thinking a particular way is going to lead to anything different. Or feeling different, you know?

THERAPIST: I think I'm understanding you. It feels like an intellectual exercise. Superficial.

PATIENT: Yes. I'm sorry, I . . .

THERAPIST: Well, that's your experience and that's important feedback. This is really helpful to know. Your experience of this is not all that uncommon. My quick glance at some of your questionnaire responses also seem to give a picture of being stuck. If we are on the same page about the importance of these different parts of yourself, and please let me know if we are or are not, we have other options for exploring these different parts.

PATIENT: Yes. The parts feel true to me. Definitely a struggle that I have become more aware of.

THERAPIST: I have an idea about how to work on this from a different angle that may seem less superficial and distant to you.

The therapist then introduced the idea of a two-chair exercise, as self-splits are a marker for two-chair work in EFT (Elliott et al., 2004). Although not labeled as a self-split, the cognitive manual and homework exercise in question address different parts of the self and encourage the client to identify and explicate the anxious and coping parts. At times, homework such as this can seem superficial and experience-distant to clients, particularly if they are prone to intellectualizing and motivated to be a "good client." From a principle-based perspective, the anxious-coping dialogue and two-chair approaches served the similar function of facilitating a new perspective/awareness of self (as well as possibly a corrective emotional experience). Given the client's expressed frustration with the dialogue strategy, the therapist introduced the option of assimilating a different strategy in what remained a broadly CBT approach. Further, there is accumulating evidence for the effectiveness of EFT for social anxiety (Elliott et al., 2013). The experiential quality of the two-chair work fit well within the broader CBT approach, and the client was able to engage relatively seamlessly. The client continued to respond more favorably to behavioral-oriented interventions and homework (rather than those that were more cognitively oriented), such as exposures and behavior experiments. Although speculative, the cognitive strategies were used as a "logic game" to help control negative emotion, while the exposures and behavior experiments focused on responding differently to negative emotions and refraining from experiential avoidance.

Although the client's earlier verbal and nonverbal behavior communicated frustration regarding the tasks of the therapy, as well as diminished expectations regarding the helpfulness of the particular approach, the decision to be responsive through assimilation was also prompted by the feedback from progress monitoring, which indicated that relatively few gains had been achieved staying the course. Integrative training, flexibility, and a principle-driven if–then rationale facilitated appropriate responsiveness in this instance.

THE INTERSECTION OF RESPONSIVITY AND DIVERSITY

Integrative therapies are designed to enhance responsiveness to individual differences, eschew a one-size-fits-all mentality, and go hand-in-hand with multiculturally informed psychotherapy. As noted, specific techniques are not the only method of assimilation. An assimilative therapist can integrate concepts, relational stances, and adjunctive strategies that best fit a given client. For example, clients with salient religious/spiritual beliefs endorse a preference for working with therapists who integrate this domain in their practice (Vieten et al., 2013), which may otherwise be a standard CBT protocol.

The importance of responsiveness can be found in the tension that exists between cultural relativism, cultural universality, and cultural adaptation perspectives of culturally informed psychotherapy. In reality, whether working from a single orientation or an integrative approach, diversity-oriented psychotherapy is a mixture of these components (Pedersen et al., 2008). This recognition underscores the potential limitations of relying solely on a *competence*-based model, which seems to imply that there is a static benchmark that a clinician either achieves or does not. An integrative clinician recognizes that clients vary in their preferences and responses to interventions. Even a client who identifies as religious, for example, may prefer a psychotherapy that minimally focuses on religious and spiritual themes.

We believe a multicultural orientation (MCO) is most conducive to responsive practice with diverse clients, as well as most consistent with an integrative spirit. MCO comprises three dimensions of client–therapist interaction: cultural humility, cultural opportunities, and cultural comfort (Owen, 2013). *Humility* is marked by a curious stance toward culture and potential cultural differences between client and therapist. *Opportunities* are moments in session when culturally relevant content is presented and there is potential for exploration. *Comfort* represents the therapist's calm or ease during culturally salient moments in session. Owen et al. (2017) found that therapists' cultural comfort partially accounted for racial–ethnic outcome disparities within their caseloads. A therapist may possess a certain degree of cultural humility and comfort that is either pancontextual or unique to a given cultural context (e.g., gender vs. religious unmatched dyads). From a marker-driven, CRPI perspective, a multiculturally oriented therapist is able to notice and make therapeutic use of cultural opportunities (in part, by responding with a certain degree of comfort and humility; if–then). If such an opportunity is bungled, a responsive therapist is also able to notice this and shift into rupture-repair mode (Eubanks et al., 2018). Accumulating research on racial/ethnic bias in health care interactions underscores the critical importance of attunement with diverse patients (Hall et al., 2015).

IMPLICATIONS FOR TRAINING TO MAXIMIZE CLINICIAN RESPONSIVENESS

We believe that integrative training intrinsically maximizes clinician responsiveness. The need for responsivity should follow from recognizing the relative strengths and limitations of single models, including their inability to universally understand and treat the diversity of individuals and presenting problems. Historically, integrationists have grappled with the assumption that one cannot integrate what one does not know well. Recalling our first clinical example, the therapist would have been unable to offer the suggested treatment augmentation without prior knowledge of the theory and application of CBT and interoceptive exposure. In our view, a clinician's ability to be responsive is severely limited if trained within a single, narrowly defined model. Consequently, exposure to multiple orientations and strategies is deemed important for responsive practice.

We have emphasized throughout this chapter that integrative therapies are diverse and dynamic. Routes to integrative practice intersect and a given therapist may shift back and forth from a home orientation and an exogenous model, both within and between clients. Integrative therapists often state that they tend to use what works best for the client—different combinations of techniques as well as different decisional processes. This leaves a virtually infinite number of integration pathways that would need to be studied and harnessed for training and practice. As such, from a training perspective, we are somewhat skeptical of the utility of manualized integrative therapies. Such an approach potentially undermines the spirit of integration and clinical responsiveness. With some exceptions (e.g., Westra et al., 2016), comparative trials involving treatment components or integrative versus standard versions of a therapy yield mixed or equivalent outcomes (see Boswell et al., 2019). Perhaps this is in large part due to the "obstacle" of responsiveness in psychotherapy outcome research.

We believe frameworks such as the CRPI are a more fruitful approach to psychotherapy training, particularly for those espousing an integrative orientation. Common principle and marker-driven approaches to clinical practice and training would help delimit the universe of therapeutic methods and enhance the feasibility of systematically determining what might be optimally employed for a given client and context.

CONCLUSION

As articulated throughout this volume, psychotherapy must reckon with the reality of responsiveness. From a comparative outcomes research perspective, this presents major obstacles. However, it also highlights exciting opportunities for moving psychotherapy practice, training, and research forward. It is difficult to conceive of a scenario that does not require an appeal to psychotherapy integration, and integrative therapists are at a major advantage to capitalize on accumulating research on appropriately responsive psychotherapy (Boswell, 2017).

REFERENCES

Ahn, H.-n., & Wampold, B. E. (2001). Where oh where are the specific ingredients? A meta-analysis of component studies in counseling and psychotherapy. *Journal of Counseling Psychology, 48*(3), 251–257. https://doi.org/10.1037/0022-0167. 48.3.251

Barlow, D. H., Ellard, K. K., Fairholme, C. P., Farchione, T. J., Boisseau, C. L., Allen, L. B., & Ehrenreich-May, J. (2011). *Unified protocol for transdiagnostic treatment of emotional disorders: Workbook.* Oxford University Press.

Beck, A. T. (1991). Cognitive therapy as the integrative therapy. *Journal of Psychotherapy Integration, 1*(3), 191–198. https://doi.org/10.1037/h0101233

Bell, E. C., Marcus, D. K., & Goodlad, J. K. (2013). Are the parts as good as the whole? A meta-analysis of component treatment studies. *Journal of Consulting and Clinical Psychology, 81*(4), 722–736. https://doi.org/10.1037/a0033004

Beutler, L. E., Consoli, A. J., & Lane, G. (2005). Systematic treatment selection and prescriptive psychotherapy: An integrative eclectic approach. In J. C. Norcross & M. R. Goldfried (Eds.), *Handbook of psychotherapy integration* (2nd ed., pp. 121–144). Oxford University Press. https://doi.org/10.1093/med:psych/ 9780195165791.003.0006

Beutler, L. E., Edwards, C., & Someah, K. (2018). Adapting psychotherapy to patient reactance level: A meta-analytic review. *Journal of Clinical Psychology, 74*(11), 1952–1963. https://doi.org/10.1002/jclp.22682

Beutler, L. E., & Harwood, T. M. (2000). *Prescriptive psychotherapy: A practical guide to systematic treatment selection.* Oxford University Press. https://doi.org/10.1093/ med:psych/9780195136692.001.0001

Boswell, J. F. (2017). Psychotherapy integration: Research, practice, and training at the leading edge. *Journal of Psychotherapy Integration, 27*(2), 225–235. https://doi.org/10.1037/int0000055

Boswell, J. F., Castonguay, L. G., & Wasserman, R. H. (2010). Effects of psychotherapy training and intervention use on session outcome. *Journal of Consulting and Clinical Psychology, 78*(5), 717–723. https://doi.org/10.1037/a0020088

Boswell, J. F., & Goldfried, M. R. (2010). Psychotherapy integration. In I. B. Weiner & W. E. Craighead (Eds.), *The Corsini encyclopedia of psychology* (4th ed., pp. 1384–1387). John Wiley & Sons. https://doi.org/10.1002/9780470479216.corpsy0753

Boswell, J. F., Newman, M. G., & McGinn, L. K. (2019). Outcome research on psychotherapy integration. In J. C. Norcross & M. R. Goldfried (Eds.), *Handbook of psychotherapy integration* (3rd ed., pp. 405–431). Oxford University Press.

Boswell, J. F., Sharpless, B. A., Greenberg, L. S., Heatherington, L., Huppert, J. D., Barber, J. P., Goldfried, M. R., & Castonguay, L. G. (2010). Schools of psychotherapy and the beginnings of a scientific approach. In D. H. Barlow (Ed.), *Oxford handbook of clinical psychology* (pp. 98–127). Oxford University Press.

Busch, F. N., & Milrod, B. L. (2013). Panic-focused psychodynamic psychotherapy-extended range. *Psychoanalytic Inquiry, 33*(6), 584–594. https://doi.org/10.1080/07351690.2013.835166

Castonguay, L. G., & Hill, C. E. (2012). *Transformation in psychotherapy: Corrective experiences across cognitive behavioral, humanistic, and psychodynamic approaches.* American Psychological Association. https://doi.org/10.1037/13747-000

Castonguay, L. G., Nelson, D. L., Boswell, J. F., Nordberg, S. S., McAleavey, A. A., Newman, M. G., & Borkovec, T. D. (2012). Corrective experiences in cognitive behavior and interpersonal–emotional processing therapies: A qualitative analysis of a single case. In L. G. Castonguay and C. E. Hill (Eds.), *Transformation in psychotherapy: Corrective experiences across cognitive behavioral, humanistic, and psychodynamic approaches* (pp. 245–279). American Psychological Association.

Constantino, M. J., Boswell, J. F., Bernecker, S. L., & Castonguay, L. G. (2013). Context-responsive psychotherapy integration as a framework for unified clinical science: Conceptual and empirical considerations. *Journal of Unified Psychotherapy and Clinical Science, 2,* 1–20.

Constantino, M. J., Coyne, A. E., & Muir, H. J. (2019). Evidence-based therapist responsivity to disruptive clinical process. *Cognitive and Behavioral Practice, 27*(4), 405–416.

Constantino, M. J., Vîslă, A., Coyne, A. E., & Boswell, J. F. (2018). A meta-analysis of the association between patients' early treatment outcome expectation and their posttreatment outcomes. *Psychotherapy, 55*(4), 473–485. https://doi.org/10.1037/pst0000169

Elliott, R., Greenberg, L. S., Watson, J., Timulak, L., & Freire, E. (2013). Research on humanistic–experiential psychotherapies. In M. J. Lambert (Ed.), *Bergin & Garfield's handbook of psychotherapy and behavior change* (6th ed., pp. 495–538). John Wiley & Sons.

Elliott, R., Watson, J. C., Goldman, R. N., & Greenberg, L. S. (2004). *Learning emotion-focused therapy: The process-experiential approach to change.* American Psychological Association. https://doi.org/10.1037/10725-000

Eubanks, C. F., Muran, J. C., & Safran, J. D. (2018). Alliance rupture repair: A meta-analysis. *Psychotherapy, 55*(4), 508–519. https://doi.org/10.1037/pst0000185

Fisher, A. J., & Boswell, J. F. (2016). Enhancing personalization of psychotherapy with dynamic assessment and modeling. *Assessment, 23*(4), 496–506. https://doi.org/ 10.1177/1073191116638735

Frank, J. D. (1961). *Persuasion and healing: A comparative study of psychotherapy.* Schocken Books.

Garfield, S. L. (1980). *Psychotherapy: An eclectic-integrative approach.* John Wiley & Sons.

Goldfried, M. R. (1980). Toward the delineation of therapeutic change principles. *American Psychologist, 35*(11), 991–999. https://doi.org/10.1037/0003-066X. 35.11.991

Goldfried, M. R., Newman, M. G., Castonguay, L. G., Fuertes, J. N., Magnavita, J. J., Sobell, L., & Wolf, A. W. (2014). On the dissemination of clinical experiences in using empirically supported treatments. *Behavior Therapy, 45*(1), 3–6. https:// doi.org/10.1016/j.beth.2013.09.007

Goldfried, M. R., Raue, P. J., & Castonguay, L. G. (1998). The therapeutic focus in significant sessions of master therapists: A comparison of cognitive-behavioral and psychodynamic-interpersonal interventions. *Journal of Consulting and Clinical Psychology, 66*(5), 803–810. https://doi.org/10.1037/0022-006X.66.5.803

Greenberg, L. S. (1995). *Process experiential psychotherapy: An emotion-focused approach.* American Psychological Association.

Hall, W. J., Chapman, M. V., Lee, K. M., Merino, Y. M., Thomas, T. W., Payne, B. K., Eng, E., Day, S. H., & Coyne-Beasley, T. (2015). Implicit racial/ethnic bias among health care professionals and its influence on health care outcomes: A systematic review. *American Journal of Public Health, 105*(12), e60–e76. https://doi.org/ 10.2105/AJPH.2015.302903

Heard, H. L., & Linehan, M. M. (2019). Dialectical behavior therapy for borderline personality disorder. In J. C. Norcross & M. R. Goldfried (Eds.), *Handbook of psychotherapy integration* (3rd ed., pp. 257–283). Oxford University Press.

Hope, D. A., Heimberg, R. G., & Turk, C. L. (2010). *Managing social anxiety: A cognitive-behavioral therapy approach: Workbook* (2nd ed.). Oxford University Press.

Hull, C. L. (1939). Modern behaviorism and psychoanalysis. *Transactions of the New York Academy of Sciences, 1*(5 Series II), 78–82. https://doi.org/10.1111/ j.2164-0947.1939.tb00007.x

Katz, M., Hilsenroth, M. J., Gold, J. R., Moore, M., Pitman, S. R., Levy, S. R., & Owen, J. (2019). Adherence, flexibility, and outcome in psychodynamic treatment of depression. *Journal of Counseling Psychology, 66*(1), 94–103. https://doi.org/10.1037/ cou0000299

Lambert, M. J. (Ed.). (2013). *Bergin & Garfield's handbook of psychotherapy and behavior change* (6th ed.). John Wiley & Sons.

Liff, Z. A. (1992). Psychoanalysis and dynamic techniques. In D. K. Freedheim, H. J. Freudenberger, J. W. Kessler, S. B. Messer, D. R. Peterson, H. H. Strupp, & P. L. Wachtel (Eds.), *History of psychotherapy: A century of change* (pp. 571–586). American Psychological Association. https://doi.org/10.1037/10110-016

Linehan, M. M. (2015). *DBT skills training manual* (2nd ed.). Guilford Press.

Messer, S. B. (2001). Introduction to the special issue on assimilative integration. *Journal of Psychotherapy Integration, 11*(1), 1–4.

Newman, M. G., Castonguay, L. G., Borkovec, T. D., Fisher, A. J., Boswell, J. F., Szkodny, L. E., & Nordberg, S. S. (2011). A randomized controlled trial of cognitive-behavioral therapy for generalized anxiety disorder with integrated techniques from emotion-focused and interpersonal therapies. *Journal of Consulting and Clinical Psychology,* *79*(2), 171–181. https://doi.org/10.1037/a0022489

Norcross, J. C., & Goldfried, M. R. (Eds.). (2005). *Oxford series in clinical psychology. Handbook of psychotherapy integration* (2nd ed.). Oxford University Press.

Owen, J. (2013). Early career perspectives on psychotherapy research and practice: Psychotherapist effects, multicultural orientation, and couple interventions. *Psychotherapy, 50*(4), 496–502. https://doi.org/10.1037/a0034617

Owen, J., Drinane, J., Tao, K. W., Adelson, J. L., Hook, J. N., Davis, D., & Fookune, N. (2017). Racial/ethnic disparities in client unilateral termination: The role of therapists' cultural comfort. *Psychotherapy Research, 27*(1), 102–111. https://doi.org/10.1080/10503307.2015.1078517

Pedersen, P. B., Draguns, J. G., Lonner, W. J., & Trimble, J. E. (Eds.). (2008). *Counseling across cultures* (6th ed.). Sage Publications.

Prochaska, J. O., & Norcross, J. C. (2002). Stages of change. In J. C. Norcross (Ed.), *Psychotherapy relationships that work: Therapist contributions and responsiveness to patients* (pp. 303–313). Oxford University Press.

Prochaska, J. O., & Norcross, J. C. (2014). *Systems of psychotherapy: A transtheoretical analysis* (8th ed.). Cengage Learning.

Rogers, C. R. (1951). *Client-centered therapy, its current practice, implications, and theory.* Houghton Mifflin.

Rosenzweig, S. (1936). Some implicit common factors in diverse methods of psychotherapy. *American Journal of Orthopsychiatry, 6*(3), 412–415. https://doi.org/10.1111/j.1939-0025.1936.tb05248.x

Stiles, W. B. (2009). Responsiveness as an obstacle for psychotherapy outcome research: It's worse than you think. *Clinical Psychology: Science and Practice, 16*(1), 86–91. https://doi.org/10.1111/j.1468-2850.2009.01148.x

Stiles, W. B., Honos-Webb, L., & Surko, M. (1998). Responsiveness in psychotherapy. *Clinical Psychology: Science and Practice, 5*(4), 439–458. https://doi.org/10.1111/j.1468-2850.1998.tb00166.x

Vieten, C., Scammell, S., Pilato, R., Ammondson, I., Pargament, K. I., & Lukoff, D. (2013). Spiritual and religious competencies for psychologists. *Psychology of Religion and Spirituality, 5*(3), 129–144. https://doi.org/10.1037/a0032699

Wachtel, P. L. (2014). *Relational perspectives book series. Cyclical psychodynamic and the contextual self: The inner world, the intimate world, and the world of cultural and society.* Routledge.

Watson, G., Adler, A., Allen, F. H., Bertine, E., Chassell, J. O., Durkin, H., Rogers, C. R., Rosenzweig, S., & Waelder, R. (1940). Areas of agreement in psychotherapy: Section meeting, 1940. *American Journal of Orthopsychiatry, 10*(4), 698–709. https://doi.org/10.1111/j.1939-0025.1940.tb05736.x

Weinberger, J. (1995). Common factors aren't so common: The common factors dilemma. *Clinical Psychology: Science and Practice, 2*(1), 45–69. https://doi.org/10.1111/j.1468-2850.1995.tb00024.x

Westra, H. A., Constantino, M. J., & Antony, M. M. (2016). Integrating motivational interviewing with cognitive-behavioral therapy for severe generalized anxiety disorder: An allegiance-controlled randomized clinical trial. *Journal of Consulting and Clinical Psychology, 84*(9), 768–782. https://doi.org/10.1037/ccp0000098

PART **III** INTEGRATION AND CONCLUSIONS

14

MEETING THE CHALLENGE OF RESPONSIVENESS

Synthesizing Perspectives

JEANNE C. WATSON AND HADAS WISEMAN

Responsiveness is ubiquitous to human interaction and is an essential aspect of positive and satisfying relationships (Reis, 2012). Nonresponsive environments are experienced as deleterious to our well-being. In this volume, Stiles (Chapter 1) and Hatcher (Chapter 2) see responsiveness as integral to all theoretical approaches with therapists continually adapting and adjusting to tailor their treatments to meet their clients' needs and characteristics. The aim of this book is to examine the concept of responsiveness in psychotherapy drawing on multiple perspectives and the wisdom of numerous research clinicians. We draw on the rich and diverse talent of our contributors to clarify its meaning, refine our understanding of the concept, and we identify some of the signals to which therapists attend when they are being responsive to inform theory, research, training, and practice. This chapter thus synthesizes material from all the chapters to provide a more elaborate map of the interpersonal terrain and a cohesive set of guidelines to inform theory, research, practice, and training.

https://doi.org/10.1037/0000240-015
The Responsive Psychotherapist: Attuning to Clients in the Moment, J. C. Watson and H. Wiseman (Editors)

FRAMING THE PROBLEM

The first two chapters of this volume frame the problem of responsiveness for researchers, clinicians, and trainees. Stiles (Chapter 1) sees appropriate responsiveness as the essence of good therapy, and defines it as doing what is right and necessary for the client at the right time, while being cognizant of the clients' needs, the emerging context, and their therapeutic approach (Kramer & Stiles, 2015). Hatcher (Chapter 2) defines responsiveness in therapy as mutual influence in the emerging context of a relationship and closely linked to the alliance. Drawing on Bacal's (1998) work, he differentiates between appropriate and optimal responsiveness. While the former emphasizes clinicians doing the right thing, optimal responsiveness sees clinicians as able to draw on an unlimited number of techniques to take advantage of emerging opportunities in the moment to facilitate clients' process and effect positive outcomes. He suggests that optimal responsiveness could provide an antidote to the potential rigidity of treatment protocols if clinicians were able to draw on an unlimited range of interventions. However, he recognizes that specific treatment approaches and protocols provide frameworks for clinicians to facilitate the realization of treatment goals and that responsiveness can be disruptive for these treatment models.

Both Stiles and Hatcher observe that therapists' responsiveness has been hiding in plain sight without being fully acknowledged or recognized by researchers. On this basis, responsiveness in psychotherapy might be likened to the elephant that is described differently by blind men, each of whom perceives but a small aspect of the whole. These two authors argue that therapists' ongoing adjustments to treatment are especially problematic for randomized controlled trials (RCTs) as they potentially change each treatment protocol, making it unique for each client. The continually evolving nature of responsiveness over the course of treatment, and the mutual influence of client and therapist, not only violate the required independence between dependent variables (DVs) and independent variables (IVs), but differential levels of therapists' responses make it impossible to establish accurate dose–effect relationships or apply quantitative measurement to determine process–outcome correlations. Additional complexity is generated by the observation that responsiveness in the moment can have multiple impacts across multiple time scales—from microseconds to months or years—and at multiple levels.

TRANSTHEORETICAL FRAMEWORKS FOR RESPONSIVENESS

In the next two chapters, Wiseman and Egozi (Chapter 3) and Eubanks et al. (Chapter 4) present two models—attachment theory and the working alliance, respectively—as transtheoretical frameworks to inform our understanding of responsiveness in psychotherapy.

Attachment Theory

Wiseman and Egozi (Chapter 3) consider responsiveness through the lens of attachment theory, seeing it as a way of building connections between the science of relationships more generally and psychotherapy relationships more specifically (Wiseman, 2017). Drawing on research in developmental psychology, the authors emphasize the centrality of responsiveness to relationships between caregivers and children and the importance of providing a secure base for the development of socioemotional regulation in infancy and childhood, positive working models of self and other, and coregulation. They note that infants are sensitive to caregiver cues of availability and responsiveness.

They advocate that attachment theory can provide an integrative framework to better understand clients' needs moment to moment in the session and across the trajectory of therapy. An attachment-informed approach to conceptualizing the therapeutic relationship postulates that it is likely to reactivate clients' long-standing expectations about the availability and responsiveness of others. To be optimally responsive in psychotherapy, they suggest that therapists regulate therapeutic distance in relation to clients' attachment needs. In addition, attachment theory offers a useful framework for research with a strong empirical base, developmental framework, and theory of affect regulation.

Working Alliance

Eubanks et al. (Chapter 4) examine responsiveness within the framework of the working alliance. These authors see responsiveness as inextricably part of the alliance-building process. They conceptualize it as mutual influence that requires a two-person perspective and adjustments to shifts in process. They suggest that responsiveness is crucial to alert therapists to ruptures and to repairing them when they occur in the session. Ruptures, defined as subtle misattunements, are identified using two markers, including confrontation and withdrawal. The rupture–repair paradigm provides a framework relevant to various theoretical orientations to enhance therapists' responsiveness in the moment.

RESPONSIVENESS ACROSS DIFFERENT TREATMENT APPROACHES

Responsiveness provides an integrative framework for moving beyond specific theoretical approaches and techniques to develop a science of relationship that cuts across specific approaches. An important objective of this volume is to identify the signals to which therapists attend in the moment in order to be responsive and how they use this information to fit their interventions to their clients and their treatment models (Stiles & Horvath, 2017).

A review of the different treatment approaches reveals a rich diversity of thinking that speaks to the plurality of lenses and ways of working to facilitate and support clients' goals in psychotherapy. In this section, we provide an overview of the similarities and differences across approaches with respect to responsiveness to elaborate a more fine-grained understanding as well as facilitate greater precision to guide research, training, and practice. We review how responsiveness is conceptualized across different approaches and specify the information as well as the specific signals or markers that therapists use to guide them in order to respond optimally in the moment. Finally, we focus on specific recommendations for training and research.

Definition and Conceptualization

Across all approaches covered in this volume, there is a recognition that to be optimally responsive, therapists need to be attentive, flexible, and sensitive as well as willing to adjust their behavior and treatment protocols to find the right response for their client in the session and over the course of psychotherapy. This requires that therapists be carefully attuned moment to moment in the session. However, there are differences in terms of the time frames that therapists use and their focus of attention moment to moment in the session across treatment approaches. For some, responsiveness starts before treatment begins to ensure treatment fit (Chapters 7 and 13); continues moment to moment during the session (Chapters 3–6 and 8–13); and over various stages of treatment, including immediately following an episode within a session, after a single session, over the course of several sessions, and at the end of treatment. The many different timelines to assess responsiveness across treatment approaches echoes Stiles's observation that treatment impact can occur on multiple timescales from microseconds to months or years and at multiple levels.

Two different models have been proposed to conceptualize responsiveness in psychotherapy. One, a two-person model (Schore, 2019; see also Chapters 1–5 and 8 in this volume), requires clinicians and researchers to consider what is happening within the therapist and the client and what is being communicated by each person in the interaction. The second model, identified by Hatcher (Chapter 2), sees therapists as goal-directed, responsive agents. The difference between the two models is more of degree than kind and reflects the differences among therapists in terms of how they balance their treatments with clients' needs and goals. The different emphases in each model highlight different perspectives. In the first, therapists are more focused on trying to *understand* clients' experiences and provide a corrective emotional or relational experience in the moment (see Chapters 3–6 and Chapters 8–11). While in the second model, therapists are more intent on *persuading and encouraging* clients to revise their thinking, beliefs, feelings, and behavior (see Chapters 7, 12, and 13). The former focus more on process and following clients' goals and objectives, while the latter focus more on outcomes and treatment goals.

SIGNALS THAT INFORM THERAPIST RESPONSIVENESS

One of the primary goals of this book is to gather the various signals or markers that alert clinicians to be more responsive across and within different treatment approaches. Therapists' responsiveness is informed by three primary sources of information: first, information that resides within *the therapist* including their theoretical lens, diagnostic indicators, treatment goals and objectives, their characteristics and reactions; second, information from *the client* that is communicated or observed during sessions, including clients' characteristics, behaviors, emotions, needs, and goals; and third, information that is *interpersonal*, pertaining to the quality of the interaction, the therapeutic relationship, the alliance, specific feedback, and diversity and differences between clients and therapists. These sources of information provide signals to guide therapists about how to intervene optimally during the session. The different sources of information are not mutually exclusive but jointly influence and amplify each other with different aspects foregrounded at different times. Indeed, appropriate or optimal responsiveness may require therapists to take account of the information from all three sources at any one time as they work at multiple levels.

Therapist Signals

These are signals that refer to the knowledge, information, theoretical perspectives as well as personal feelings and experiences that therapists draw on to guide their responsiveness moment to moment in the session. These include the therapist's theoretical lens, specific diagnostic markers, therapists' characteristics, and therapists' reactions.

Theoretical Lens

Therapists' understanding of how to respond optimally is informed by their theoretical perspectives. These can vary widely, leading some to emphasize the importance of relationship and attachment histories with a greater focus on process (see Chapters 3, 5, 6, 8, 10, and 11), while others emphasize cognitions and behaviors along with highly structured treatment agendas and outcomes (see Chapters 7, 12, and 13).

The authors who are more relationship focused see the self as socially constructed and emphasize the importance of the family system as a crucible for subsequent development and current functioning. They see therapy as providing a corrective relational and emotional experience and use enactments to structure the therapeutic process. Wiseman and Egozi (Chapter 3) use the lens of attachment theory to assess and negotiate clients' needs for interpersonal distance and closeness to provide a novel relationship context and support change. Tishby (Chapter 5), looking through the lens of relational psychodynamic theory, has the goal of promoting authenticity and differentiation in relationship, thus making room for the needs of self and other. Silberschatz (Chapter 6), using the plan formulation method and drawing on cognitive–psychodynamic–relational theory, seeks to provide a corrective experience that will disprove patients' negative expectations of close relationships. Watson (Chapter 8), sees the provision of a positive relational experience, characterized by understanding, prizing, and acceptance, as providing an antidote to negative relationships with self and others leading to the development of more positive behaviors, including self-compassion, self-protection and self-soothing, as well as enhanced emotional processing and regulation. Diamond et al. (Chapter 10) use enactments (in-session corrective attachment/identity episodes) in the context of family therapy to facilitate positive and novel interactions among family members thereby providing a corrective relational and emotional experience to enhance family functioning and connection between nonaccepting parents and their sexual and gender minority adult children. Kramer (Chapter 11), similar to Silberschatz (Chapter 6), uses Plan Analysis in the treatment of personality disorders (Caspar, 2019; Grawe, 1992) to identify and respond to clients' underlying motives and plans rather than to their presenting behaviors, thereby reducing the intensity of the latter to promote new learning and the emergence of other styles of relating. Ribeiro et al. (Chapter 9) use the Innovative Moments in Psychotherapy Scale to monitor shifts in clients' understanding of problematic experiences in narrative therapy in order to guide therapists and support changes in their clients.

Authors who focus more on changing behaviors with highly structured treatment agendas have their sights set on specific outcomes over the course of therapy. They are concerned with matching clients and therapists based on the beliefs of the former and the strengths of the latter to identify what clients need in order to progress optimally in therapy. These clinicians attend to whether treatment is "on track" and whether therapists need to deviate from their protocol to get "back on track." To guide their treatments, they constantly monitor the alliance and effectiveness of different treatment modules while paying close attention to clients' motivational language. Constantino et al. (Chapter 7) see the first step in being responsive as assessing clients' readiness to engage in therapy as well as therapists' strengths in order to facilitate matching of clients and therapists. During treatment they attend to the alliance, monitoring agreement on tasks and goals to ensure the treatment plan fits. When clients show resistance, deviations from the treatment protocol are considered and implemented in order to try to get the treatment back on track. Bedics and McKinley (Chapter 12), in their presentation of dialectical behavior therapy (DBT), emphasize that the hierarchical structure of the treatment modules guides therapists' responsiveness, as they can be rearranged or eliminated depending on clients' responses to treatment. Boswell et al. (Chapter 13) present an integrative treatment framework that requires therapists to be competent across a number of treatment approaches to find the one that best fits each client. These authors identify two metaframeworks for guiding clinicians' choice of techniques or approach, the principles of change approach developed by Goldfried (1980), which identifies the core ingredients of change that therapies have in common that account for treatment outcomes and can inform treatment decisions, and context responsive psychotherapy integration, which relies on specific markers to guide clinicians.

Diagnostic Markers

Some authors use specific diagnostic categories like trauma or addiction to guide how they respond to their clients (see Chapters 7 and 11–13). Kramer (Chapter 11) refers to "disorder-specific" responsiveness (as separate from "generic" responsiveness and "individualized" responsiveness) to distinguish being responsive to processes underlying specific disorders. Focusing on personality disorders and especially borderline personality disorder (BPD), he suggests that mentalization-fostering interventions, in the context of mentalization-based therapy, represent optimal responsiveness. Bedics and McKinley (Chapter 12) delineate principles of DBT treatment (Linehan, 1993) that were developed for the treatment of suicidal behavior and BPD. For example, in standard DBT (S-DBT), therapist interventions are delivered to clients that meet diagnostic criteria for BPD in a way that matches the interpersonal, emotional, and cognitive challenges faced by clients for whom stabilization is a priority.

Therapist Characteristics

As Hatcher (Chapter 2) notes, therapists are more than their techniques; they are persons with distinct personalities, characteristics, and histories. To be responsive, therapists need to be open and willing to be flexible and deviate from their course in order to align what they are doing with their clients' focus, direction, and goals. This requires them to develop a high level of competence balanced with humility so that they allow sufficient space for clients to express their concerns freely and do not make themselves central to the process.

Therapist Reactions

In the process of attending to their clients, therapists monitor their own reactions, positive and negative, and learn how to contain them so they can use them effectively to enhance responsiveness in the moment and over the course of therapy. Therapists' feelings of tension, boredom, irritation, or disconnection can alert them to ruptures (Chapter 4). Responsive therapists manage these negative feelings to successfully repair ruptures and minimize their occurrence and are aware that repair is more than metacommunication. Responsive therapists remain curious, practice patience at times when they are experiencing negative reactions, and consider repair strategies that fit with clients' relationship histories in order to choose one that will offer a corrective experience (Chapters 3–6 and 8). Responsive therapists are aware of their own relational patterns. Wiseman and Egozi (Chapter 3) suggest that to be appropriately or optimally responsive, therapists need to regulate their relational needs and attend to how these are impacting their treatments. Other reactions that therapists attend to for information about how things are going include feelings of acceptance or rejection and a sense of session momentum (Chapter 8). Both positive and negative feelings provide feedback to the therapist that can guide their choice of technique or direct their focus of attention in the session (Chapters 4 and 8).

Client Signals or Markers

Leiman and Stiles (2001) proposed that for clients to assimilate problematic experiences, therapists needed to work within clients' therapeutic zone of proximal development (TZPD). They suggested that if therapists' interventions exceed clients' TZPD, then clients are likely to falter and be unable to work at a higher level. However, if therapists remain within clients' TZPD, they will be more likely to master different levels and successfully integrate problematic experiences. The term "zone of proximal development" (ZPD) was coined by Vygotsky (1978) as a framework for understanding children's cognitive development. In this model, Vygotsky suggested that psychological functions that the child acquired developed first between the child and adult and subsequently were internalized by the child. Leiman and Stiles (2001) proposed that an analogous process occurs in psychotherapy with certain psychological functions developing between the client and therapist before being internalized by the client.

The concept of clients' ZPD provides a useful framework for evaluating clients in terms of different psychological functions and capacities over the course of treatment in order to guide therapists' responsiveness moment by moment in the session. A number of different ZPDs have been identified in this volume, including clients' relational maps, their self-states and self-organizations, their emotional processing and regulation capacity, and their understanding of different problematic issues as revealed in their narratives.

Clients' Relational Maps
Clients' relational or interpersonal maps are rooted in their attachment histories (Chapters 3–6, 8, 10, and 11). These maps include clients' interpersonal behavior, their attachment experiences, their beliefs and expectations about relationships with self and other, and their degree of differentiation. These approaches work directly with clients' relational maps to respond optimally to their behavior in the session. Some therapists try to relate to their clients in noncomplementary ways in order to facilitate new ways of interacting with others and cultivate alternative self-states (Chapters 3, 5,

6, 8, 10, and 11), while other therapists suggest specific techniques to shift clients' relationships with self and other using chair dialogues or enactment tasks (Chapters 8 and 10). Understanding client's attachment histories and how they impact their relationships with self and others as well as their emotional processing capacity is central to guiding therapists' responsiveness in some approaches. To apprehend clients' relational and interpersonal maps, relationally oriented therapists listen for the themes that occur in clients' narratives related to their attachment histories and their relationships with self and others (Chapters 3, 5, 6, and 8–10) to guide their choice of technique moment to moment and session to session over the course of therapy.

Clients' Self-States and Self-Organization

Client self-states serve as markers to therapists about how to respond appropriately or optimally in the session. These self-states include dreams, dissociated self-states, defensiveness (Chapters 5, 6, 10, 11, and 13), and negative self-organizations (Chapters 5 and 8). Therapists attend to these states to promote greater self-awareness of what is happening in the moment and provide new experiences within the session to facilitate better integration and access to alternative self-states in their clients, for example, greater self-compassion, self-assertiveness, and self-soothing as well as enhanced understanding of themselves, their needs, and goals. Watson (Chapter 8) suggests that therapists in emotion-focused therapy (EFT) be alert to clients' collapsing during chair dialogues, for example, when they are unable to access self-compassion, regulate their affect, or be more self-protective, to inform them of where to focus in the session. Tishby (Chapter 5) endeavors to make clients more aware of shut off aspects of their experience, while Silberschatz (Chapter 6) and Kramer (Chapter 11) seek to change clients' views of themselves in relationship with others. Other negative self-states identified by Diamond et al. (Chapter 10) in working with families include defensiveness in the face of negative emotion expressed by others and being resistant and fearful of coercion to feel or act differently towards others. Boswell et al. (Chapter 13), using an integrative perspective, suggest that clients' expressions of self-striving indicate a need for self-verification or validation.

Clients' Emotional Expression

To remain attuned to their clients, responsive therapists attend and attune to clients' emotional states during the session. Therapists attend to shifts and changes in clients' emotions and affective states to guide their choice of technique and assess resolution of specific tasks, as well as the successful attainment of certain stages or goals in therapy. Clients' emotional expression alerts therapists about where to focus their attention moment to moment in the session. Tishby (Chapter 5) attends to clients' shifts in affect to assist with the formulation of warded off self-states and defenses. Watson (Chapter 8) notes that EFT therapists attend to clients' expressions of pain and distress and whether they are aware of and able to symbolize their emotional experience in the session in order to guide differential responding. Responsive therapists are attentive to the painful experiences revealed in clients' attachment histories, their memories of events, and their nonverbal behavior in the session. Signs of pain include verbal and nonverbal expressions of sadness, fear, vulnerability, and helplessness as well as intensity of expression. Bedics and McKinley (Chapter 12) point out that clients' emotional processing is an important goal in DBT, so monitoring and following it in the session provides useful feedback about choice of treatment modules.

Shifts from negative to positive emotions are important in most therapeutic approaches, as they provide feedback about whether therapy is progressing well and specific techniques are appropriate. For example, Watson (Chapter 8) notes that clients' expressions of relief and lightness at the end of a chair dialogue in EFT are important signals that something important has shifted in terms of their relationships with the self and/or others. Similarly, Bedics and McKinley (Chapter 12) observe that in DBT, expressions of fulfillment and joy are recognized as indicators of successful treatment.

In contrast, expressions of negative emotion serve as cues and indicators in most approaches that therapists need to be more responsive both with respect to the state of the alliance and to clients' more immediate needs and goals in the session. For example, Diamond et al. (Chapter 10), suggest that to carefully manage multiple therapeutic alliances, therapists monitor the emotional expressions of each family member and pay special attention to clients' expressions of pain and defeat as well as signs that they are giving up during enactments in family therapy. Watson (Chapter 8) and Bedics and McKinley (Chapter 12) are alert to clients' emotional processing capacity and the extent to which they are able to regulate it both in and out of the session. Watson (Chapter 8) notes that in EFT, responsive therapists attend to clients' capacity to be aware of their organismic experience, label it, and regulate their levels of arousal and expression. While Bedics and McKinley (Chapter 12), from a DBT perspective, work to facilitate clients' capacity to effectively regulate their negative emotions especially during the first stage of treatment.

Clients' Shifts in Understanding

A number of approaches attend to shifts in clients' understanding of themselves, others, and problematic experiences as reflected in their narratives.

Responsive therapists use these shifts as a guide to how to respond appropriately and/or optimally in the session. Ribeiro et al. (Chapter 9), using the therapeutic collaboration model in narrative therapy, assess clients' TZPD to decide whether to offer more challenging or supportive interventions. Their assessment is facilitated by the Innovative Moments Scale. These authors see therapeutic responsiveness that reflects therapists' sensitivity to their clients' actual and potential developmental level with respect to their understanding of different problematic issues as a way to enhance collaboration and the attainment of treatment goals. In EFT, the coherence and elaborated quality of clients' narratives serve as cues to therapists about the extent to which clients understand themselves and their experiences (Chapter 8). Specific narrative markers, including changes in clients' innovative moments and levels of assimilation, orient therapists' attention and focus moment to moment in the session and across treatment (Chapters 1, 8, and 9).

Clients' Problematic and Self-Injurious Behaviors

This category includes clients' suicidal and self-injurious behaviors, threats of self-harm, and other negative behaviors. While suicidal and self-injurious behavior was only explicitly mentioned by Bedics and McKinley (Chapter 12) as an important sign to inform treatment planning in the session in DBT, it is likely that all therapists are attentive to these markers. To be appropriately or optimally responsive at these critical moments, DBT practitioners are encouraged to strike a balance between being overly restrictive and too accommodating to these behaviors. These markers assume priority in Stage 1 of their treatment approach and are prioritized over other treatment goals. Other negative behaviors that are markers to which therapists attend in the session include client hostility and impatience (Chapter 4) and maladaptive blaming and defensiveness in emotion and attachment-based family therapy (Chapter 10). At these moments, it is suggested that therapists change tack and concentrate on working through the negative behavior with their clients.

Clients' Nonverbal Behavior

Clients' facial expressions, body language, posture, and vocal quality are additional signals to guide therapists' responsiveness in the moment. Responsive therapists attend to clients' nonverbal behavior to gather information about their self-states, the quality of their engagement in the session, their emotional processing capacity, as well as various interpersonal pulls and expectations. Clients' nonverbal behavior pulls therapists' attention and is a useful guide about what to respond to in the moment as well as how to respond. Tishby (Chapter 5) suggests that relational psychodynamic therapists might attend to clients' nonverbal behavior to refine their understanding of the transference or their clients' dissociated self-states. While Silberschatz (Chapter 6) and Kramer (Chapter 11) attend to clients' nonverbal behavior to guide their responses to clients' specific interpersonal styles. In experiential therapy, when clients' body language displays defeat and vulnerability, conveyed by a sinking diaphragm and heaviness in the torso, experiential therapists usually respond with support (Chapters 8 and 10). Alternatively, they may try to deepen clients' experience in the moment, to increase their awareness of and access to their felt sense as they work with them to shift to alternative states. For example, if a client is slouching, the therapist might suggest they sit up and see how that feels, or alternatively if the client's voice is timid and quiet, the therapist might suggest they speak louder to experience being more assertive.

Interpersonal Signals

These signals refer to the interactions between client and therapist, including the quality of the working alliance and the presence of ruptures, specific client feedback about the treatment, as well as the differences between client and therapist in order to take account of each client's diversity and uniqueness.

Alliance Rupture Markers

All authors spoke about continuously monitoring the alliance and attending to signals that indicated there were breaks in collaboration. The objective was to maintain an agreed upon therapeutic focus and engagement in certain tasks. Rupture markers of withdrawal and confrontation (Chapter 4) were identified as markers by several authors. It was suggested that while ruptures often can be resolved with negotiation, this might not always be appropriate or effective. Clients' interpersonal styles are an important factor to consider when attempting to resolve alliance ruptures. Successful negotiation might depend on clients' levels of secure attachment, as more insecure clients tend to avoid or minimize the contribution of the therapist (Chapters 3 and 5) and thus may not profit from rupture resolution dialogues as much as more secure clients.

When monitoring the alliance, therapists were aware of clients' TZPD and capacity to engage with the therapist and the treatment approach based on their clients' relational and interpersonal maps. Responsive therapists were sensitive to moments when their clients were capable of engaging in certain ways and took account of their clients' flexibility, cognitive complexity, and capacity for change and integration (Chapters 5–9 and 11). Therapists were alert to markers signifying readiness to engage in treatment (Chapters 7–9, 12, and 13). Constantino et al. (Chapter 7) listen to clients' motivational language to gauge their readiness. Watson (Chapter 8) notes that EFT therapists attend to task markers to gauge readiness as well as their clients' expressed willingness to engage in specific tasks like chair dialogues or focusing.

Responsive therapists across all approaches were alert to signs of client resistance to specific techniques or ways of working, including therapists' interpretations or engaging in experiential tasks like chair work or family enactments. Responsive therapists attend to moments when their clients' express ambivalence about the treatment approach or share low outcome expectations as a guide for when to be less directive. At these times, responsive therapists work to negotiate whether to continue on the same track or do something different. Ribeiro et al. (Chapter 9) suggest that for therapists to be optimally responsive they may need to "relocate" their interventions within clients' TZPD.

Client Feedback

Attending to clients' feedback is recommended within all approaches and by all contributors. To be optimally responsive, therapists listen to clients' feedback in the session, and some proactively gather information using specific measures in order to decide whether to stay or change course and offer something different to their clients. Ribeiro et al. (Chapter 9) propose that in narrative therapy, clients' negative and positive comments provide feedback to guide therapists' choice of more challenging or more supportive interventions in the context of the therapeutic collaboration model. While the overall goal is to help clients to further develop within their TZPD, they are sensitive to their clients' responses and adjust and correct their interventions if a previous intervention is observed to be outside their client's TZPD. Most approaches emphasize the importance of clients' agreement to indicate that a technique or intervention is within the clients' TZPD (Chapters 4, 7–10, and 12). Constantino et al. (Chapter 7) suggest that clients' agreement with the therapists' direction and choice of technique is evidence that the client believes in the treatment.

More formal feedback is obtained when therapists actively solicit it using various measures and outcome indices including clients' ratings of the alliance and possible ruptures (Chapters 4 and 5), assessments of in-session process, and evaluations about how the client is responding to the treatment after each session and at various stages over the course of treatment (Chapters 6, 7, and 11–13). Therapists' attention to and acknowledgment of clients' responses and feedback to them in terms of how they are feeling in the relationship with the therapist, the appropriateness of the specific interventions, and their overall satisfaction with progress are essential if they are to remain connected and work well together (Chapter 9).

Clients' Diversity and Uniqueness

Being attuned to and responsive with diverse populations requires therapists be open and receptive to cultural diversity and express cultural humility (Owen et al., 2016). Eubanks et al. (Chapter 4) emphasize that both client and therapist factors can contribute to ruptures in cross-cultural dyads with research showing that demographic differences can lead to more frequent alliance ruptures. Responsive therapists are attuned to issues of diversity. They are sensitive to differences between therapists and clients on a continuum of factors, including but not limited to race, sex, gender, class, religion, identity, and culture and are willing to discuss these openly (Chapters 4, 5, 7, 8, 10, and 11). Responsive therapists are aware when their clients feel invalidated in the session and are sensitive to those behaviors that might be experienced as microaggressions.

Constantino et al. (Chapter 7) and Eubanks et al. (Chapter 4) observe that misalignment in the session may not only have to do with feelings of ambivalence and treatment credibility but may reflect cultural misattunements and microaggressions. Diamond et al. (Chapter 10) suggest that it is important to be sensitive to clients' cultural beliefs about identity and the tensions between self-expression and self-actualization that might exist in families and larger cultural groupings. Similarly, Watson (Chapter 8) encourages therapists to be sensitive to emotional expression rules that vary across individuals, families, and cultures, and support clients to find the modes of expression that work best for them within their specific contexts. Kramer (Chapter 11) encourages therapists to be careful when applying diagnostic categories to clients from diverse populations, as they may not fit clients' cultural and spiritual frameworks or be appropriate or relevant to them.

Integrating Therapist, Client, and Interpersonal Signals

In closing, we have attempted to provide a preliminary map of the markers or signals that therapists attend to as they navigate the interpersonal terrain of psychotherapy. Table 14.1 outlines the three categories of signals according to whether they originate with the therapist, the client, or the interpersonal

TABLE 14.1. Signals That Guide Responsiveness Across Different Therapeutic Approaches

Signal categories	Specific signals	Examples of signals
Therapist signals	Theoretical lens	Relationship focused, behavior focused
	Diagnostic markers	Trauma, addiction, personality disorders
	Therapists' characteristics	Personalities, qualities, attachment history
	Therapists' inner reactions	Negative feelings (e.g., boredom, tension), relational needs, positive feelings (e.g., acceptance)
Client signals	Clients' relational maps	Interpersonal behavior, attachment histories, beliefs, expectations, level of differentiation of self and other
	Clients' self-states and self-organizations	Dreams, dissociated self-states, defensiveness, negative self-organizations, self-striving
	Clients' emotional expression	Shifts in emotion, expressions of pain, distress, sadness, fear, helplessness, vulnerability, intensity of expression, positive emotion
	Clients' shifts in understanding	Views of self, of other, and of problems; narrative coherence; changes in innovative moments; levels of assimilation
	Clients' problematic and self-injurious behavior	Self-harm, suicidal intent, hostility, maladaptive blaming and defensiveness
	Clients' nonverbal behavior	Facial expressions, body language, posture, vocal quality
Interpersonal signals	Alliance ruptures	Confrontation, withdrawal, client readiness, client engagement, client resistance, client ambivalence, clients' low outcome expectations, therapist microaggressions
	Client feedback	Informal signals: negative comments, positive comments, agreement
		Formal signals: measures of in-session and postsession processes, outcome indices
	Client diversity and uniqueness	Race, culture, gender, class, religion, identity, beliefs, cultural rules, conflicting expectations, self-expression, emotional expression rules

process, as well as the specific signals identified by our contributors to guide therapists' responsiveness in different approaches. Though numerous, these therapist, client, and interpersonal signals are but the tip of the iceberg of all the information that therapists attend to and synthesize to be appropriately and optimally responsive to their clients in treatment. As we began to wrestle with the concept of responsiveness in psychotherapy and identify the myriad signals that guide therapists' responsiveness moment to moment and over the course of treatment, it sometimes felt as if we were trying to contain an ocean in a teacup. We started to question "how we manage to get it right at all." But then, that might be said of all our relationships.

TRAINING FOR RESPONSIVENESS

Ongoing training is vital to enhance therapists' responsiveness. With respect to training, the authors acknowledge that responsiveness is hard to teach, as it cannot be specified in advance. However, it is vital that trainees and practitioners be sensitized to the importance of responsiveness to optimize treatment outcomes across diverse approaches. Therapists can be taught to be aware of internal and external signs as well as possible obstacles to enhance their sensitivity. As numerous authors note throughout this volume, responsiveness is not a matter of being competent in the delivery of specific techniques only. Rather, it is a sensitively choreographed dance that occurs between therapist and client to facilitate positive treatment outcomes. There is no "one size fits all," but instead therapists must learn to attend and attune to a variety of signals and markers to enable them to be more sensitive to their clients, assess their needs moment to moment in the session, and manage the interpersonal and therapeutic process even as they work within specific treatment parameters. Boswell et al. (Chapter 13), using an integrative approach, strongly encourage therapists to gain competence in a variety of treatment approaches and maximize the number of tools and ways of responding to different clients at their disposal.

To enhance therapists' sense of efficacy with respect to understanding and following clients' relational and interpersonal maps, Kramer (Chapter 11) and Silberschatz (Chapter 6) suggest using Plan Analysis or the Plan Formulation method. Wiseman and Egozi (Chapter 3) suggest that acquiring an understanding of clients' attachment styles can serve as a useful guide to therapist responsiveness in therapy especially with respect to clients' needs for interpersonal distance or closeness. Tishby (Chapter 5) suggests that teaching trainees theater improvisational skills might enhance their creativity and spontaneity in the moment and help them to think on their feet when engaged in the relational dance with their clients.

Numerous authors emphasize the need for therapists at different stages of development to learn how to manage negative affect in the session (Chapters 4, 5, 8, 10, and 12), both their own and their clients. Therapists' negative reactions can occur in response to clients' behaviors like hostility or withdrawal, intense expressions of pain and hopelessness, or their own feelings of incompetence. Most important, training needs to focus on the identification of specific signals or markers that indicate that therapists might need to change focus, reassess their direction, or reconnect with their clients in the session. Too much emphasis on technical expertise alone comes at the expense of a focus on therapist and client factors, as well as the interpersonal aspects of treatment. Training to enhance responsiveness includes therapists listening for spontaneous informal feedback from their clients, as well being more systematic in their efforts to actively solicit feedback from them.

FUTURE DIRECTIONS FOR RESEARCH ON RESPONSIVENESS

Robert Sapolsky, a neuroendocrinologist who has studied the effects of hierarchical social organizations on stress levels in baboons, sagely observed that science can provide information about patterns and general trends and expectations, but it cannot tell us what each individual neuron or person will do moment to moment (Sapolsky, 2004, 2017). This individual variability encapsulates the problem posed by therapist responsiveness for psychotherapy researchers. Stiles (Chapter 1) and Hatcher (Chapter 2) argue that responsiveness is problematic for RCTs and empirically supported treatments insofar as it interferes with the uniform delivery of techniques and treatment adherence. The focus of outcome research has been to identify what works for most people and has overlooked individual variations and the adjustments therapists make to tailor their treatments to each individual client at different moments over the course of psychotherapy. They argue that no single approach is ever delivered in the same way twice given the vagaries of clients, therapists, and emerging contexts. The demand to adhere to treatment manuals in RCTs is at odds with therapists' being optimally responsive in the moment and trying to do the "right thing at the right time" for their clients as the need arises.

The problem of responsiveness is especially acute for research carried out within a positivistic tradition that privileges prediction, independence between IVs and DVs, and quantitative measurement over qualitative description and observation. As an alternative to current research paradigms, Stiles (Chapter 1) suggests that psychotherapy researchers studying responsiveness focus on achievements instead of quantifiable actions. Referring to the "Pirsig phenomenon," he notes that while it is hard to specify quality in advance, it is easy to recognize its presence. Thus, he suggests a shift in focus to describe and measure sequences and specify process outcomes. Stiles (Chapter 1) suggests that researchers need to better understand and study responsiveness in psychotherapy in order to build robust explanatory theories of change. He encourages researchers to address the following questions: "What kinds of signals are they [therapists] tuned to, and how do they use this information to make the intervention better fit the client and the circumstances?" (Stiles & Horvath, 2017, p. 80). We hope that the chapters in this book may provide some answers to these questions.

As they study responsiveness, Stiles suggests that researchers engage in more fine-grained description of psychotherapy processes, use case studies as well as conversational analysis, and focus on immediate effects to better understand its role in therapy with the aim of building explanatory theories. He notes that measures of responsiveness already exist in the form of evaluative process measures, including the working alliance (Horvath & Greenberg, 1989), empathy (Barrett-Lennard, 1962), responsiveness (Elkin et al., 2014), etc. These are some of the same factors identified by Norcross and Wampold (2019) as the components of psychotherapy relationships that are effective and necessary. Stiles (Chapter 1) encourages researchers to unpack evaluative process measures to identify good process and try to specify what contributes to these outcomes. For example, what contributes to a client feeling understood and valued moment to moment and overall in psychotherapy?

Qualitative inquiry and research would be one way to investigate clinicians' and clients' subjective experiences and intentions during moments of responsive interaction to further map the interpersonal terrain (Chapters 1 and 8). Qualitative research is useful to elaborate how participants experience and perceive interactions (Levitt et al., 2016; Rennie, 1994). Questions to address include "What contributes to therapists being responsive?" "What do therapists working within different approaches experience and perceive in the moment that signals them to change their interactions?" and "How do they respond?" One of the objectives of this book is to begin to identify and catalogue these signals or markers; however, this is just the beginning. There is much that needs to be elaborated and clarified. Moreover, as we have seen, different approaches work with different definitions and conceptualizations of responsiveness; some are more focused moment to moment (Chapters 4–6 and 8–10), while others use a broader timescale starting with improved treatment matching at the beginning of therapy and ongoing assessments of outcome at varying time points over the course of treatment (Chapters 7, 12, and 13).

Another method that might be useful to enhance our understanding of responsiveness in psychotherapy and extrapolate principles for practice would be to identify and study treatment anomalies or times when therapists vary in their delivery of different treatments and subject these to intensive study and analysis. Isolating and describing small sequences of interaction in psychotherapy has been done successfully using task analysis (Rice & Greenberg, 1984; Greenberg, 1991). This method has been used to develop performance models of specific tasks in EFT (Greenberg et al., 1993) and to illuminate different types of therapeutic ruptures as well as ways to resolve them effectively in therapy (Safran & Muran, 2000; Eubanks et al., Chapter 4, this volume). As Stiles (Chapter 1) suggests, studying moments when therapists are optimally responsive and identifying *what* they are responding to and *how* they are responding and then measuring more proximate as well as more distal outcomes could provide important information that would contribute to building a more comprehensive theory of change.

A number of the authors have emphasized the need to research and identify therapist characteristics that contribute to responsiveness (Chapters 2, 3, 5–7, 10, 11, and 13). Wiseman and Egozi (Chapter 3) highlight the potential impact of therapist attachment styles on how to respond to clients' needs. Others have underlined the role of therapists' emotions, both positive and negative, in facilitating responsiveness in the moment, including managing countertransference reactions (Chapter 5) and negative feelings of incompetence and rejection (Chapters 4, 5, 8, and 10). These authors suggest that positive emotions such as feelings of confidence and acceptance can serve as a measure that things are going well. Kramer (Chapter 11) highlights the need to investigate the impact of positive and negative therapist behaviors, including reassurance and criticism, on responsiveness with different populations. Another question that has been highlighted is "What are the personal characteristics of responsive therapists?" Research on the training and development of psychotherapists (Orlinsky et al., 2015) for appropriate responsiveness (Hatcher, 2015) is also needed. Hatcher (Chapter 2) and Silberschatz (Chapter 6) suggest that the study of "supershrinks" might be a productive avenue of inquiry to investigate questions like "How do they adapt their treatments?" "When do they adapt?" and "What enables them to be optimally responsive across a wide range of patients?"

In addition to therapist factors, research should focus on client characteristics that not only elicit therapists' responsiveness but also enable them to be receptive to therapists' responsive behaviors. Researchers are attempting to identify client characteristics (Cohen & DeRubeis, 2018; Norcross & Wampold, 2019) as well as treatment markers. Cohen and DeRubeis (2018) proposed the Personalized Assessment Index as a method for identifying what works for whom in the treatment of depression, while Norcross and Wampold (2019) identified client factors, including attachment style, coping, gender identity, spirituality, reactance level, and preferences as client factors that contribute to outcome in psychotherapy.

Kramer (Chapter 11) notes that it is important for research on client factors to go beyond a narrow focus on specific diagnostic criteria. Constantino et al. (Chapter 6) and Boswell et al. (Chapter 13) continue to work to identify and map treatment by aptitude interactions to facilitate the matching of clients to treatments to enhance responsiveness in psychotherapy. Other client factors identified by authors in this volume include culture, class, identity, cultural rules, beliefs and expectations about identity, self-expression, and emotional expression.

Another important factor identified by Stiles (Chapter 1) is clients' zones of proximal development. Several different client capacities and functions have been identified as ZPDs that can be useful to guide responsiveness in different treatment approaches. These include clients' relational maps and interpersonal styles, their self-states and self-organizations, their emotional processing and regulation capacity, and their understanding and assimilation of problematic experiences (Chapter 1, 5, 8, and 9). Silberschatz (Chapter 6), Tishby (Chapter 5) and Kramer (Chapter 11) point to the usefulness of clients' relational maps and expectations to guide therapists' responsiveness with different clients. These client variables warrant further investigation and elaboration to better understand responsiveness in psychotherapy as well as factors that affect outcome.

To advance the field, numerous authors have suggested a new research paradigm informed by a two-person psychology that takes account of both participants as well as the interaction between client and therapist (Chapters 2, 4, 5, 7, 8, and 11). Hatcher (Chapter 2) posits a full responsiveness model that takes account of two people mutually influencing each other in contrast to a model that privileges the therapist as a goal-directed agent and fails to adequately account for the client as similarly goal-directed in psychotherapy. Some of the questions that need to be addressed within a two-person framework include "What do responsive interactions in psychotherapy look like?" and "How are they different from unresponsive interactions?" Tishby (Chapter 5) suggests that we need more studies that examine the role of mutuality. She notes that congruence between therapist and client in terms of emotional experience in the session as well as ratings of the therapeutic alliance is associated with good outcomes. Interpersonal circumplex models

(Benjamin, 1974; Horowitz et al., 2000) also provide useful frameworks and measurement tools for examining interactions between clients and therapists, as well as how clients relate to their own experience and interact with others. Tishby (Chapter 5) and Constantino et al. (Chapter 7) suggest that researchers need to rate both therapists and clients on the same measures to better mirror and capture the mutuality between them.

To develop a comprehensive theory of change, better maps of the interpersonal terrain are necessary to enhance our treatments (Watson, 2018; Wiseman, 2017). An exclusive focus on technical expertise is insufficient to adequately meet the needs of many clients. Clinicians need to acquire technical expertise as well as knowledge of how to respond appropriately and optimally across a range of clients and emerging contexts if they are to be maximally competent and effective. A goal espoused by a number of authors is to develop a science of relationship for psychotherapy (Chapters 1–3 and 5) that is informed by relationship science (Chapter 2), developmental psychology (Chapters 1, 3, 8, and 9), and psychotherapy theories, research, and practice. To map this terrain, it will be important to use a variety of methodologies and to focus on immediate in-session processes and successful episodes of interaction while continuing to build links between more proximal and more distal outcomes including within the session, immediately postsession, at intervals across treatment, at the end of therapy, and longer term (Watson, 2018).

FINAL THOUGHTS

Our contributors have enriched and expanded our thinking about what it means to be responsive in psychotherapy. We hope that this book will provide practitioners and researchers with a preliminary map indicating different routes to enhance their responsiveness in the session and across the treatment trajectory. In keeping with the concept of responsiveness, this map is best thought of as interactive and evolving, as researchers and clinicians continue to discover new routes and ways of adapting and tailoring treatments and techniques for each client's journey, while taking account of changing conditions and emerging contexts—like explorers and hikers forging new paths while attending to the conditions of the terrain, the weather, and the seasons. Although as therapists and researchers we have gained valuable information on how to enhance therapist responsiveness, we encourage researchers to continue to engage in theory building, unpack existing measures, and develop new measures and methods to accumulate research on how "to get it right" and be optimally responsive for the sake of our clients and enhanced treatment outcomes.

REFERENCES

Bacal, H. A. (1998). *Optimal responsiveness: How therapists heal their patients* (H. A. Bacal, Ed.). Jason Aronson.

Barrett-Lennard, G. T. (1962). Dimensions of therapist response as causal factors in therapeutic change. *Psychological monographs: General and applied, 76*(43), 1–36. https://doi.org/10.1037/h0093918

Benjamin, L. S. (1974). Structural analysis of social behavior. *Psychological Review, 81*(5), 392–425. https://doi.org/10.1037/h0037024

Caspar, F. (2019). Plan analysis and the motive-oriented therapeutic relationship. In U. Kramer (Ed.), *Case formulation for personality disorders: Tailoring psychotherapy to the individual client* (pp. 265–290). Academic Press. https://doi.org/10.1016/B978-0-12-813521-1.00014-X

Cohen, Z. D., & DeRubeis, R. J. (2018). Treatment selection in depression. *Annual Review of Clinical Psychology, 14*(1), 209–236. https://doi.org/10.1146/annurev-clinpsy-050817-084746

Elkin, I., Falconnier, L., Smith, Y., Canada, K. E., Henderson, E., Brown, E. R., & McKay, B. M. (2014). Therapist responsiveness and patient engagement in therapy. *Psychotherapy Research, 24*(1), 52–66. https://doi.org/10.1080/10503307.2013.820855

Goldfried, M. R. (1980). Toward the delineation of therapeutic change principles. *American Psychologist, 35*(11), 991–999. https://doi.org/10.1037/0003-066X.35.11.991

Grawe, K. (1992). Komplementäre Beziehungsgestaltung als Mittel zur Herstellung einer guten Therapiebeziehung [Complementary therapeutic relationship as a mean for the establishment of a good therapeutic relationship]. In J. Margraf & J. C. Brengelmann (Eds.), *Die Therapeut-Patient-Beziehung in der Verhaltenstherapie* [The therapist-patient relationship in behavior therapy] (pp. 215–244). Röttger-Verlag.

Greenberg, L. S. (1991). Research on the process of change. *Psychotherapy Research, 1*(1), 3–16. https://doi.org/10.1080/10503309112331334011

Greenberg, L. S., Rice, L., & Elliott, R. (1993). *Facilitating emotional change: The Moment-by-Moment Process.* Guilford Press.

Hatcher, R. L. (2015). Interpersonal competencies: Responsiveness, technique, and training in psychotherapy. *American Psychologist, 70*(8), 747–757. https://doi.org/10.1037/a0039803

Horowitz, L. M., Alden, L. E., Wiggins, J. S., & Pincus, A. L. (2000). *Inventory of Interpersonal Problems manual.* The Psychological Corporation.

Horvath, A. O., & Greenberg, L. S. (1989). The development and validation of the Working Alliance Inventory. *Journal of Counseling Psychology, 36*(2), 223–233. https://doi.org/10.1037/0022-0167.36.2.223

Kramer, U., & Stiles, W. B. (2015). The responsiveness problem in psychotherapy: A review of proposed solutions. *Clinical Psychology: Science and Practice, 22*(3), 277–295. https://doi.org/10.1111/cpsp.12107

Leiman, M., & Stiles, W. B. (2001). Dialogical sequence analysis and the zone of proximal development as conceptual enhancements to the assimilation model: The case of Jan revisited. *Psychotherapy Research, 11*(3), 311–330. https://doi.org/10.1080/713663986

Levitt, H. M., Pomerville, A., & Surace, F. I. (2016). A qualitative meta-analysis examining clients' experiences of psychotherapy: A new agenda. *Psychological Bulletin, 142*(8), 801–830. https://doi.org/10.1037/bul0000057

Linehan, M. (1993). *Cognitive behavioral treatment of borderline personality disorder.* Guilford Press.

Norcross, J. C., & Wampold, B. E. (Eds.). (2019). *Psychotherapy relationships that work* (3rd ed., Vol. 2). Oxford University Press.

Orlinsky, D. E., Strauss, B., Rønnestad, M. H., Hill, C., Castonguay, L., Willutzki, U., & Carlsson, J. (2015). A collaborative study of development in psychotherapy trainees. *Psychotherapy Bulletin, 50*(4), 21–25.

Owen, J., Tao, K. W., Drinane, J. M., Hook, J. N., Davis, D. E., & Kune, N. F. (2016). Client perceptions of therapists' multicultural orientation: Cultural (missed) opportunities and cultural humility. *Professional Psychology: Research and Practice, 47*(1), 30–37. https://doi.org/10.1037/pro0000046

Reis, H. T. (2012). Perceived partner responsiveness as an organizing theme for the study of relationships and well-being. In L. Campbell & T. J. Loving (Eds.), *Interdisciplinary research on close relationships: The case for integration* (pp. 27–52). American Psychological Association. https://doi.org/10.1037/13486-002

Rennie, D. L. (1994). Clients' deference in psychotherapy. *Journal of Counseling Psychology, 41*(4), 427–437. https://doi.org/10.1037/0022-0167.41.4.427

Rice, L. N., & Greenberg, L. S. (Eds.). (1984). *Patterns of change: Intensive analysis of psychotherapy process.* Guilford Press.

Safran, J. D., & Muran, J. C. (2000). *Negotiating the therapeutic alliance: A relational treatment guide.* Guilford Press.

Sapolsky, R. M. (2004). *Why zebras don't get ulcers: The acclaimed guide to stress, stress-related diseases, and coping-now revised and updated* (3rd ed.). Holt Paperbacks.

Sapolsky, R. M. (2017). *Behave: The biology of humans at our best and worst.* Penguin Press.

Schore, A. N. (2019). *The development of the unconscious mind.* W. W. Norton.

Stiles, W. B., & Horvath, A. O. (2017). Appropriate responsiveness as a contribution to therapist effects. In L. G. Castonguay & C. E. Hill (Eds.), *How and why are some therapists better than others? Understanding therapist effects* (pp. 71–84). American Psychological Association. https://doi.org/10.1037/0000034-005

Vygotsky, L. (1978). *Mind in society: The development of higher psychological processes.* Harvard University Press.

Watson, J. C. (2018). Mapping patterns of change in emotion-focused psychotherapy: Implications for theory, research, practice and training. *Psychotherapy Research, 28*(3), 389–405. https://doi.org/10.1080/10503307.2018.1435920

Wiseman. H. (2017). The quest for connection in interpersonal and therapeutic relationships. *Psychotherapy Research, 27*(4), 469–487. https://doi.org/10.1080/10503307.2015.1119327

Index

A

AAI (Adult Attachment Interview), 74–75
Abductions, 29
ABFT. *See* Attachment-based family therapy
"Abstract communication" withdrawal marker, 86, 98
Acceptable plans and behaviors, Plan Analysis, 242–243
Acceptance
    in attachment-based family therapy, 221
    attending to therapist's own feelings of, 185
    dialectic of acceptance versus change, 267–268
    in therapeutic relationship for EFT, 172, 175
Accommodation, 184
Acculturation, 250
Acknowledgment, 240
Active assessment of client needs, 171
Active passivity versus apparent competence (dialectical dilemma), 266, 271
Active therapeutic stance, 143
Actual development level, 196–198
Adams, K. E., 188
Adherence
    competence vs., 152, 153, 241–242
    and optimal responsiveness, 44–46, 316
    outcome research on, 42–44, 152, 153
    perseverative, 153
    and therapist responsiveness, 45–47, 273
Adolescents, resistance from, 230–231

Adult Attachment Interview (AAI), 74–75
Adverse childhood experiences, 135
Affective state
    "content/affect split" withdrawal markers, 86, 90
    management/regulation of therapist's, 190, 316
    tailoring interventions to client's, 4–5, 171–172
AFT (alliance-focused training), 99–100, 127
Agency, 88–89, 175
Aggressive behavior, 89, 238, 239
Ainsworth, M. D. S., 59, 60, 62
Alignment
    feelings as indicator of, 176
    on perceptions of working relationship, 156
    on treatment-related beliefs, 155
Alliance. *See* Therapeutic alliance; Working alliance
Alliance convergence, 153
Alliance-focused training (AFT), 99–100, 127
Alternative meanings, rehearsing, 201–202
Alternative self-narratives, consolidation of, 202–203
Altman, N., 97
Ambivalence, in context-responsive psychotherapy integration, 157, 160–161, 286
American Indian population, 274

American Psychological Association (APA), 125, 151

Amplification, of unique outcomes, 202

Anger, in attachment-based family therapy, 223–224

Anxiety, attachment, 65, 73, 74, 221

Anxious-self-coping-self dialogue, 289, 290

APA (American Psychological Association), 125, 151

APES (Assimilation of Problematic Experience Scale), 188

Apparent competence, 266, 271

"Appeasing" withdrawal marker, 86

Appropriate responsiveness, 40–42
   in attachment-based family therapy, 220–221, 223–228
   as common factor, 49–50
   defined, 16, 41, 220, 277
   descriptive measures of, 21–22
   developing and enhancing, 51–53
   for effective therapists, 16–17
   evaluative measures of, 20–24, 27
   in framing of responsiveness problem, 300
   and history of therapeutic relationship, 77
   as integral part of treatment, 20
   optimal responsiveness vs., 44–45, 300
   research focusing on immediate effects of, 27–28
   in rupture repair, 83–84
   short-term client discomfort and, 23
   in therapeutic collaboration model, 198–199
   in treatment of personality disorders, 239
   undermining of process–outcome model by, 18–19
   and working alliance, 49

Approval, empathy and validation vs., 226–227

Aptitude-treatment-interaction approach, 25, 258

Aron, L., 117

Arousal, modulation of, 177

As-needed telephone consultation, 258

Assessment, as responsiveness, in EFT, 172, 174–175

Assimilation model, 196

Assimilation of Problematic Experience Scale (APES), 188

Assimilation theory, 29

Assimilative integration, 281–283, 289–291

Attachment and identity episodes, ABFT, 221–223, 227–228

Attachment anxiety, 65, 73, 74, 221

Attachment avoidance, 65, 73–76, 221

Attachment-based family therapy (ABFT), 9, 219–234
   initiation of, 219
   research on responsiveness in, 230–232
   and responsiveness to intersectionality, 228–230
   therapeutic tasks of, 221–223
   therapist responsiveness to challenges in, 223–228
   training and supervision to enhance therapist responsiveness in, 232–233

Attachment history, relational maps and, 307–308

Attachment style
   as client factor in therapy relationship, 4
   and language use, 74–75
   rupture frequency/resolution and client, 123
   and self-organization, 178
   of therapist, 318
   understanding client's, 315

Attachment theory, 59–77, 304
   and attachment dynamics in therapeutic relationship, 64–65, 74
   closeness markers in client–therapist relational narratives, 67–72
   as explanatory theory of responsiveness, 29, 301
   infant–parent interaction research on coregulation, 61–62
   and in-session measures of responsiveness, 72–76
   internal working models and relationship representations in, 63–64
   regulating therapeutic distance, 65–67
   responsiveness concept in, 60
   secure base in, 62–63
   therapeutic tasks in, 64

Attending
   to client feedback, 183–184
   in emotional processing by clients, 177
   to moment-to-moment behavior, 5
   to multiple family members, in ABFT, 220–221

to primary behavioral targets, in DBT, 264–265, 267
to therapist's own feelings, 184–185
Attentiveness, 240, 241
Attitude
for addressing ruptures, 87–88
in experiential therapy, 173
Attuned responsiveness, measuring, 22
Attunement
assessment of, 75–76
attachment theory and, 59
to client's diversity and uniqueness, 187, 313
to dissociated self-states, 119–121
in emotion-focused therapy, 172, 174–175
empathic, 76–77
in exploratory resolution strategies, 91–92
goal-corrected empathic, 76–77
for identifying alliance ruptures, 84
in metacommunication, 95
to motivational language, 155, 157, 162–163
in mutual recognition, 109
to poignancy of language, 182
research on need for, 153
and responsiveness, 3, 5, 172
for secure attachment, 60
training to increase, 126
to transference–countertransference patterns and self-disclosure, 114–116
Atzil-Slonim, D., 122
Authenticity, 48, 70–72
Autonomic nervous system, 4
Autonomy, 63, 72, 73, 173
Aversive behavior, DBT, 272
Aviram, A., 43, 164
Avoidance, attachment, 65, 73–76, 221
Awareness, 93, 112
Axis I personality disorders, 257

B

Bacal, H. A., 7, 44–45, 300
Baldwin, S. A., 43
Ballistic assumption, 38, 273
Barber, J. P., 44
Beck, Aaron, 51–52
Behavioral skills, as primary target in S-DBT, 264

Behavioral targets of S-DBT
increasing dialectical behavioral patterns as, 263–264
primary, 264–265, 267
secondary, 265–267
Behaviorism, 278
Beliefs
cultural, about identity, 229, 313
pathogenic, 134–135, 137–138
religious/spiritual, 4, 229–230, 291
treatment-related, 155, 157, 159
Belongingness, 48
Benjamin, J., 109
Berthoud, L., 243
Biases, 64, 87, 232
Bisexual clients, ABFT with, 229
Blaming, 223–224
Border-crossing behavior, 238, 239
Borderline personality disorder (BPD)
DBT for treatment of, 10, 257, 261, 280
disorder-specific responsiveness to clients with, 246
external focus for clients with, 238–239
individualized responsiveness to clients with, 246–250
mentalization-based therapy for treatment of, 241–242
research on responsiveness, alliance, and outcomes in, 244–247
therapist signals in treatment of, 306
Bordin, E. S., 49, 84
Boston Change Process Study Group, 109–110
Boswell, J. F., 43, 282
Bottom-up training, 166
Bowlby, J., 7, 59, 60, 62–64
Breaks, in therapeutic collaboration, 208–210
Brief psychodynamic therapy, 243
Brief strategic family therapy (BSFT), 230
Bromberg, P. M., 108
Bush, M., 138

C

Caregiver responsiveness, 60–63
Case analysis, in countertransference research, 124–125
Case formulation
individualized responsiveness based on, 242–243, 248

and responsiveness as doing more of
the same, 156, 163
training in, 147
Case management strategies, 270–272
Case-specific plans, 136
Case studies, responsiveness research
using, 26
Caspar, F., 24, 246
Caston, J., 138
Castonguay, L. G., 44, 59, 282, 285
CBT. *See* Cognitive behavioral therapy
CCRT. *See* Core conflictual relationship
theme
CCT. *See* Counter change-talk
Central object relations patterns, 114
Ceremonies, consolidation phase,
202–203
CFI–R (Countertransference Factors
Inventory Revised), 128
Challenging of client perspectives
balance of offering support and, 211
and deconstructing problematic
self-narratives, 203
by nonresponsive therapists, 208–210
in therapeutic collaboration model,
197–198, 204, 206–207
Change
common principles of change
framework, 10, 284–285, 287–288
dialectic of acceptance versus,
267–268
readiness for, 4, 312
Change-oriented treatment, 157
Change processes
alliance on, 83
in attachment-based family therapy,
222–223
in narrative therapy, 200–210
Change-talk (CT), 155, 157, 160, 162
Change theory
in assimilation model, 196
comprehensive, 318, 320
in innovative movements model, 196
in narrative therapy, 200
stages of change theory, 281
Child development, responsiveness
research in, 24
Choice, client, 46
Choice points for context-dependent
resolution strategies, 92–93
Clark, M. S., 47–48
Client-centered therapy, 239, 278

Client diversity. *See also* Diverse client
populations
attunement to, 313, 314
tailoring interventions to, 198–199
Client factors
outcome research on, 152
in receptiveness to therapist
responsiveness, 165, 318–319
in therapy relationship, 4
Client responsiveness, 50
Client self-disclosure paradox, 17–18
Client signals and markers, 303, 307–311,
314
emotional expression, 308–309
integrating therapist and interpersonal
markers with, 313, 315
nonverbal behavior, 310–311
problematic and self-injurious behavior,
310
relational or interpersonal maps, 307–308
self-states and self-organization, 308
shifts in understanding, 309–310
Client stabilization, 258
Client–therapist relational narratives,
67–72, 77
Clinical departure
in cognitive behavioral therapy, 158–161
in context-responsive psychotherapy
integration, 152
due to cultural misattunement, 161–162
research on, 153, 163–165
responsiveness as, 156–158, 163–164
Clinical supervision, 27
Clinicians, responsiveness concept for,
5–6, 237
Closeness markers, in relational narratives,
67–72
Close relationships, 37, 47–48
Cognitive analytic therapy, 91
Cognitive behavioral therapy (CBT), 278
adherence research on, 43, 44
alliance-focused training in, 127
assimilative integration of EFT with,
289–291
client responsiveness and, 50
context-responsive psychotherapy
integration in, 158–161
corrective experiences in, 285
credibility and outcome expectation
with, 283
cultural misattunement with traditional,
161–162

IEP interventions in, 281–282
motivational interviewing integrated with, 163–164, 281–283, 286
task analysis of rupture repair in, 91
third-wave, 278
for treatment of panic, 287, 288
Cognitive modification, 269–270
Cognitive–psychodynamic–relational theory, 134, 304
Cognitive revolution, 278
Cognitive state, tailoring interventions to, 4–5, 171–172
Cognitive therapy, 20, 51–52, 203
Cohen, Z. D., 52, 319
Cohesion, group, 21, 23
Collaboration. *See also* Therapeutic collaboration model (TCM)
in alliance, 110
in narrative therapy, 199
on therapy goals, 21, 49
Collaborative problem-solving, 223
Collyer, H., 43
Combs, G., 202
Comfort, cultural, 162, 291, 292
Common factor(s)
common principles of change vs., 284
CRPI vs. interventions based on, 164
outcomes of therapists focusing on, 282
as pathway to integration, 283
responsiveness as, 49–50, 278
Common principles of change framework, 10, 284–285, 287–288, 305
Communication. *See also* Metacommunication
about DBT with modified delivery, 261–262
abstract, as withdrawal marker, 86, 98
attachment and patterns of, 74–75
irreverent communication strategies, 270
reciprocal communication strategies, 270
of responsiveness, 191
in therapeutic collaboration model, 198
Compassion, in rupture repair, 87
Competence
apparent, 266, 271
in attachment-based family therapy, 232
outcome research on, 42–43, 152
responsiveness vs., 240, 315
as therapist signal, 306
Competence-based models, 291
Complementary interventions, MOTR-based therapy, 248–250

Comprehensive theory of change, 318, 320
Concerns of parents, in ABFT, 226–227
Confidence, 181
Confirmation bias, 87
Conflict, 127, 134–135
Confrontational approach, 144, 184
Confrontational coping, 96
Confrontation ruptures, 84, 123
exploratory resolution strategies for, 91
recognizing, 84, 86
relational needs associated with, 89
resolution choice points with, 92–93
Conjoint corrective attachment/identity episodes, 222–223, 227–228
Connolly Gibbons, M. B., 25
Consensus, on goals of therapy, 21, 49, 220
Consolidation of self-narratives, 202–203
Constantino, M. J., 53, 286
Constructionism, 199
Consultation, in dialectical behavior therapy, 258, 270–272
Consultation team, 258, 270, 272
"Content/affect split" withdrawal markers, 86, 90
Context-responsive psychotherapy integration (CRPI), 10, 151–166, 305
case examples, 158–161
in cognitive behavioral therapy, 158–161
combining common principles of change with, 287–288
for culturally diverse client populations, 161–162
defined, 154–158
markers in, 53
as metaframework, 285–286
research across treatment lifespan on, 162–165
and research on responsivity/ attunement in psychotherapy, 152–153
training to maximize responsivity and attunement in, 165–166, 293
Contextual model of psychotherapy, 45, 90–93
Contingencies, 25, 85
Contingency management, 269
Control-mastery theory, 24, 26, 133–148
clinical study of therapist effects, 143–146
with diverse client populations, 146–147
overview of, 134–137

process and outcome research on interventions using, 137–140
and responsiveness to client plan formulation, 135–137
on therapist effects and responsiveness, 140–143
training implications of, 146
Convergence, alliance, 153
Conversational analysis, 26
Coping behaviors
anxious-self-coping-self dialogue, 289, 290
as client factor in therapy relationship, 4
in response to microaggressions, 96, 97
Core conflictual relationship theme (CCRT), 67
in countertransference management, 128
countertransference research on, 124–125
negotiation over, 110–112
Coregulation, 61–62, 87, 89
Corrective experience(s)
in attachment-based family therapy, 221–223, 227–228
in common principles of change framework, 284–285
rupture repair as, 88–90, 286
in two-person model of responsiveness, 303
Counter change-talk (CCT)
ambivalence signaled by, 157, 160
and change readiness, 155
and outcome of therapy, 162–163
Countertransference
attunement to, 114–116
managing, 125, 127–128, 318
process and outcome research on, 124–125
Countertransference Factors Inventory Revised (CFI–R), 128
Coutinho, J., 123
COVID-19 pandemic, 11
Cox, A., 18
Coyne, A. E., 153
Credibility
building, in current treatment, 163
and first-step responsiveness, 155, 162
and outcome of CBT approaches, 283
CRPI. *See* Context-responsive psychotherapy integration
CT. *See* Change-talk

Cultural adaptation, as client factor, 4
Cultural beliefs, about identity, 229, 313
Cultural comfort, 162, 291, 292
Cultural competence, 146–147
Cultural context
in delivery of DBT, 273–274
for therapeutic collaboration, 211–212
for therapist responsiveness, 250
Cultural humility, 162, 291, 292
Culturally-informed family-based treatments, 231
Cultural opportunity, 162, 291, 292
Cultural ruptures, 95–98, 313
Curiosity mind-set, 87, 199
Curtis, R. C., 117
Cyclical psychodynamics model, 279

D

Dahl, H. J., 124
Danger perception, 135
DBT. *See* Dialectical behavior therapy
DBT diary card, 264–265
DBT-Linehan Board of Certification, 273
DBT® Skills Training Manual, 2nd ed. (Linehan), 263
Deactivating strategies, 65, 67
Debt, enactment with client in, 117–119
Deconstruction of problematic self-narratives, 200–201, 203, 207
Defensiveness, 224, 308
"Deferential and appeasing" withdrawal marker, 86
Delgado-Romero, E. A., 96
Departure models. *See* Clinical departure
DeRubeis, R. J., 52, 319
Descriptive variables, 21
Detachment, 68
Developmental model of the self, 9, 175
Developmental psychology, 301
Diagnosis, therapy selection based on, 133–134, 146, 147
Diagnostic and Statistical Manual of Mental Disorders (DSM), 133
Diagnostic interview styles, 18
Diagnostic markers, 306, 313, 314
Dialectical behavioral patterns, 263–264, 267
Dialectical behavior therapy (DBT), 10, 257–274, 305
client signals in, 308, 310
four modes of S-DBT, 259

four stages of, 258–259
future research on responsivity in, 273–274
modifications of S-DBT to enhance responsiveness, 259–262
responsive outpatient individual therapy, 262–272
structural strategies promoting responsivity in, 263–267
theoretical integration in, 280
training to enhance responsivity in, 272–273
treatment strategy selection and delivery in, 267–272
Dialectical dilemmas, 266, 271
Dialectical treatment strategies, 267–268
Dialogue(s)
anxious-self-coping-self, 289, 290
in attachment-based family therapy, 222–223, 227–228
empty chair, 173–174, 189
self-soothing, 179
two-chair, 178–179, 189, 290
Diamond, G. M., 230, 231
Differential treatment outcomes, tests of, 19–20
Differentiation, of self from other, 175, 180–181
Direct immediate resolution strategies, 91–93
Disagreements, client–emotion-focused therapist, 185–186
Discomfort, appropriate responsiveness and, 23
Discovery-oriented treatments, 157
Disembedding, for rupture resolution, 112
Disempowered populations, alliance with members of, 95
Dismissive attachment, 123
Disorder-specific responsiveness, 306
defined, 240
empirical research on, 245–246
in personality disorder treatment, 241–242
Dissociated self-states, 108, 119–121
Dissociative model of mind, 108
Distress
interpersonal distance during, 66
as micromarker, 182
self-disclosure as adaptive response to, 17

Diverse client populations. *See also* Client diversity
alliance ruptures and repairs with, 95–99
context-responsive psychotherapy integration with, 161–162
control-mastery theory in work with, 146–147
family therapy with, 231
integrative therapies with, 291–292
narrative therapy with, 211–212
personality disorder treatments with, 250–251
psychodynamic relational psychotherapy with, 121
responsive emotion-focused therapy with, 187–188
responsiveness to, 5
Diversity-oriented psychotherapy, 291
Doan, R. E., 202
"Dodo Bird" verdict, 15–17, 19, 41
"Doing more of the same," responsiveness as, 155–156, 158, 163
"Doing the right thing" domain, of appropriate responsiveness, 41
and adherence to treatment approach, 43–44, 316
client responsiveness and, 50
in context-responsive psychotherapy integration, 154, 164
evaluative assessment of, 29
in framing of responsiveness problem, 300
and history of therapeutic relationship, 77
in personality disorder treatment, 237, 240, 245, 252
in therapeutic collaboration model, 198
"Doing what is required" domain, of appropriate responsiveness, 41–42, 300
Doran, J. M., 110
Dose-effect relations, 19, 300
Dropout rate
generic therapist responsiveness and, 241
integrative movement as response to, 279
responsiveness of treatment model and, 46
rupture recognition and, 85
therapist responsiveness and, 22
therapist responsiveness in TCM and, 210–211

Drug abstinence module, S-DBT with, 260
DSM (*Diagnostic and Statistical Manual of Mental Disorders*), 133
During-session responsiveness, in CRPI, 155–158, 163–164
Dyadic process research, 122

E

Eagle, M. N., 63
Eames, V., 123
Early termination. *See* Dropout rate
EBP (evidence-based practice), 151, 251
Eclecticism, technical, 280–281, 283
ECR (Experiences in Close Relationships Scale), 73
Effect sizes, 19, 262, 300
EFT. *See* Emotion-focused therapy
Elkin, I., 21–22, 241, 244
Emotional attunement training, 76–77, 126
Emotional connection, assuming too much, 69–70
Emotional development, 4
Emotional experiencing, as goal of DBT, 258
Emotional expression
   as client signal/marker, 308–309, 314
   cultural rules of, 313
Emotional learning, 4, 5
Emotional presence, 227–228
Emotional processing
   developing capacity for, 177–178, 188
   in developmental model of self, 175
   as goal of DBT, 258
   and positive self-organization, 178–179
   as priority in EFT, 186
Emotional regulation, 175, 177–178, 259–261
Emotional vulnerability versus self-invalidation (dialectical dilemma), 266
Emotion-focused therapy (EFT), 26, 49, 171–192
   assimilative integration of CBT with, 289–291
   attachment-based family therapy and, 221
   challenging strategies in, 203
   client signals in, 308–310
   with diverse client populations, 187–188

micromarkers of therapist responsiveness in, 181–187
research on responsiveness in experiential therapy, 188–189
responsiveness concept in, 172–175
task analyses in, 91, 318
task markers to enhance responsiveness in, 175–176
therapeutic zones of proximal development in, 176–181
training to enhance responsiveness in, 189–191
Emotion schemes, 177, 180
Emotions of clients. *See also* Negative feelings; *specific types*
   as micromarkers, 181–182
   responding to parents' emotions in ABFT, 226–227
   self-attending to, 177
   vulnerable, 223–224
Empathic attunement, 76–77
Empathy, 164
   approval vs., 226–227
   as evaluative process variable, 21, 23
   in generic therapist responsiveness, 240–241
   and responsiveness in EFT, 172, 189
   shifting from blaming to, 223–224
   in therapeutic relationship, 172, 175
Empirically supported treatment (EST)
   appropriate responsiveness in, 42
   client responsiveness to, 50
   and diagnosis-based therapy selection, 133
   responsiveness-based adjustments to, 316
   with therapeutic collaboration model, 197
   training in delivery of, 146
Empirical research
   on dialectical behavior therapy, 262
   on disorder-specific responsiveness, 245–246
   on engagement strategies of ABFT, 231
   on generic responsiveness, 244–245
   on individualized responsiveness, 245–246
Empty chair dialogues, 173–174, 189
Enactments, 304
   in attachment-based family therapy, 220–223, 227–228
   client signals in, 309

in narrative therapy, 201
in psychodynamic relational
psychotherapy, 117–119
Engagement
and appropriate responsiveness, 22
on measures of therapeutic distance,
72, 73
strategic structural-systems, 230
Environmental intervention strategies, in
DBT, 270–272
Epston, D., 202
Equivalence theory, 52
EST. *See* Empirically supported treatment
Evaluative measures, 317
of appropriate responsiveness, 20–24,
27
describing good process with, 23–24
of outcome, 23n1
in process–outcome research, 23–24
unpacking, 27
Evaluative variables, 20–21, 240
Everyday problems in living, 258
Evidence-based practice (EBP), 151, 251
Expectations. *See also* Outcome
expectation (OE)
setting realistic, in ABFT, 225–226
therapeutic task of exploring, 64
Experience level, therapist effects and,
142
Experiences in Close Relationships Scale
(ECR), 73
Experiential awareness, 93
Experiential therapy. *See also* Emotion-
focused therapy (EFT)
integration and, 278
nonverbal behavior in, 311
presence in, 172
questioning in, 174
research on responsiveness in, 188–189
therapist attitude in, 173
Expertise, technical, 316, 320
Expert knowledge, 199–200
Explanatory theories of responsiveness,
28–29
Exploratory rupture resolution strategies,
90–94, 97
Exploring scale, PACS, 75
Exposure therapy, 133, 260, 269–270
External focus, clients with, 238–239
Externalization, 200–201
Extraordinary treatment, clients requesting,
238, 239

F

Facial expressions, 182, 191
Facilitative skills, 27
Family members, attending/responding to
multiple, 220–221
Family therapy, 221, 230–231
Fatter, D. M., 127–128
Fear, in attachment-based family therapy,
225, 226
Feedback
for developing therapist responsiveness,
51
micromarkers/signals in client,
183–184, 312–314
noncontingent, 61
soliciting, about source of rupture, 97
training therapists to listen for, 316
Feedback loops, 49
Feelings of therapists, 86–87, 184–185.
See also Negative feelings
Feeling Word Checklist (FWC), 124
Felt flow, 185–186
Ferreira, A., 210
Finkel, E. J., 47
First-step responsiveness, 154–155, 158,
162–163
Flexibility, therapist. *See* Therapist
flexibility
Flow, as micromarker, 185–186
Focusing technique, 177–178
Following client's direction, responsiveness
as, 172–174
Frank, J. D., 284
Frawley-O'Dea, M. G., 126
Freedman, J., 202
Freud, S., 52, 278
Friedlander, M. L., 27
Fuertes, J. N., 187
Fulfillment, as goal DBT, 258
FWC (Feeling Word Checklist), 124

G

GAD. *See* Generalized anxiety disorder
Gaete, J., 26
Gassner, S., 138
Gaztambide, D. J., 97
Gender identity, as client factor, 4
Gender minority individuals. *See* Sexual
and gender minority individuals
Genderqueer clients, ABFT with, 229

Generalized anxiety disorder (GAD)
IEP interventions in CBT for, 281–282
resistance from patient with, 157
standard CBT for treatment of, 164
Generic therapist responsiveness, 240–241,
244–245
Genuineness, in therapeutic relationship,
172, 175
"Getting off on the right foot,"
responsiveness as, 154–155, 162–163
Global quality of interaction, 245
Goal-corrected empathic attunement,
76–77
Goal-oriented responsiveness, 39, 46, 303
Goals of therapy
in attachment-based family therapy,
221–222, 232
consensus and collaboration on, 21,
49, 220
in dialectical behavioral therapy, 258,
263
responsiveness based on, 232
rupture resolution based on, 92
in therapeutic collaboration model, 197
Goldfried, M. R., 284, 305
Gonçalves, M. M., 188
Good psychiatric management, 251
Gorkin, M., 115
Greenberg, L., 175, 188, 189
Grieving, inhibited, 266
Grosse-Holtforth, M., 24
Group cohesion, 21, 23
Group skills training, 258–261, 269, 270
Gunderson, J. G., 251
Gupta, S., 126–127

H

Hatcher, R. L., 24
Hayes, J. A., 127–128
Hayes, S. C., 52
Hebrew University, 126
Hierarchical approach, in DBT, 258–259,
264–266
Higham, J., 230
Highly-structured treatment agendas, 305
Hill, C. E., 126–127
Hippocrates, 133
Hirsch, I., 117
Hofmann, S. G., 52
Holbrook, D., 18
Holmes, J., 60, 76

Homogeneity myth, 146
Honos-Webb, L., 38
Horowitz, L. M., 137
Horvath, A. O., 41, 88, 100, 171, 317
Humanistic therapy, 164
Humility
cultural, 162, 291, 292
for optimal responsiveness, 190
in rupture repair, 87
Hyperactivating strategies, 65–67
Hypothalamic–pituitary axis, 4

I

Identity
corrective attachment/identity episodes,
221–223, 227–228
cultural beliefs about, 229, 313
and problematic self-narratives, 202
IEP (interpersonal and emotional
processing) interventions, 281–282,
285
If-then guidance system of CRPI
for clinical departures, 156–158
for cognitive behavioral therapists,
158–161
reducing decision-making errors with,
285–286
research on, 164
Imel, Z. E., 43
Immediacy, 125, 126–127
Immediate disclosure, 125
Immediate effects, responsiveness research
on, 27–28
Immediate rupture resolution strategies,
90, 91
Implicit knowledge, 5, 109–110
Inappropriate responsiveness, 282–283
Inattention, experience of, 68
Incomplete narratives, 179–180
Inconsistent interventions, 145–146
Independent variable, 19–20, 300
India, 250
Indirect immediate resolution strategies,
91, 92
Individualized responsiveness
at beginning of BPD treatment,
247–250
defined, 240
empirical research on, 246–247
in personality disorder treatment,
242–243

Individual therapy, in DBT, 262–272
  as mode of S-DBT, 258
  modification of module for, 260
  responsive selection and delivery of,
    267–272
  structural strategies in, 263–267
Infant–parent interaction research, 60–62,
    109–110, 301
Inhibited grieving, 266
Innovative Moment in Psychotherapy
    Scale, 305, 310
Innovative moments model, 196, 202
Insecure attachment
  empathic attunement to clients with,
    76–77
  IWMs and relationship representations
    with, 63–64
  rupture resolution for clients with, 123
In-session measures of responsiveness,
    72–76
Integration. *See also* Context-responsive
    psychotherapy integration (CRPI)
  assimilative, 281–283, 289–291
  four pathways of, 278–284
  of signals informing therapist
    responsiveness, 313–315
  theoretical, 279–280
Integrative movement, 279
Integrative therapies, 277–293, 302,
    305. *See also* Context-responsive
    psychotherapy integration (CRPI)
  case examples, 287–291
  with diverse client populations,
    291–292
  four pathways of integration, 278–284
  immediate self-disclosure in, 125
  metaframeworks to facilitate
    responsiveness in, 284–286
  self-states in, 308
  training to maximize therapist
    responsiveness in, 292–293
Interactive matrix, 108
Internal working models (IWMs), 63–64
Interoceptive exposures, 288
Interpersonal and emotional processing
    (IEP) interventions, 281–282, 285
Interpersonal circumplex models, 319–320
Interpersonal dysfunction, for clients with
    personality disorders, 238
Interpersonal interactions, responsiveness
    in, 3
Interpersonal maps, 307–308, 314, 319

Interpersonal processes, in developmental
    model of self, 175
Interpersonal pulls, 186–187
Interpersonal signals or markers, 303,
    311–315
  alliance ruptures, 85–86, 311–312
  attunement to diversity and uniqueness,
    313
  client feedback, 312–313
  integrating therapist and client markers
    with, 313, 315
Interpersonal therapy
  client responsiveness in, 50
  rupture repair in, 91, 164
  therapist MOTR and client plans in, 243
  therapist responsiveness in, 239
Interpretations, 18–19
Intersectionality, 97–98, 228–230
Intersubjective negotiation, of relational
    needs, 90
Intersubjective therapy process, 107
Intimacy, client experience of, 69
Intrapersonal markers of alliance ruptures,
    86–87
Irreverent communication strategies, 270
IWMs (internal working models), 63–64

J

Joyful life, as goal DBT, 258

K

Karterud, S., 242, 245
Katz, M., 43
Kelley, H. H., 47
Kramer, U., 24–27, 40, 41, 49, 243

L

Language
  attachment style and, 74–75
  motivational, 155, 157, 162–163
  in narrative therapy, 200
  poignancy of, 182
Learning, emotional, 4, 5
Leiman, M., 175, 196, 307
Lesbian, gay, and bisexual individuals, 96.
    See also Sexual and gender minority
    individuals
Lietaer, G., 239
"Lifespan," treatment, 9, 162–165
Linehan, M., 258, 263, 266, 268

M

Madigan, Stephen, 195, 203–210
Maiwald, L. M., 43
Maladaptive blaming, 223–224
Mallinckrodt, B., 66, 72
Manualized therapies. See Treatment
    manuals
Markers to enhance responsiveness,
    303–315
    client signals or markers, 303, 307–315
    in cognitive behavioral therapy, 158–161,
        282
    in CRPI, 154–156, 163–164, 286
    defined, 25
    in emotion-focused therapy, 175–176,
        178–180
    integration of, 313–315
    interpersonal signals, 311–315
    in personality disorder treatments,
        240–243
    research on, 52–53
    in standard dialectical behavioral
        therapy, 263–266
    therapist signals, 304–307, 313–315
    training therapists to recognize, 316
Maroda, K. J., 114
Matching
    of clients and therapists, 155, 163
    of clients and treatments, 143–146, 319
MBT (mentalization-based therapy),
    241–242, 245–246
McCluskey, U., 76
McLeod, B. D., 43
McLeod, J., 199
Meditation, 127, 128
Memory consolidation, 179, 180
Mendes, I., 188
Mentalization-based therapy (MBT),
    241–242, 245–246
Messer, S. B., 281
Meta-analyses, effect sizes reported in, 262
Metacommunication
    and common principles of change
        framework, 285
    in marker studies, 53
    in psychodynamic relational
        psychotherapy, 112–113
    in rupture resolution, 93–95, 99
Metaframeworks, 284–286
Microadjustments, for rupture resolution,
    164

Microaggressions, 96, 97, 313
Microanalytic studies of responsiveness,
    188
Microinvalidations, 96
Micromarkers, 181–187
Microprocesses, in DBT, 273
Miller-Bottome, M., 123
Mindfulness, 127
Mirroring, 183
Modulation, of arousal and emotional
    expression, 177
Moment-by-moment clinical maps, 232
Moment-to-moment behavior, 5, 84
Motivational interviewing (MI), 43
    CBT integrated with, 163–164, 281–283,
        286
    in CRPI, 160–161
    marker studies of, 53
    pretreatment, 155
Motivational language, 155, 157, 162–163
Motive-oriented therapeutic relationship
    (MOTR), 24
    complementary interventions using,
        248–250
    individualized responsiveness and,
        242–244, 246
Mount Zion Brief Therapy Research
    project, 139–140
Multicultural orientation, 291–292
Multidimensional family therapy, 221, 230
Muran, J. C., 53, 89, 91, 96, 110, 123
Mutuality, 25, 319, 320
Mutual recognition
    in psychodynamic relational
        psychotherapy, 109, 110
    and self-disclosure of
        countertransference, 114–115
    training to increase, 126
Mutual regulation model, 62. See also
    Coregulation

N

Narratives
    making sense of experience with,
        179–180
    shifts in, 188
Narrative therapy (NT), 195–213
    change process in, 203–210
    client signals in, 310
    cultural and diversity issues in, 211–212
    interpersonal signals in, 312

research on responsiveness and TCM in, 210–211
responsiveness in, 199–203
and therapeutic collaboration model, 196–199, 203
and training in TCM, 212–213
National Institute of Mental Health, 21–22
Native Alaskan population, 274
Naturalistic studies, 25
Natural phenomenon, responsiveness in, 38–39
Needs, relational, 88–90, 306–307
Needy self-state, 119–121
Negative affect, therapist's regulation of, 190
Negative feedback, 183–184
Negative feelings
  as client signal, 309
  as indicator of misalignment, 176
  in rupture repair, 87
  therapist's attending to own, 185
  as therapist signal, 306
  therapist's managing of, 190, 318
Negative interactions, 45
Negative life experiences, 4
Negative self-statements, 175
Negotiations in alliance, 110–112, 311
Nelson, M. L., 127
Neo-Freudians, 278
New behavioral skills, as primary target in S-DBT, 264
Newman, M. G., 281–282, 285
Nonaccepting parents of sexual and gender minority youth. *See also* Attachment-based family therapy (ABFT)
  initiation of therapy by, 219
  resistance to therapy for, 231
  responding to feelings and concerns of, 226–227
  working alliance between therapist and, 222
Nonassertiveness problems, 162
Noncontingent feedback, 61
Nonimmediate disclosure, 125
Nonimprovement rates, treatment model responsiveness and, 46
Nonresponsiveness, 3, 208–210
Nonverbal behavior
  as client signal/marker, 310–311, 314
  as micromarker, 182–183

in motive-oriented therapeutic relationship, 243, 246
for optimal responsiveness, 191
Norcross, J. C., 4, 21, 24, 133–134, 317, 319
Norouzian, N., 53
NT. *See* Narrative therapy

O

Objective truth, 108
O'Brien, K. M., 62
Observer-rated measure of generic responsiveness, 241
OE. *See* Outcome expectation
One-person psychology, 107–108
Openness, 189–190
Opportunity, cultural, 162, 291, 292
Optimal responsiveness, 22
  and adherence, 44–46, 316
  appropriate responsiveness vs., 44–45, 300
  as common factor, 49–50
  consultation to therapist for, 272
  in control-mastery theory, 137, 138, 144
  defined, 44–45
  developing and enhancing, 51–53
  for emotion-focused therapists, 172, 189–191
  and supportive responsiveness, 48
Osatuke, K., 27
Outcome expectation (OE)
  for CBT approaches, 283
  change in, as clinical departure marker, 157
  in CRPI, 286
  first-step responsiveness and, 155, 162
Outcome measures
  in CRPI, 156, 157
  evaluative, 23n1
Outcome monitoring, 286
Outcome research
  on adherence and competence, 42–44, 152, 153
  on alliance, 83, 244–247
  on client self-disclosure, 17–18
  on control mastery theory, 137–140
  on countertransference, 124–125
  Dodo's verdict in, 15–17, 19
  on first-step responsivity, 162–163
  on responsiveness in BPD treatment, 244–247

on responsiveness in integrative
therapies, 292
responsiveness undermining, 19–20
on rupture repair, 84, 123
on therapist effects, 140–141
on therapist flexibility, 282
Outpatient individual therapy, 262–272
Owen, J., 97, 291

P

PACS (Patient Attachment Coding
System), 74–75
Pain, as micromarker, 182
Panic-focused psychodynamic
psychotherapy, 287–288
Pantheoretical framework, of CRPI,
154–158, 285
Parents. *See also* Nonaccepting parents of
sexual and gender minority youth
infant–parent interaction research,
60–62, 109–110, 301
as secure base, 62–63
Parry, A., 202
Participant observer role, of therapist, 117
Partner responsiveness, 47–48
Passive coping, 96
Passive therapeutic stance, 143
Past, seeing, as therapeutic task, 64
Pathogenic beliefs, 134–135, 137–138
Patience, in rupture repair, 87–88
Patient Attachment Coding System (PACS),
74–75
Patient-focused interventions, 143–146
Patient's Experience of Attunement and
Responsiveness (PEAR) Scale, 22
Perceptual control theory, 28
Performance indices, provider, 155, 163
Perseverative adherence, 153
Personality disorder treatment, 237–252
brief psychodynamic therapy, 243
case example of individualized
responsiveness, 247–250
disorder-specific therapist
responsiveness in, 241–242
generic therapist responsiveness in,
240–241
importance of responsiveness in, 238–239
individualized therapist responsiveness
in, 242–243
research on responsiveness, alliance,
and outcomes in BPD, 244–247

and therapist competence vs.
responsiveness, 240
therapist responsiveness with diverse
client populations, 250–251
training to enhance responsiveness in,
251
Personalized Advantage Index, 52
Personalized Assessment Index, 319
Personalized treatment approaches, 52
Personal reactions, of therapists, 184–185
Person-centered treatment, 157
Pessoa, Fernando, 195
Pirsig, Robert, 24
Pirsig phenomenon, 24, 27, 317
Plan Analysis
in case example of BPD treatment, 248
enhancing responsiveness with, 315
individualized responsiveness with,
242–243
as responsive treatment approach, 26, 305
training in, 251
Plan compatibility, 137–140, 142–143, 156
Plan formulation method, 8, 304, 315
misconstrual of, 145
outcome research on, 137–140,
142–143
responsiveness to, 135–137
scientific mindedness in, 147
training in, 147
Pluralistic psychotherapy, 26
Poignancy of language, 182
Political activism, 199
Positive feedback, 183, 184
Positive feelings, 185, 309
Positive psychology, 316–317
Positive regard, 21
Positive reinforcement, validation as, 269
Positive therapeutic atmosphere, 241
Postpsychological therapy, 199
Posttraumatic stress disorder (PTSD), 133,
260, 261
Posture, as micromarker, 182
Potential development level, 196–198, 204
Power differential, 96, 199–200
Preferences, as client factor, 4
Preoccupied attachment, 75, 76, 123
Presence, 172, 227–228
Primary behavioral targets, 264–265, 267
Prioritization, of DBT treatment goals, 258
Problematic behavior
as client signal/marker, 310, 314
conceptualization of, in DBT, 269

Problematic self-narratives, 200–203, 207
Problem formulation, 176, 200
Problem-solving
   in attachment-based family therapy, 223
   balancing validation and, 267–268
   in standard dialectical behavior therapy, 268–270
Problem states, markers of, 175
Procedural knowledge, 5
Process-based therapies, 52
Process–outcome research
   evaluative measures in, 23–24
   on plan compatibility, 139–140
   responsiveness and, 15–19
Process research
   on control mastery theory, 137–140
   on countertransference, 124–125
Process variables, 21
Protective coping, 96
Provider performance indices, 155, 163
Psychoanalysis, 37, 63, 278
Psychodynamic psychotherapy
   adherence research from, 43–44
   appropriate responsiveness in, 77
   challenging strategies in, 203
   integration of behaviorism and, 278
   plan compatibility research from, 138–140
   task analysis of rupture repair in, 91
Psychodynamic relational psychotherapy, 107–128
   client signals in, 311
   dissociated self states in, 119–121
   enactment identification and processing, 117–119
   mutual recognition and implicit relational knowing, 109–110
   negotiations in alliance in, 110–112
   research on attunement and responsiveness in, 122–126
   and responsiveness in two-person paradigm, 107–109, 121–122
   ruptures and resolution in, 112–113
   theoretical lens of, 304
   training in responsiveness in, 126–128
   transference–countertransference patterns and self-disclosure in, 114–116
Psychopathology, 4
Psychotherapy Relationships That Work (Norcross), 4
PTSD. *See* Posttraumatic stress disorder
"Push where it moves" principle, 17, 198

Q

Qualitative research, 25–26, 143–146, 317–318
Quality, recognizing, 24
Quality of life, behavior interfering with, 264
Questioning
   about unique outcomes, 202
   in experiential therapy, 174
   in externalization, 200–201
   in narrative therapy, 200, 204

R

Racial and ethnic minority clients, ruptures with, 95–97. *See also* Diverse client populations
Randomized clinical trials (RCTs)
   of DBT modes as stand-alone interventions, 260
   and diagnosis-based therapy selection, 133
   responsiveness-based adjustments to treatment in, 300, 316
   of standard dialectical behavior therapy, 258
   training in therapies supported by, 146
   of validation strategies in DBT, 269
RAP (relationship anecdotes paradigm) interviews, 67–72
Reactance level, 4, 280–281
Readiness for change, 4, 312
Reciprocal causation, 49
Reciprocal communication strategies, 270
Reconstruction of self-narratives, 201–202, 207
Reflecting behavior, 183
Reflection, 173, 187–188
Reflexive questions, 26
Regressive wishes, in enactments, 119
Rehearsal, of alternative meanings, 201–202
Reis, H. T., 47–48, 60, 64
Rejection, 185, 221
Relatedness needs, 88–90
Relational corrective experiences. *See* Corrective experience(s)
Relational health, 156, 163
Relational maps, 307–308, 314, 319
Relational narratives, client–therapist, 67–72, 77

Relational needs, 88–90, 306–307
Relational psychoanalysis. *See*
    Psychodynamic relational
    psychotherapy
Relational responsiveness, 48–50, 281
Relational rupture in family, ABFT to
    address, 221–222
Relational supervision, 126–127
Relational therapy approaches, 283,
    304–305, 308
Relationship anecdotes paradigm (RAP)
    interviews, 67–72
Relationship building goal of ABFT
    challenges with establishing, 225–226
    establishing, 221–222
    shifting from blaming to empathy for,
        223–224
Relationship factors, 24, 152
Relationship representations, in attachment
    theory, 63–64
Relationship science, 47–50, 320
Religious beliefs
    assimilative integration of, 291
    as client factor, 4
    therapist sensitivity to, 229–230
Repetition of ruptures, 123
Resistance
    from adolescents, 230–231
    in CRPI, 157, 159–161
    cultural misattunement as cause of,
        161–162
    in marker studies, 52–53
    motivational interviewing to reduce, 164
    signs of, 312
    treatment methods to overcome, 51–52
Resonating with client experience, 184
Responsibility for rupture, 96–98
Responsiveness. *See also specific types*
    and attunement, 3, 5
    competence vs., 240, 315
    defined, 16, 76, 133, 300
    demonstrating, 25
    in-session measures of, 72–76
    in relationships, 299
    research aspects undermined by, 18–20
    in research on ruptures, 84–85
    training to enhance, 99
    transtheoretical frameworks for, 301–302
Responsiveness concept, 3, 37–53
    appropriate responsiveness, 40–42
    and appropriate vs. optimal
        responsiveness, 44–45

in attachment theory, 60
client responsiveness, 50
in emotion-focused therapy, 172–175
in psychotherapy, 37, 38
relational responsiveness, 48–50
for researchers vs. clinicians, 237
specifying nature and scope of, 38–40
supportive responsiveness, 47–48
therapist responsiveness, 51–53
in treatment approaches, 42–44,
    302–303
in treatment models, 45–47
Responsiveness in psychotherapy research,
    4–5, 15–29
    appropriate responsiveness concept for
        research, 41–42
    with attachment-based family therapy,
        230–232
    and client self-disclosure paradox,
        17–18
    with CRPI across treatment lifespan,
        162–165
    evaluative measures of appropriate
        responsiveness, 20–24
    with experiential therapy, 188–189
    future directions for, with DBT, 273–274
    future research directions, 27–29,
        316–320
    historical methods of addressing, 24–27
    with psychodynamic relational
        psychotherapy, 122–126
    research aspects undermined by
        responsiveness, 18–20
    research on need for responsiveness and
        attunement, 152–153
    research on responsiveness, alliance,
        and outcomes in BPD, 244–247
    and responsiveness concept, 38, 40
    on TCM in narrative therapy, 210–211
Responsiveness problem
    engaging with, 25–27
    formulating, 17–18, 237
    framing of, 300
Responsive rupture resolution, 88–95
    with clients from diverse backgrounds,
        95–99
    context-dependent strategies in, 90–93
    intersecting relational needs in, 88–90
    metacommunication in, 93–95
Ribeiro, E., 188
Rice, L. N., 182, 189
Right brain functioning, 4

Risk, tolerable, 198, 212
Rogers, C. R., 3, 24, 49, 172, 173, 178, 278
Roth, A., 123
Rubel, J. A., 124
Rupture markers, 314
  future research on, 100
  interpersonal, 85–86, 311–312
  intrapersonal, 86–87
  in psychodynamic relational psychotherapy, 112
Rupture Resolution Rating System (3RS), 85
Ruptures, 83–100, 301–302
  with clients from diverse backgrounds, 95–99
  context-dependent strategies for resolving, 90–93
  in CRPI, 157–158, 286
  cultural, 95–98, 313
  defined, 112
  felt flow indicating, 185
  future research on, 100
  intersecting relational needs underlying, 88–90
  metacommunication and, 93–95
  microadjustments to address, 164
  in psychodynamic relational psychotherapy, 112–113
  repairing, as responsive process, 27
  research on, 84–85, 123–124
  as resistance markers, 53
  task analysis of repair of, 189
  therapist attitudes for addressing, 87–88
  training to prevent/repair, 99–100
Rutter, M., 18

S

Sachse, R., 188
Safran, J. D., 53, 89, 91, 96, 110, 112, 123, 127
Sameness, myth of, 146
"Same old story," 180
San Francisco Psychotherapy Research Group, 134, 135
Santisteban D. A., 230
Sapolsky, Robert, 316
Sarnat, J. E., 126
Schore, A. N., 4, 188
Scientific mindedness, 146–147

S-DBT. *See* Standard dialectical behavior therapy
Secondary behavioral targets, DBT, 265–267
Secure attachment, 60
  IWMs and relationship representations with, 63
  language/communication patterns of clients with, 74–75
  rupture resolution for clients with, 123, 311
  TASc scores of therapists with, 75–76
Secure base
  in attachment theory, 62–63, 301
  regulating therapeutic distance to establish, 66–67
  therapeutic task of providing, 64
A Secure Base (Bowlby), 62
Security scale, PACS, 75
Self
  in assimilation model, 196
  developmental model of, 9
  differentiation of, 175, 180–181
  in psychodynamic relational psychotherapy, 108
Self-awareness, for rupture-marker monitoring, 112
Self-compassion, 179
Self-definition need, 90
Self-disclosure
  client self-disclosure paradox, 17–18
  of countertransference, 114–116
  research on impact of, 125–126
Self-governance, 175, 181
Self-harming (self-injurious) behaviors
  as client signal/marker, 310, 314
  by clients with personality disorders, 238–239
  perceptions of therapist dialectics and, 268
Self-invalidation, 266
Self-narratives
  consolidation of alternative, 202–203
  deconstruction of problematic, 200–201, 203, 207
  in innovative moments model, 196
  reconstruction of, 201–202, 207
Self-organization
  as client signal/marker, 308, 314
  developing positive, 178–179
  in developmental model of self, 175
Self-regulation, 48, 180–181

Self-soothing dialogues, 179
Self-states
    as client signal/marker, 308, 314
    dissociated, 108, 119–121
Self-strivings, 286
Sense making, narratives for, 179–180
Session-level monitoring and feedback, 27
Sexual and gender minority individuals.
    See also Attachment-based family
        therapy (ABFT)
    family therapy with, 231
    initiation of therapy by, 219, 231
    working alliance between therapist and,
        222
Sexual orientation, as client factor, 4
Sheffield psychotherapy project, 19
Shelton, K., 96
"Shifting topic away" withdrawal marker,
    86
Shock trauma, 135
Shut off aspects of experience, 308
Signals informing therapist
    responsiveness. *See* Markers to
    enhance responsiveness
Silberschatz, G., 22, 135, 137–141
Silence, in relational narratives, 68–69
Skills training, 258–261, 269, 270
Smedslund, J., 26
Snyder, J., 22
Soothing, 179, 224
Specificity theory, 26
Spiritual beliefs, 4, 291
Stage-process model, 89–90, 123
Stages of change theory, 281
Standard dialectical behavior therapy
    (S-DBT)
    defining direction of individual sessions
        in, 263–267
    four modes of, 259
    intervening with responsivity in,
        267–272
    outpatient individual therapy in,
        262–272
    responsive modifications to, 259–262
Standardized treatments, 151
Stiles, W. B., 7, 24–27, 37–42, 45, 46, 49,
    83, 88, 100, 171, 175, 196, 240, 277,
    307, 317
Still-face procedure, 24, 61–62
Strange situation procedure, 60, 66
Strategic structural-systems engagement,
    230

Stress trauma, 135
Structural family therapy, 221
Structural strategies of DBT, 263–267
    addressing secondary behavioral
        targets, 265–266
    attending to primary behavioral targets,
        264–265
    increasing dialectical behavioral
        patterns, 263–264
Strupp, Hans, 23n1
STS (systematic treatment selection),
    280–281
Stylistic treatment strategies, 270
Substance use disorder, 260, 261, 274
Sue, S., 146–147
Suicidal behavior
    client signals in, 310
    by clients with personality disorders,
        238–239
    DBT for treatment of, 257
    as primary behavioral target, 264
"Supershrinks," 51, 140–141, 143–144,
    318
Supervision, 27, 126–127, 232–233
Supportive approach
    balance challenging approach and, 211
    control-mastery theory on use of, 144
    in narrative therapy, 204, 205
    in therapeutic collaboration model,
        197–198, 203
Supportive–expressive psychotherapy,
    110–112, 124
Supportive responsiveness, 47–48
Surko, M., 38
Symbolization, 177, 180
Symptom reduction, individualized
    responsiveness and, 247
Systematic evocative unfolding, 189
Systematic treatment selection (STS),
    280–281, 283
Systemic therapies, 220
Szapocznik, J., 230

T

Talia, A., 74–76
Targeting, in S-DBT, 264
TASc (Therapist Attunement Scales),
    75–76
Task analysis
    of attachment-based family therapy, 232
    of markers of problem states, 175

of productive episodes in experiential therapy, 189
of responsiveness, 26, 318
Task maps, 175
Task markers, in emotion-focused therapy, 175–176
TCCS. *See* Therapeutic Collaboration Coding System
TCM. *See* Therapeutic collaboration model
TDS (Therapeutic Distance Scale), 72–73
TDS–O (Therapeutic Distance Scale Observer version), 73
Technical eclecticism, 280–281, 283
Technical expertise, 316, 320
Technical responsiveness, 281
Technique-focused interventions, 144–146
Telephone consultation, 258
Testing of therapist, by client, 137–138
T-GRAF (therapeutic gratification, relief, anxiety, or frustration) model, 66, 74
Theater improvisational skills, 126, 315–316
Theoretical integration, 279–280
Theoretical orientation
    and integrative therapies, 277
    knowledge of, for responsiveness, 292
    therapist signals through lens of, 304–305, 314
    training in, 165
Theory-based techniques, 42
Theory-building research strategy, 29, 210
Therapeutic alliance. *See also* Working alliance
    as accomplishment, 88
    adolescent resistance to, 230–231
    BPD treatment outcome research on, 244–247
    defined, 83
    with disempowered client populations, 95
    as evaluative process variable, 21, 23
    and generic responsiveness, 244–245
    and global quality of interaction, 245
    and individualized responsiveness, 246
    in mentalization-based therapy, 245–246
    negotiations in, 110–112, 311
    outcome research on, 83, 244–247
    in relational therapy approaches, 283
    research consistent with two-person psychology on, 122
    ruptures in. *See* Ruptures

and therapeutic zones of proximal development, 311–312
    within-therapist variation in, 122
Therapeutic change processes. *See* Change processes
Therapeutic Collaboration Coding System (TCCS), 203, 204, 212–213
Therapeutic collaboration model (TCM), 196–199
    and breaks in collaboration, 208–210
    client signals with, 310
    diversity and intercultural context for, 211–212
    future research on, 213
    and narrative therapy, 203
    research on, 210–211
    therapist responsiveness in, 203–210
    training in, 212–213
Therapeutic distance
    appropriate, 70–72
    assessment of, 72–74
    regulating, 65–67, 301
    relational narratives for studying, 77
    too little, 69–70
    too much, 68–69
Therapeutic Distance Scale (TDS), 72–73
Therapeutic Distance Scale Observer version (TDS–O), 73
Therapeutic gratification, relief, anxiety, or frustration (T-GRAF) model, 66, 74
Therapeutic relationship. *See also* Motive-oriented therapeutic relationship
    appropriate responsiveness and history of, 77
    assessing strength of, 186
    attachment dynamics in, 64–65, 301
    client factors in, 4
    in dialectical behavior therapy, 268
    in emotion-focused therapy, 171, 172, 175
    felt flow of, 185
    in narrative therapy, 199
    in psychodynamic relational psychotherapy, 110
    relating parenting experience to, 64
    in supportive–expressive psychotherapy, 124
    treatment model and, 46
    in two-person model of psychology, 108–109
Therapeutic responsiveness
    control-mastery theory on, 134, 138–139
    defined, 83, 195

in narrative therapy, 199–203
in therapeutic collaboration model,
    198–199
Therapeutic tasks
in attachment-based family therapy,
    221–228
in attachment theory, 64
Therapeutic zone of proximal development
    (TZPD), 176–181
Therapeutic zones of proximal
    development (TZPD), 9
and alliance, 311–312
and client feedback, 312
client signals related to, 307–311
diversity and intercultural issues in
    negotiation of, 212
in emotion-focused therapy, 175
interventions not responsive to limit of,
    208–210
research on responsiveness to, 210–211
responsiveness as working within, 213
and therapeutic collaboration model,
    197–199
Therapist Attunement Scales (TASc),
    75–76
Therapist effects (therapist factors)
clinical study of, 143–146
control-mastery theory on, 140–143
outcome research on, 152
in perceived responsivity, 165
Therapist flexibility
in context-responsive psychotherapy
    integration, 151, 154
in emotion-focused therapy, 171–172
outcome research on, 153, 282
process research on, 153
Therapist-offered conditions, 49
Therapist responsiveness. *See also*
    Appropriate responsiveness; Optimal
    responsiveness
and adherence to treatment model,
    45–47
attachment theory as framework for,
    59–77
to challenges in attachment-based
    family therapy, 223–228
and client's feelings about therapy, 140
competence vs., 240
control-mastery theory on, 147
developing and enhancing, 51–53
disorder-specific, 241–242
with diverse client populations, 250–251

generic, 240–241, 244–245
importance of, in personality disorder
    treatment, 238–239
to intersectionality, 228–230
markers to enhance. *See* Markers to
    enhance responsiveness
micromarkers of, 181–187
in narrative therapy, 203–210
and regulation of therapeutic distance,
    65–67
training to enhance. *See* Training to
    enhance responsiveness
and treatment approach, 42–44
Therapists
attitudes of, 87–88, 173
characteristics of, 306, 314, 318
competence of. *See* Competence
reactions by, 184–185, 306–307, 314
relational needs of, 90, 306–307
rupture recognition by, 85
Therapist signals, 303–307, 314
diagnostic markers, 306
integrating client and interpersonal
    markers with, 313, 315
theoretical lens, 304–305
therapist characteristics, 306
therapist reactions, 306–307
Therapy-interfering behavior, 264
Therapy relationship. *See* Therapeutic
    relationship
Third Interdivisional American
    Psychological Association Task Force
    on Evidence-Based Relationships and
    Responsiveness, 125
Third-wave cognitive-behavioral therapy,
    278
Thomas Aquinas, 143
3RS (Rupture Resolution Rating System),
    85
Time scale, for responsiveness, 16,
    154–158, 300–303
Timing, of stylistic strategies, 270
Tishby, O., 69, 124–125
Tolerable risk, 198, 212
Top-down training, 166
Toukmanian, S., 188
Tracking, responsiveness as, 172–174
Training (generally)
alliance-focused, 99–100, 127
bottom-up, 166
responsiveness in, 24
on rupture prevention/repair, 99–100

skills, 258–261, 269, 270
top-down, 166
Training to enhance responsiveness,
    315–316
  in attachment-based family therapy,
      232–233
  in context-responsive psychotherapy
      integration, 165–166
  control-mastery theory in, 146
  in CRPI, 165–166
  in dialectical behavior therapy, 272–273
  in emotional attunement, 76–77, 126
  in emotion-focused therapy, 189–191
  in integrative therapies, 292–293
  in personality disorder treatment, 251
  in psychodynamic relational
      psychotherapy, 126–128
  therapeutic collaboration model in,
      212–213
Transference
  attunement to, 114–116
  client responsiveness and, 50
  implicit relational knowing vs., 110
  progress and plan compatibility vs., 138
Transference–countertransference matrix,
    114–116
Transgender clients, 229. *See also* Sexual
    and gender minority individuals
Transtheoretical frameworks, 197, 299,
    301–302
Traumatic experiences, in control-mastery
    theory, 135
Treatment delivery for DBT
  communication about modified,
      261–262
  heterogeneity of, 262
  responsivity in, 267–272
  for stand-alone modules, 260–261
Treatment focus, negotiation on, 110–112
Treatment hierarchy, in S-DBT, 258–259,
    264–266
Treatment "lifespan," 9, 162–165
Treatment manuals
  for attachment-based family therapy,
      232
  for dialectical behavior therapy, 267,
      272–273
  for integrative therapies, 292
Treatment-related beliefs, 155, 157, 159
Treatment strategy, responsive selection of,
    267–272
Treatment theories, 28–29

Tronick, E., 61, 62
Truth, objective, 108
Two-chair dialogues, 178–179, 189, 290
Two-person psychology, 8
  dissociated self states in, 119
  model of responsiveness in, 121–122,
      303, 319
  in psychodynamic relational
      psychotherapy, 107–109
  research consistent with, 122, 188
  rupture resolution in, 124
  transference and countertransference
      in, 114
TZPD. *See* Therapeutic zones of proximal
    development

U

Uckelstam, C.-J., 122
Unconscious biases, 64
Understanding
  checking of, 173
  of lived experience, 175, 179–180
  shifts in, as client marker, 309–310, 314
Unfinished business, statements of, 175
Unformulated dissociated self states, 119
Uniqueness, attunement to client's, 187,
    313
Unique outcomes, in narrative therapy,
    202
University of Miami, 230
Unrelenting crises versus inhibited
    grieving (dialectical dilemma), 266
Unsatisfactory responses, research on, 44

V

Validation
  approval vs., 226–227
  in attachment-based family therapy,
      224–226, 230
  balancing problem-solving and,
      267–268
  in cultural rupture resolution, 99
  microinvalidations, 96
  in S-DBT, 268–269
  self-invalidation, 266
  supportive responsiveness and, 48
Van Kessel, W., 239
Verbal component, of MOTR, 243, 246
Verbal feedback, 183
Verbal fluency, 189–190

Verbal techniques, adjusting, 18
Videotape supervision, 233
Vocal quality, 182, 191
Vulnerable emotions, in ABFT, 223–224
Vygotsky, L., 196, 307

W

Wachtel, P. L., 279
WAI (Working Alliance Inventory), 122, 244
Wampold, B. E., 45, 133–134, 317, 319
Waning beliefs, client expressing, 157, 159
Warmth, in therapeutic relationship, 175
Wasserman, R. H., 282
Watson, J. C., 175
Weak, clients presenting as, 238, 239
Webb, C. A., 42–43
Weiss, J., 135, 138
Werbart, A., 26
Westra, H. A., 53, 281–283, 286
White, M., 199, 200, 202
Wiseman, H., 69, 124–125
Withdrawal ruptures, 84
    defined, 123
    with diverse client populations, 96, 98
    exploratory resolution strategies for, 91–92

markers of, 86, 90, 98
    recognizing, 85
    relational needs associated with, 89–90
    resolution choice points with mixed rupture, 92–93
Working alliance. *See also* Therapeutic alliance
    in attachment-based family therapy, 222, 226–227
    with parents, in ABFT, 222, 226–227
    and relational responsiveness, 48–50
    responsiveness and quality of, 40, 300
    as transtheoretical framework for responsiveness, 301–302
    with young adult, in ABFT, 222
Working Alliance Inventory (WAI), 122, 244
Working relationship, alignment on perceptions of, 156

Z

Zajonc, R. B., 24
Zeifman, D. M., 61, 62
Zilcha-Mano, S., 122
Ziv-Beiman, S., 125
Zone of proximal development (ZPD), 307, 319. *See also* Therapeutic zone of proximal development (TZPD)

About the Editors

Jeanne C. Watson, PhD, is a professor in the Department of Applied Psychology and Human Development, OISE, University of Toronto, Ontario, Canada. A major exponent of humanistic–experiential psychotherapy, she has contributed to the development of emotion-focused therapy (EFT). Dr. Watson has conducted psychotherapy process and outcome studies to examine the effectiveness of different psychotherapy approaches and to identify the active ingredients of change. She is coauthor and coeditor of eight books, including *Emotion-Focused Therapy for Generalized Anxiety* with Leslie Greenberg. Dr. Watson, an APA Fellow, was president of the International Society for Psychotherapy Research in 2014–2015 and was awarded the Distinguished Research Career Award from the society in 2020. She is a certified clinical psychologist in private practice in Toronto and regularly conducts workshops in EFT around the world.

Hadas Wiseman, PhD, is a professor in the Department of Counseling and Human Development, Faculty of Education, University of Haifa, Israel. Her scholarly work and research focus on the psychotherapy process, the therapeutic relationship, attachment in psychotherapy, personal and professional development of psychotherapists, and intergenerational trauma and interpersonal relationships in families of Holocaust survivors. She coauthored *Echoes of the Trauma: Relational Themes and Emotions in Children of Holocaust Survivors* (with Jacques P. Barber) and coedited *Developing the Therapeutic Relationship: Integrating Case Studies, Research, and Practice* (with Orya Tishby). She was president of the International Society for Psychotherapy Research (in 2013–2014). Dr. Wiseman is a certified clinical psychologist in private practice in Kiryat Tivon, Israel.